PROGRESS IN PATHOLOGY
Volume Three

EDITED BY

NIGEL KIRKHAM MD FRCPath

Consultant Histopathologist,
Royal Sussex County Hospital, Brighton, UK

NICHOLAS R. LEMOINE MD PhD MRCPath

Professor of Molecular Pathology,
Imperial Cancer Research Fund Oncology Unit, Royal Postgraduate Medical School,
Hammersmith Hospital, London, UK

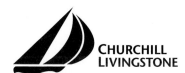

CHURCHILL
LIVINGSTONE

NEW YORK EDINBURGH LONDON MADRID MELBOURNE AND TOKYO 1997

CHURCHILL LIVINGSTONE
Medical Division of Pearson Professional Limited

Distributed in the United States of America by
Churchill Livingstone Inc., 650 Avenue of the Americas, New York,
N.Y. 10011, and by associated companies, branches and
representatives throughout the world.

First published 1997

ISBN 0 443 05583 1

British Library Cataloguing in Publication Data
A catalogue record for this book is available from the British Library.

Library of Congress Cataloging in Publication Data
A catalog record for this book is available from the Library of Congress.

The
publisher's
policy is to use
paper manufactured
from sustainable forests

Printed in Singapore

Contents

Preface

According to Kealey[1] the concept of Progress was invented by Francis Bacon less than 500 years ago. He tells us that Bacon defined Progress, in *Advancement of Learning*, as the addition of new knowledge to old, to promote the creation of yet more. That same concept of Progress has been applied by us in selecting topics for this volume.

In the *Journal of Pathology* a reviewer of Volume 2 suggested that in our quest to explore the 'growing edge' of Pathology we had demonstrated that it had a diffusely infiltrative margin rather than a pushing edge.[2] We have chapters in the present volume that support both cases. Contributions on microsatellite instability, on the role of stroma in tumour growth and on genomic imprinting point towards some of the areas of growth in our knowledge of mechanisms.

The current status of the autopsy is reviewed and its place in clinical research is emphasized in the chapter that challenges some old chestnuts in our understanding of the morbid anatomy of hypertension. We have excellent reviews of some problematic diagnostic areas including blistering and inflammatory skin diseases, hepatitis, trophoblastic disease, synovial fluid and the spleen.

The volume also includes an article on mathematical modelling, a review of developments in microbiology and speculations about Pathology in the 21st century. We have had many favourable comments from readers of the first two volumes. We feel sure that Volume 3 builds well on the success that they have achieved and offers more than enough new knowledge to add to the old and to be a stimulus to further Progress.

Brighton   N.K.
London   N.R.L.
1997

1 Kealey T. The economic laws of scientific research. London: Macmillan, 1996
2 McManus D T. J Pathol 1996; 179: 223

Contributors

Tina Bocker MD
Kimmel Cancer Institute, Thomas Jefferson University, Philadelphia, USA

Lorenzo Cerroni MD
Associate Professor of Dermatology, Department of Dermatology, University of Graz, Graz, Austria

Dennis W. K. Cotton BSc PhD BM MD FRCPath
Reader in Pathology and Honorary Consultant, Department of Pathology, University of Sheffield Medical School, Sheffield, UK

Susan E. Davies MB BS MRCPath
Consultant Pathologist, Department of Histopathology, Royal Free Hospital, London, UK

Harold Fox MD FRCPath FRCOG
Emeritus Professor of Reproductive Pathology, Department of Pathological Sciences, University of Manchester, Manchester, UK

Ferdinand Hofstädter MD
Professor, Institute of Pathology, University of Regensburg, Regensburg, Germany

Alan G. Jardine BSc MD MRCP
Lecturer in Nephrology, Department of Medicine and Therapeutics, University of Glasgow, Western Infirmary, Glasgow, UK

Nigel Kirkham MD FRCPath
Consultant Pathologist, Histopathology Laboratory, Royal Sussex County Hospital, Brighton, UK

El-Nasir Lalani BSc(Hons) MB ChB PhD
Senior Lecturer, Department of Histopathology, Royal Postgraduate Medical School, Hammersmith Hospital, London, UK

Nicholas R. Lemoine MD PhD MRCPath
Professor of Molecular Pathology, Imperial Cancer Research Fund Oncology
Unit, Royal Postgraduate Medical School, Hammersmith Hospital, London,
UK

George B. M. Lindop BSc MB ChB FRCP FRCPath
Senior Lecturer and Consultant in Histopathology, Department of Pathology,
University of Glasgow, Western Infirmary, Glasgow, UK

N. P. Mapstone MB ChB MRCPath
Senior Lecturer in Pathology, University of Leeds and Honorary Consultant
Pathologist, Leeds General Infirmary, Leeds, UK

John Paul MRCPath
Consultant Medical Microbiologist and Director, Brighton Public Health
Laboratory, Royal Sussex County Hospital, Brighton, UK

Phil Quirke MB BS PhD MRCPath
Reader in Gastrointestinal Pathology, University of Leeds and Honorary
Consultant Pathologist, Leeds General Infirmary, Leeds, UK

Suzanne Rogers BSc MB ChB MRCPath
Consultant Histopathologist, Department of Pathology, Doncaster Royal
Infirmary, Doncaster, UK

Josef Rüschoff MD
Professor, Institute of Pathology, University of Regensburg, Regensburg,
Germany

Gordon W. H. Stamp MB ChB FRCPath
Department of Histopathology, Royal Postgraduate Medical School,
Hammersmith Hospital, London, UK

R. D. Start MD MRCPath
Consultant Histopathologist, Chesterfield Royal Hospital, Chesterfield, UK

Benjamin Tycko MD PhD
Associate Professor of Pathology, Columbia University College of Physicians
and Surgeons, New York, New York, USA

Bridget S. Wilkins DM PhD MRCPath
Senior Lecturer in Pathology, University Department of Pathology,
Southampton General Hospital, Southampton, UK

1

Microsatellite instability – an indicator of a new mechanism in carcinogenesis

T. Bocker   J. Rüschoff   F. Hofstädter

The mismatch repair system and mismatch repair defects

Errors easily occur in normal DNA replication – misincorporation or slippage frequently takes place, especially in microsatellites. Microsatellites consist of short DNA motifs up to 8 bases long, which are tandemly repeated several hundred times. However, they do not code for protein and their function is not fully understood. The most common microsatellite in eukaryotes, $(CA)_n$, can be found at more than 150 000 loci all over the genome. Other frequent microsatellites are tri-, tetra- or pentanucleotide repeats, or iterations of a single base as poly(A) tracts. When a replication error (RER) occurs, the incorrect bases are detected, excised and corrected by the mismatch repair system that seems to function homologously in various bacteria, yeast and humans (Fig. 1.1). In *Escherichia coli*, mismatch repair is initiated by binding of MutS to base mispairs and to loops of up to four unpaired nucleotides. After binding to this heteroduplex, the MutS–DNA complex is bound by the *mutL* gene product and the excision of a tract of single-stranded DNA containing the mismatched nucleotides follows:[1] activation of a latent GATC endonuclease, which is associated with the MutH protein, causes the incision of the unmodified strand at the hemimethylated d(GATC) sequence on either side of the mismatch and subsequently the incorrect DNA strand is excised and corrected (Fig. 1.2).

The human mismatch system consists of four known proteins: hMSH2, hMLH1, hPMS1 and hPMS2, which show high homology to both the bacterial and yeast mismatch repair system and have been cloned during the last few years.[2-6]

The first proof of the proposed functional similarity of the human mismatch repair system to the well described system in *E. coli* came from Fishel

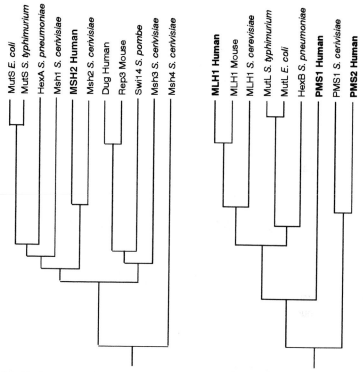

Fig. 1.1 Evolutionary relatedness of MutS and MutL homologues. Sequence homologies were used to build a family tree in which divergence of lines indicates nearest relatives (reproduced with permission of Current Opinion in Genetics & Development)[51]

et al[7] who were able to demonstrate that purified human MSH2 protein binds to DNA containing mismatched nucleotides. The specificity of binding was tested by competition with unlabelled homoduplex DNA, which had to be added in an excess of 50–100-fold until homoduplex DNA was bound in a significant amount. Saturation occurred at a protein:DNA ratio of 4:1. At these concentrations a 'supershift' band appeared, which can be interpreted as a homopolymeric multimer of hMSH2 bound to the mismatched oligonucleotide. This phenomenon has also been observed in yeast, when the yeast MLH1 and PMS1 proteins have been added to yeast MSH2 bound to a mismatched DNA substrate.[8] These authors suggested that a ternary complex containing MSH2–MLH1–PMS1 is formed, whereas Fishel discussed the alternative that the super-shift in yeast is an oligomeric form of MSH2, while MLH1 and PMS1 promote its formation at lower MSH2 protein concentrations.

However, the role of hMSH2 in binding to insertion/deletion mismatches remains to be assessed. Whereas in *E. coli* only insertions forming loops of more than 4 consecutive unpaired bases[9,10] can be repaired, human cell extracts with an intact mismatch repair system can correct

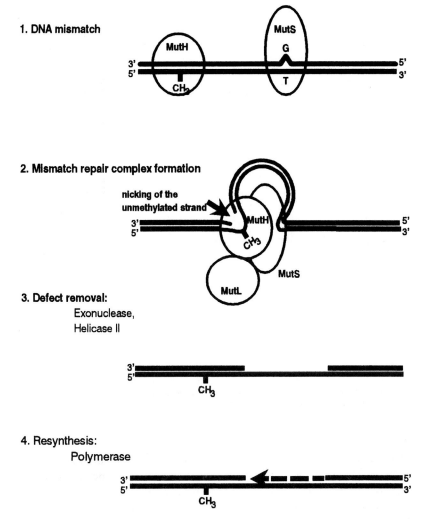

1. **DNA mismatch**

2. **Mismatch repair complex formation**

nicking of the
unmethylated strand

3. **Defect removal:**
   Exonuclease,
   Helicase II

4. **Resynthesis:**
   Polymerase

Fig.1.2 Mismatch repair in *E. coli*. Base mismatches are detected by MutS; MutH recognizes and nicks the unmethylated strand at hemimethylated GATC sites and a MutHLS complex forms. Subsequently, ATP. dependent helicase UvrD and a single-stranded exonuclease lead to the excision of the newly synthesized strand. The gap is filled with the help of the polymerase III holoenzyme complex.

heteroduplexes containing mismatches 1–16 extra bases. Extracts of the human colorectal cancer (CRC) cell line LoVo, a cell line with deletions in both *hMSH2* alleles, have been shown to have lost the capability to repair DNA containing mispaired or unpaired bases. HCT116, a CRC cell line without detectable wild-type *hMLH1* gene product, is unable to repair DNA containing 1 to 4 mismatched or unpaired bases but the same extract can correct heteroduplexes containing 5, 8, or 16 unpaired bases, depending on the sequence context.[11] Qualitative as well as quantitative differences in the stability of various microsatellite alleles in tumour cells and tumour cell lines have been described,[12,13] and the identification of extracts defective in the repair of loops but not of mismatches suggests different requirements for mismatch and loop repair.

Mutations in the mismatch repair system have been reported to lead to a 13-fold increase of microsatellite instability in *E. coli*, when MutS and MutL are affected. In yeast the microsatellite mutation rate rises by a factor of 100–700-fold when MSH2, MLH1 or PMS1 are defective.[14] In different human colorectal carcinoma cell lines with mutations of the mismatch repair genes the mutation rate at different microsatellite loci was elevated more than 1000-fold in comparison to cell lines with intact mismatch repair which have an estimated rate of 10^{-4} per allele per cell replication.[12]

Hereditary non-polyposis colorectal carcinoma (HNPCC) – a cancer syndrome characterized by microsatellite instability

Colorectal cancer is the second most common malignant tumour in men and women, representing about 15% of all cancers diagnosed in the USA. The majority of CRC consists of sporadic cancers with regard to the family history and is thought to be largely dependent on environmental factors. However, several familial cancer syndromes have been described which constitute about 15% of the total incidence of CRC. Thereby, (1) syndromes with pre-existing adenomatous polyps have to be distinguished from (2) syndromes without pre-existing polyps.[15]

Syndromes with pre-existing polyps

Familial adenomatous polyposis (FAP) patients present with hundreds of polyps distributed all over the large bowel and virtually all affected individuals develop CRC at a young age. FAP results from inheritance, in an autosomal dominant fashion, of mutations of the *APC* gene. FAP represents 1% of CRC and the prevalence of the gene is 1:10000 of the population. Other adenomatous polyposis syndromes such as Gardner's, Oldfield's or Turcot's syndromes are even less frequent.

Syndromes without pre-existing polyps

The hereditary non-polyposis colorectal cancer syndrome (HNPCC) or Lynch Syndrome is the most frequent of CRC syndromes without pre-existing polyps accounting for about 10% of total CRC and thus representing the most frequent hereditary cancer syndrome in humans with an allele frequency that has been estimated to be as high as 1 in 200.[5] A large family with a strong history of gastrointestinal cancer and endometrial cancer was first described 80 years ago by Aldred Warthin,[16] and the hereditary non-polyposis syndrome was later defined clinically by

Table 1.1 Lynch-syndrome

Amsterdam criteria (strict criteria) (Lynch 1988)

Type I
- At least three relatives with histologically verified CRC; one of them a first degree relative of the other two, FAP excluded
- Two successive generations affected
- Age of onset under 50 years (one of the three relatives)

Type II
Additional extracolonic cancer in the family history such as endometrial cancer or small bowel cancer

Copenhagen criteria (loose criteria)
Any one diagnosis of the 'strict' set of cancers plus ovarian cancer diagnosed before age 50 years, stomach cancer diagnosed before age 50 years, hepatobiliary cancer, pancreatic cancer, transitional cell carcinoma of the bladder, ureter or kidney, or the diagnosis of any two of these cancers at any age

---

Henry Lynch:[17] For the diagnosis to be made clinically, three first degree relatives from two generations have to be affected and least one of them has to develop CRC under the age of 50 years. In addition in about 30% of cases, other cancers such as small bowel, endometrial, breast, gastric, transitional cell or hepatopancreatic cancer occur in the family and this syndrome is classified as Lynch II (Table 1.1). In the patients affected, synchronous and metachronous carcinomas at different sites are also found in a high percentage. Other related colon cancer syndromes without preexisting adenomatous polyps are Muir-Torre's Syndrome and the hereditary flat adenoma syndrome. Muir-Torre's syndrome consists of at least one visceral malignant tumour and a dermatological lesion, usually a sebaceous tumour. Patients with the hereditary flat adenoma syndrome present with up to 100 flat adenomas that are predominantly localized in the proximal colon, the age of onset being higher than in HNPCC patients.

Genetic analysis of hereditary colorectal caranomia

The genetic background for the hereditary CRC syndromes without preexistent polyps has only been elucidated during the last 2 years – the underlying mechanism is a defect in DNA repair that causes numerous mutations. Ionov et al[18] were the first to describe ubiquitous somatic mutations in simple repeated sequences as characteristic for a subset of colorectal carcinomas, which seem to occur independently from the multistep carcinogenesis model set up by Fearon and Vogelstein.[19] The above-mentioned mutations were reductions of poly(A) tracts and other simple repetitive sequences in tumour DNA compared with the constitutional DNA of the same patient. Meanwhile, a variety of microsatellites on multiple chromosomes have been analysed, and deletions as well as insertions of one or a few repeat motifs have been found. This phenomenon has been called the mutator phenotype

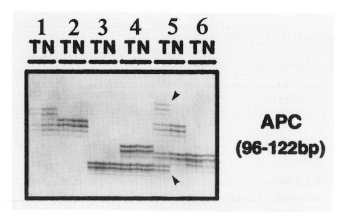

Fig.1.3 Microsatellite instability in colorectal carcinomas. Microsatellite analysis of DNA from six colorectal carcinomas (T) and corresponding normal mucosa (N) at the locus D5S346. Allele shifts can be seen in tumour DNA from patient 5 (see arrowheads).

or replication errors-positive (RER positive) phenotype (Fig. 1.3). However, until now it has not been clear how many microsatellite loci must show instability in order to qualify as the mutator phenotype. Some tumours exhibit replication errors in virtually all simple repetitive loci analysed, others show the microsatellite instability phenotype in only one or two of the investigated loci. At least five loci should therefore be analysed in order to reliably assess microsatellite instability – if microsatellite alterations are found at none or only one of the loci, the number of loci should be further increased. The RER positive phenotype with alterations at more than two microsatellite loci has been detected in a variety of malignant and premalignant lesions. Interestingly, the RER positive phenotype is observed in approximately 15% of sporadic colorectal carcinomas compared with 90% in HNPCC tumours.[20]

The connection between microsatellite instability, mismatch repair defects and HNPCC has been clearly shown. Aaltonen et al[20] described replication errors to be characteristic for CRCs of HNPCC patients compared with sporadic CRC Linkage analyses of large HNPCC kindreds were carried out and revealed mutations of hMSH2 as an underlying factor.[20] At the same time, Fishel et al[2] identified hMSH2 via its homology to the bacterial MutS and proposed the association with HNPCC. Later, hMLH1, hPMS1 and hPMS2 were also found to be mutated in HNPCC families.[4,5] Surprisingly, even in phenotypically normal human cells from HNPCC patients, microsatellite instability has been detected in single-cell equivalents of Epstein-Barr virus-transformed lymphoblasts and from non-neoplastic colon tissue.[21] The alterations were observed predominantly in the lymphoblastoid cells and in colon mucosa by comparison to the non-epithelial fraction such as muscularis propria. Depending on the microsatellite loci investigated, up to 53% of single-cell equivalents of colon mucosa exhibited microsatellite instability, whereas in non–epithelial colon tissue the maximal rate was 10%. This indicates that in phenotypically normal cells the RER positive phenotype is expressed predominantly in rapidly regenerating tissue.

In sporadic CRC with microsatellite instability, however, it could be demonstrated that factors other than germline mutations or somatic mutations must also be involved, as in 10 patients with sporadic CRC only one had a germline mutation of *hMLH1* and the other three mismatch repair genes were not affected. Moreover only three of seven sporadic tumour cell lines with microsatellite instability had somatic mutations in a mismatch repair gene. Therefore, it must be concluded that other factors in addition to the four human mismatch repair genes described so far are responsible for microsatellite instability.[22] For example, exonuclease-deficient variants of the polymerase delta have been shown to cause microsatellite instability in colorectal cancer cell lines without defects in the mismatch repair system. The mechanism appears to be an increase of replication errors which exceeds the repair capacity of the mismatch repair system.[23]

Microsatellite instability, mismatch repair defects and carcinogenesis

The mechanism of carcinogenesis in tumours with the replication error phenotype is far from clear. As the simple repetitive sequences are located mainly within introns and between genes[24] the microsatellite alterations found in HNPCC tumours are probably not directly involved in tumorigenesis. However, in the colorectum they seem to be an early event in carcinogenesis, occurring in adenomas.[12] Several factors may play a role in malignant transformation, selection and clonal expansion:

1. mutations in oncogenes and tumour–suppressor genes;
2. escape from immune surveillance;
3. alterations in the reactions towards chemicals as alkylating substances;
4. different response to other environmental factors.

Mutations in oncogenes and tumour–suppressor genes

One hypothesis is that the DNA repair defects lead to oncogenic changes in transforming genes. The spontaneous mutation rate at the hypoxanthine phosphoribosyl transferase locus (*HPRT*) has therefore been determined in RER positive and RER negative tumour cell lines. The functioning of HPRT is indicated by the ability of cells to grow in 6-thioguanine. In the study by Battacharyya et al[25] it was shown that the mutation rate is increased 200–600-fold in the mismatch defective tumour cell lines HCT116, HCT15 and DLD1 compared with SV40-transformed human fibroblasts.

The *MCC, DCC* and *p53* genes being tumour–suppressor genes of particular importance for colorectal tumorigenesis, have been analysed in normal cells and nine cancers of seven HNPCC patients by single-strand conformation polymorphism and loss of heterozygosity assays (LOH). In normal cells no sequence alterations were observed and LOH was detected solely in advanced and metastatic tumours.[26] By contrast, an unusual form of multiple somatic mutations of *p53* and *APC* with predicted alterations of the translated protein was observed in two HNPCC families. Up to six mutations per gene were found, consisting either of simple nucleotide substitutions or frameshift mutations, all occuring in a stretch of repeated nucleotides.[27] In sporadic colorectal carcinomas, however, the tumour suppressor genes typically show a LOH of one allele and an inactivation of the second allele, mostly by a point mutation.[28]

Very recently it has been demonstrated that the C-terminal domain of p53 recognizes sites containing insertion/deletion mismatches, the binding activity becoming stronger with increasing size of the loop of inserted DNA and the half-life of the complexes being 2 h or more.[29] Like yeast and human MSH2, p53 has a higher affinity for insertion/deletion mismatches than for mispaired bases. A highly stable p53–DNA complex at the site of a lesion could therefore activate genes responsible for apoptosis or cell cycle control or otherwise enhance the DNA repair mechanisms.[29]

Recent observations have pinned down inactivation of the type II TGF-β receptor (TGF-β RII) as playing an important role in the carcinogenesis.[30] Epithelial cell growth can be inhibited by transforming growth factor β (TGF-β), and antisense inhibition of TGF-β leads to an enhancement of tumorigenicity of tumour cells. Therefore, loss of the negative regulation by TGF-β can be expected to give a growth advantage and to contribute to tumour development. RER positive colon cancer cell lines have now been found to carry somatic mutations in small repeated sequences in the *TGF-β RII* gene, resulting in the loss of expression of the receptor. A GT insertion has been identified in a 6 base pair GTGTGT repeat at nucleotides 1931 to 1936 in the cell line VACO481 leading to a frameshift mutation. Other somatic *TGF-β RII* mutations were detected within a sequence of 10 repeating adenines between nucleotides 709 to 718 in seven other colon cancer cell lines with microsatellite instability. On the other hand, inactivation of the TGF-β receptor does not seem to be characteristic for other colon cancers so it is surmised that this could be a specific event in tumours resulting from microsatellite instability.

Escape from immune surveillance

Another interesting factor that could be relevant is the resistance of tumour cells to immune response. Three tumour cell lines with microsatellite instability and mismatch repair defects (Lo Vo, DLD1 and HCT15, the latter two established from the same tumour) shared the inability to express surface β2-microglobulin, which is essential for antigen presentation in HLA class I-mediated T-cell responses. Another RER positive cell line with normal mismatch binding capacity, SW480, also does not express β2-microglobulin. Consequently, the tumour cells could escape T-cell cytotoxicity by loss of the ability to express HLA class I antigens.[31]

Alterations in the response to alkylating agents

Repeatedly it has been observed that cells with the mutator phenotype are tolerant to alkylating agents. The human lymphoblastoid B-cell line Mt1 has been shown to be resistant to the cytotoxic effects of N-methyl-N'-nitro-N-nitrosoguanidine (MNNG) but remains sensitive to mutagenesis induced by MNNG. As the mutagenic and the cytotoxic effects of MNNG are attributed largely to its ability to alkylate the O^6 position of guanine, the resulting primary lesion in MNNG-treated cells is O^6-methylguanine. Therefore the mutations are almost exclusively G $\rightarrow$ A transitions, based on the miscoding properties of O^6-methylguanine. By contrast, spontaneous mutations consist of single-nucleotide insertions, tranversions and A $\rightarrow$ G transitions. Although MNNG is a potent mutagen, the alkylation adducts do not seem to be intrinsically toxic but the cytotoxic effects arise during the early steps of mismatch correction.[32] The sensitivity to MNNG could be restored in the human RER positive cell line HCT116 by introducing a human chromosome 3 with one copy of a normal $hMLH1$.[33] However, normally the cytotoxic effect of MNNG is dosage dependent, whereas in HCT116+ch3 cells the cell death was not immediate: first, a dosage-dependent growth arrest was observed that led to a loss of colony forming ability and consecutive cell death. De Wind et al[34] have differentiated between the $Msh2^{-/-}$ cell line dMsh2-9, the $Msh2^{+/-}$ cell line sMsh2-21 and the wild-type cell line wt-2 and found that the LD_{50} for MNNG was increased 20-fold in the $Msh2^{-/-}$ line compared with the heterozygous and the wild-type cell line.[34]

Moreover, it has been speculated that the mismatch repair genes themselves can be a mutational hotspot for certain carcinogens: in an animal model for colorectal cancer, microsatellite instability has been described in rat colon tumours induced by 2-amino-1-methyl-6-phenylimidazo (4,5-b) pyridine, whereas colon tumours induced by another heterocyclic amine, 2-amino-3-methylimidazo (4,5-f) quinoline[35] did not develop microsatellite instability. As the mutational spectra of the two heterocyclic amines differ, the mismatch repair genes may be mutational hot spots for the former carcinogen.

Environmental factors

The fact that patients with mismatch repair defects preferentially develop carcinomas located in the colorectum and other organs represented in the Lynch syndrome, whereas other organs such as the thyroid seem to be never affected, suggests that environmental factors also play an important role. Viruses have been discussed as having a direct or indirect influence, as in the Kaposi's sarcomas and non-Hodgkin's lymphomas of human immuno-deficiency virus (HIV)-infected patients microsatellite instability has also been detected, whereas in HIV-negative patients there is no evidence of instability in similar lesions.[36]

Interestingly, chronic inflammation also seems to be a predisposing factor, as microsatellite instability has been found in 27% of colorectal carcinomas and 19% of dysplasias on the background of ulcerative colitis, this rate clearly being higher than in sporadic colorectal carcinomas. However, there was no correlation with the severity of the lesion, and the mismatch repair genes have not yet been analysed in this context.[37]

Recently the mismatch repair gene *MSH2* has been knocked out in mice. The *MSH2*[-/-] and the heterozygous mice were healthy at birth but six of the 19 homozygous mice developed metastasizing T-cell lymphomas and one acquired a generalized histiocytic sarcoma. The rapid development of the immune system in the newborn mice is thereby thought to be particularly vulnerable to the first manifestations of transforming events.[34] Similar results were obtained with *MSH2* knock-out mice by another group: five mice developed T-cell lymphomas and one a lymphoma of B-cell origin. However, the haematopoietic development of the homozygous mice was shown to be normal.[38] *PMS2* was the next gene to be knocked out in mice. It turned out that *PMS2*-deficient mice are also viable, and again development of four lymphomas and of two cervical sarcomas was observed in a total of 14 *PMS2*[-/-] mice. The tumours also exhibited microsatellite instability. The wild type and heterozygous mice, by contrast, did not develop benign or malignant tumours. Interestingly, the males homozygous for the defect were sterile and showed abnormalities in chromosome synapsis during meiosis prophase I whereas the female homozygotes appeared fully fertile.[39]

Pathological implications of microsatellite instability in colorectal cancer

It has repeatedly been described that CRC which fulfil the HNPCC criteria are clinically and morphologically distinct from the tumours, following Vogelstein's concept of multistep carcinogenesis.[19] In an international co-operative study of 165 HNPCC families, a characteristic tumour phenotype has been delineated: the mean age of onset is 45 years, 60–70% of the tumours are localized proximal to the splenic flexure, adenomas are not increased in frequency but synchronous as well as metachronous carcinomas are frequently observed.[40] Histopathologically there is a preponderance of mucinous and poorly differentiated carcinomas, some of which exhibit a medullary growth pattern.[41] The host response often consists of a dense peritumoral lymphocytic infiltrate or lymphoid aggregates at the tumour margin.[42] This seems to be an indicator for a host immune response which may contribute to the favourable prognosis of HNPCC patients that has been observed. At the same time the DNA content is predominantly diploid compared to a rate of about 60% aneuploid sporadic carcinomas.[43] A diploid DNA content has also been proposed to be associated with a favourable prognosis, although in multivariate studies it is controversial whether this is an independent prognosticator.[43]

By comparative genomic hybridization (CGH) only two of six tumours

Table 1.2 Microsatellite instability in colorectal cancer[47]

	Sporadic CRC RER negative	Sporadic CRC RER positive	HNPCC RER positive
Frequency of RER	85%	15%	90%
Age (mean)	66 years	60 years	45 years
Localization: proximal colon	30–35%	80–94%	56–62%
Histology			
grade 3	7%	55%	37%
mucinous	20–30%	82%	40%
Ploidy: diploid	25%	80%	60%

with microsatellite instability showed deletions of one chromosomal segment each, whereas a variety of gains and losses were observed in tumours with stable microsatellites, especially gains on chromosomes 7, 13 and 20q and deletions on chromosome 17, 18 and 9p.[44] This again underlines the observation that tumours with microsatellite instability form a distinct tumour entity that does not follow the classical model of multistep carcinogenesis.

It appeared that sporadic CRC with microsatellite instability share the phenotypical characteristics of HNPCC tumours. They are also mostly located in the right colon, are diploid, and the histopathology is often similar to the type described above (Table 1.2).[45,46] Here again a Crohn's-like lymphocytic infiltrate is found that may represent the morphological equivalent of a different pattern of immune response compared with other colorectal tumours. Another interesting factor is the low proliferative activity of RER-positive tumours compared with RER-negative carcinomas as assessed by AgNOR staining,[46] which gives further weight to the improved prognosis that has been found.

These data suggest the existence of a distinct tumour entity that is not only characterized by the mutator phenotype but also by specific clinical and pathological findings which can be found in HNPCC and in sporadic CRC as well.

Other tumours have also been investigated with respect to microsatellite instability. Interestingly, sporadic cancers of the HNPCC spectrum may exhibit microsatellite instability as well as tumours not at all associated with HNPCC. For example, RER are also detected in small-cell lung cancer and tumour cells in the blast crisis of chronic myeloid leukaemia.[47] However, the percentage of cases with microsatellite instability is lower than that in HNPCC tumours. On the other hand, microsatellite instability is rarely found in cancers of breast, liver, testis, prostate, thyroid, bladder and squamous cell oesopha- geal cancer. In stomach cancer the RER-positive phenotype is detected mainly in poorly differentiated and non-signet cell carcinomas that are localized mainly in the distal stomach. This further substantiates the hypothesis that RER positive tumours form a distinct entity. In gastric cancer as well as in colorectal carcinomas an improved prognosis has been correlated with microsatellite instability, although this was not an independent prognostic factor.[48]

Conclusions

What are the consequences of our understanding of microsatellite instability and mismatch repair defects?

The identification of HNPCC patients is important because the follow-up of the patient has to be intensified owing to the increased risk of secondary carcinomas; therefore some authors have even proposed total colectomy in HNPCC patients with CRC. Additionally, the relatives should be screened with regular colonoscopies. Guidelines of surveillance and treatment of HNPCC patients and their families have been published by the international collaborative group on HNPCC.[49] Microsatellite analysis is useful as a screening method before the mismatch repair genes are sequenced, which is a time-and cost-consuming task. However, microsatellite analysis should only complement a detailed family history. As many families are too small for segregation analyses and as microsatellite instability is also found in sporadic carcinomas, both have to go hand in hand. The tumour phenotype mentioned above may also help to identify patients for when a search of mismatch repair gene mutations is appropriate. At present three methodological approaches can be utilized to detect hereditary mismatch repair gene defects:

1. linkage analyses, which can only be carried out in large kindreds;
2. use of an in vitro synthesized protein assay; and
3. direct sequencing of the mismatch repair genes.[50]

Functional assays of the mismatch repair capacity would be desirable for the future. When a mismatch repair gene mutation is found, the family members affected with germline mutations can be easily identified and genetic diagnosis can consequently be included in intensified tumour screening programmes.

The mechanism by which mismatch repair defects lead to cancer and the reason why the carcinomas occur preferentially in the colorectum, stomach, endometrium and others still remains to be clarified. Irrespective of the familial implications, the detection of this cancer predisposition syndrome with microsatellite instability seems to be of special clinical interest because of the improved prognosis.

Key points for clinical practice

● Microsatellite instability is found in about 15% of sporadic CRC and 90% of HNPCC as well as in various other HNPCC-related and unrelated carcinomas.
● Mutations in the human mismatch repair genes *hMSH2*, *hMLH1*, *hPMS1* and *hPMS2* have been found to cause microsatellite instability.

- Consider HNPCC when a patient presents with CRC and has a strong family history of CRC – especially if any one of the affected individuals is under the age of 50 years.
- HNPCC and sporadic CRC with microsatellite instability are characterized by a localization proximal to the splenic flexure, a diploid DNA content, a low proliferative activity and special histological features such as medullary or mucinous growth and a Crohn's-like peritumoral lymphocytic infiltrate and a tendency towards an improved prognosis.
- The exact mechanism of carcinogenesis is unknown, but mutations in the *TGF-β RII*, in *p53* and *APC* tumour suppressor genes have been described.
- Mice with knock-out of *MSH2* or *PMS2* are viable but develop lymphomas and sarcomas at an early age. Heterozygous animals resemble the wild type.

Note added in proof

A further human MutS homologue, hMSH6, has been cloned recently, which was originally designated GTBP or p160. It forms a mismatch nucleotide binding complex with hMSH2 (Drummond, *Science* 1995; **268**: 1909; Palombo, *Science* 1995; **268**: 1912; Papadopoulos, *Science* 1995; **268**: 1915). hMSH2 has also been found to form mispair binding complexes with hMSH3 (DUG1) (Palombo, *Curr Biol* 1996; **6**: 1181; Acharya, *Proc Natl Acad Sci (USA)* 1996, in press). Interestingly, MSH2 knock-out mice develop intestinal adenomatous polyps and carcinomas at an age of 6 and more months (Reitmeier, *Cancer Res* 1996; **56**: 3842).

Acknowledgement

This work was supported by the Wilhelm Sander-Stiftung, Munich, Germany (grant 93.055.2).

REFERENCES

1 Grilley M, Griffith J, Modrich P. Bidirectional excision in methyl-directed mismatch repair. J Biol Chem 1993; 268: 11830–11837
2 Fishel R, Lescoe MK, Rao MRS, et al The human mutator gene homolog MSH2 and its association with hereditary nonpolyposis colon cancer. Cell 1993; 75: 1027–1036
3 Leach FS, Nicolaides NC, Papadopoulos N et al Mutations of a MutS homolog in hereditary non-polyposis colorectal cancer. Cell 1993; 75: 1215–1235
4 Nicolaides NC, Papadopoulos N, Liu B, et al Mutations of two PMS homologues in hereditary nonpolyposis colon cancer. Nature 1994; 371: 75–80
5 Papadopoulos N, Nicolaides NC, Wie YF, et al Mutation of a MutL homolog in hereditary colon cancer. Science 1994; 262: 1625–1629
6 Bronner CE, Baker SM, Morrison PT, et al Mutation in the DNA mismatch repair gene homologue hMLH1 is associated with hereditary non-polyposis colon cancer. Nature 1994; 368: 658–661
7 Fishel R, Ewel A, Lescoe MK. Purified human MSH2 protein binds to DNA containing mismatched nucleotides. Cancer Res 1994; 54: 5539–5542

8 Prolla TA, Pang Q, Alani E, Kolodner RD, Liskay RM. MLH1, PMS1, and MSH2 interactions during the initiation of DNA mismatch repair in yeast. Science 1994; 265: 1091–1093

9 Parker BO, Marinus MG. Repair of DNA heteroduplexes containing small heterologous sequences in Escherichia coli. Proc Natl Acad Sci USA 1992; 98: 1730–1734

10 Carraway M, Marinus MG. Repair of heteroduplex DNA molecules with multibase loops in Escherichia coli. J Bacteriol 1993; 175: 3972–3980

11 Umar A, Boyer JC, Kunkel TA. DNA loop repair by human cell extracts. Science 1994; 266: 814–816

12 Shibata D, Peinado MA, Ionov Y, Malkhosyan S, Perucho M. Genomic instability in repeated sequences is an early somatic event in colorectal tumorigenesis that persists after transformation. Nature Genet 1994; 6: 273–281

13 Wooster R, Cleton-Jansen AM, Collins N, et al Instability of short tandem repeats (microsatellites) in human cancers. Nature Genet 1994; 6: 152–156

14 Strand M, Prolla TA, Liskay RM, Petes TD. Destabilisation of tracts of simple repetitive DNA in yeast by mutations affecting DNA mismatch repair. Nature 1993; 365: 274–276

15 Rustgi A. Hereditary gastrointestinal polyposis and nonpolyposis syndromes. N Engl J Med 1994; 331: 1694–1702

16 Warthin AS. Heredity with reference to carcinoma: as shown by a study of the cases examined in the pathological laboratory of the University of Michigan 1895–1913. Arch Intern Med 1913; 12: 546–555

17 Lynch HT, Watson P, Kriegler M, et al Differential diagnosis of hereditary nonpolyposis colorectal cancer (Lynch syndrome I and Lynch syndrome II). Dis Colon Rectum 1988; 31: 372–377

18 Ionov Y, Peinado MA, Malkhosyan S, Shibata D, Perucho M. Ubiquitous somatic mutations in simple repetitive sequences reveal a new mechanis for colonic carcinogenesis. Nature 1993; 363: 558–561

19 Fearon E, Vogelstein B. A genetic model for colorectal tumorigenesis. Cell 1990; 61: 759–767

20 Aaltonen LA, Peltomaki P, Leach F, et al Clues to the pathogenesis of familial colorectal cancer. Science 1993; 260: 812–816

21 Parsons R, Li GM, Longley M, et al Mismatch repair deficiency in phenotypically normal human cells. Science 1995; 268: 738–740

22 Liu B, Nicolaides NC, Markowitz S, et al Mismatch repair gene defects in sporadic colorectal cancers with microsatellite instability. Nature Genet 1995; 9: 48–55

23 da Costa LT, Liu B, El-Deiry WS, et al Polymerase delta variants in RER positive colorectal tumours. Nature Genet 1995; 9: 10–11

24 Weber JL, May PE. Abundant class of human DNA polymorphisms which can be typed using the polymerase chain reaction. Am J Hum Genet 1989; 44: 388–396

25 Bhattacharyya NP, Skandalis A, Ganesh A, Groden J, Meuth M. Mutator phenotypes in human colorectal carcinoma cell lines. Proc Natl Acad Sci USA 1994; 91: 6319–6323

26 Wu C, Akiyama Y, Imai K, et al DNA alterations in cells from hereditary non-polyposis colorectal cancer patients. Oncogene 1994; 9: 991–994

27 Lazar V, Grandjouan S, Bognel C, et al Accumulation of multiple mutations in tumor suppressor genes during colorectal tumorigenesis in HNPCC patients. Hum Mol Genet 1994; 3: 2257–2260

28 Goh HS, Chan CS, Khine K, Smith DR. p53 and behaviour of colorectal cancer. Lancet 1994; 344: 233–234

29 Lee S, Elenbaas B, Levine A, Griffith J. p53 and its 14 kDa C-terminal domain recognize primary DNA damage in the form of insertion/deletion mismatches. Cell 1995; 81: 1013–1020

30 Markowitz S, Wang J, Myeroff L, et al Inactivation of the type II TGF-β receptor in colon cancer cells with microsatellite instability. Science 1995; 268: 1336–1338

31 Branch P, Bicknell DC, Rowan A, Bodmer WF, Karran P. Immune surveillance in colorectal carcinoma. Nature Genet 1995; 9: 231–232

32 Kat A, Thilly WG, Fang WH, Longley MJ, Li GM, Modrich P. An alkylation-tolerant, mutator human cell line is deficient in strand-specific mismatch repair. Proc Natl Acad Sci USA 1993; 90: 6424–6428

33 Koi M, Umar A, Chauhan DP, et al Human Chromosome 3 corrects mismatch repair deficiency and microsatellite instability and reduces N-methyl-N'-nitro-N-nitrosoguanidine tolerance in colon tumor cells with homozygous h*MLH1* mutation. Cancer Res 1994; 54: 4308–4312

34 de Wind N, Dekker M, Berns A, Radman M, te Riele H. Inactivation of the mouse Msh2 gene results in mismatch repair deficiency, methylation tolerance, hyperrecombination, and predisposition to cancer. Cell 1995; 82: 321–330

35 Canzian F, Ushijima T, Serikawa T, Wakabayashi K, Sugimura T, Nagao M. Instability of microsatellites in rat colon tumors induced by heterocyclic amines. Cancer Res 1994; 54: 6315–6317

36 Bedi GC, Westra WH, Farzadegan H, Pitha PM, Sidransky D. Microsatellite instability in primary neoplasms from HIV+ patients. Nature Med 1995; 1: 65–68

37 Suzuki H, Harpaz N, Tarmin L, et al Microsatellite instability in ulcerative colitis associated colorectal dysplasias and cancers. Cancer Res 1994; 54: 4841–4844

38 Reitmeier AH, Schmits R, Ewel A, et al MSH2 deficient mice are viable and susceptiable to lymphoid tumours. Nature Genet 1995; 11: 64–70

39 Baker SM, Bronner CE, Zhang L, et al Male mice defective in the DNA mismatch repair gene PMS2 exhibit abnormal chromosome synapsis in meiosis. Cell 1995; 82: 309–319

40 Vasen HF, Mecklin JP, Watson P, et al Surveillance in hereditary nonpolyposis colorectal cancer: an international cooperative study of 165 families. Dis Colon Rectum 1993; 36: 1–4

41 Lynch HT, Smyrk TC, Watson P, et al Genetics, natural history, tumor spectrum, and pathology of herditary nonpolyposis colorectal cancer: an updated review. Gastroenterology 1993; 104: 1535–1549

42 Smyrk TC, Lynch HT, Watson PA, Appleman HD. Histologic features of hereditary nonpolyposis colorectal carcinoma. In: Utsunomiya J, Lynch HT, eds. Hereditary Colorectal Cancer. Tokyo: Springer, 1990: pp 357–362

43 Kouri M, Laasonen A, Mecklin JP, Jarvinen H, Franssila K, Pyrhonen S. Diploid predominance in hereditary nonpolyposis colorectal carcinoma evaluated by flow cytometry. Cancer 1990; 65: 1825–1829

44 Schlegel J, Stumm G, Scherthan H, et al Comparative genomic in situ hybridization (CGH) of colon carcinomas with replication error. Cancer Res 1995; 55: 6002–6005

45 Kim H, Jen J, Vogelstein B, Hamilton SR. Clinical and pathological characteristics of sporadic colorectal carcinomas with DNA replication errors in microsatellite sequences. Am J Pathol 1994; 145: 148–156

46 Bocker T, Schlegel J, Kullmann F, et al Genomic instability in colorectal carcinomas: comparison of different evelation methods and their tumorbiological significance. J Pathol 1996; 179: 15–19

47 Rüschoff J, Bocker T, Schlegel J, Stumm G, Hofstaedter F. Microsatellite instability: new aspects in the carcinogenesis of colorectal carcinoma. Virchows Arch 1995; 426: 215–222

48 Strickler JG, Zheng J, Shu Q, Burgart LJ, Alberts SR, Shibata D. p53 mutations and microsatellite instability in sporadic gastric cancer: when guardians fail. Cancer Res 1994; 54: 4750–4755

49 Lynch PM. Surveillance and treatment of hereditary non-polyposis colorectal cancer. Anticancer Res 1995; 14: 1641–1646

50 Marra G, Boland R. Hereditary nonpolyposis colorectal cancer: the syndrome the genes, and historical perspectives. J Natl Cancer Inst 1995; 87: 1114–1125

51 Fishel R, Kolodner RD. Identification of mismatch repair genes and their role in the development of cancer. Curr Opin Genet Dev 1995; 5: 382–395

2

Diagnosis of cutaneous blistering diseases by conventional (light) microscopy

L. Cerroni

Vesiculobullous disorders of the skin comprise a wide number of unrelated entities sharing the formation of blisters within or below the epidermis. These disorders can be classified in many different ways: most often, they are divided according to pathogenetic criteria (i.e. autoimmune, infectious, etc.). As dermatopathologists see diseases in a static, two-dimensional way, in this review I will classify cutaneous blistering disorders in a dermatopathological fashion: that is, according to what one sees through the microscope. Three main histopathological features of blistering diseases are useful for the diagnosis: 1) the anatomical level of the split (subcorneal/intracorneal, within the spinous layer, suprabasal, subepidermal and intradermal); 2) the mechanism of blister formation (spongiosis, acantholysis, ballooning, mechanic separation, dermo-epidermal separation, oedema); and 3) the features of the inflammatory infiltrate. Cutaneous blistering diseases in this survey are grouped according to the main histopathological criterion, that is, the level of blister formation.[1] It must be underlined that different diseases show similar reaction patterns. A few histopathological clues that can be helpful for the diagnosis have been added. In some cases, however, histopathology alone does not allow a definitive diagnosis. Thus, a short discussion of the clinical features of each entity, as well as of the most relevant investigations which confirm (or exclude) a given histological diagnosis, have been included.[2,3] The optimal sites for harvesting skin biopsies for direct immunofluorescence analysis are listed in Table 2.1.

Two pitfalls in the diagnosis of cutaneous blistering disease according to the histopathological pattern must be underlined: the first concerns the regeneration of the epidermis in older lesions. With time, bullae that were subepidermal may look intradermal, and, more generally, blisters may appear to be at a level higher than they formed. To avoid this pitfall, care

Table 2.1 Optimal sites of skin biopsy for direct immunfluorescence of cutaneous blistering diseases

Disease	Optimal site of the biopsy
Bullous lichen planus	Lesional
Bullous pemphigoid	Perilesional, Normal
Bullous systemic lupus erythematosus	Perilesional
Bullous vasculitis	Lesional
Chronic bullous disease of childhood	Perilesional
Cicatricial pemphigoid	Perilesional
Dermatitis herpetiformis	Perilesional, Normal
Epidermolysis bullosa	Perilesional
Epidermolysis bullosa acquisita	Perilesional
Erythema multiforme	Lesional
Herpes gestationis	Perilesional
Lichen planus pemphigoides	Perilesional
Linear IgA dermatosis	Perilesional
Pemphigus	Perilesional
Porphyria cutanea tarda	Perilesional
Toxic epidermal necrolysis	Lesional

should be taken to obtain specimens only from lesions that are very recent. The second pitfall relates to the protean nature of the diseases we seek to identify. Any single disease can show in a given case a pattern different from the rule: for example, bullous lupus erythematosus reveals subepidermal blisters that usually show a predominant neutrophilic infiltrate; in some instances, however, a predominance of lymphocytes may be found. This is due partly to the natural history of the lesions themselves (i.e. different inflammatory cells may appear at different times during the evolution of a single lesion), and partly to the differences that always exist among various patients affected by the same disease.

Intraepidermal blistering diseases

Subcorneal/intracorneal blisters

Subcorneal/intracorneal blistering diseases are characterized by a very superficial blister located within, or just below, the horny layer. Owing to the superficial location, the horny layer may be completely missing. The blister may be filled with granulocytes, or may be devoid of inflammatory infiltrate. This pattern is shared by the diseases listed in Table 2.2A. In addition, a similar pattern can be observed as an exception in cases of incontinentia pigmenti and bullous mycotic infections.

Histopathology – differential diagnostic features

Blisters caused by acantholysis are found in the superficial variants of pemphigus, namely, pemphigus erythematosus and pemphigus foliaceus

Table 2.2 Intraepidermal blistering diseases

A Subcorneal/intracorneal
   Bullous impetigo
   Erythema toxicum neonatorum
   Infantile acropustulosis
   Miliaria crystallina (sudamina)
   Pemphigus erythematosus (Senear-Usher syndrome)
   Pemphigus foliaceus
   Staphylococcal scalded-skin syndrome
   Subcorneal pustular dermatosis (Sneddon-Wilkinson)
   Transient neonatal pustular melanosis

B Within the spinous layer
   Allergic contact dermatitis
   Bullous ichtyosis (bullous congenital ichthyosiform erythroderma)
   Bullous mycotic infections
   Dyshidrotic dermatitis (pompholyx)
   Epidermolysis bullosa simplex (Weber-Cockayne subtype)
   Friction blisters
   Hydroa vacciniformis
   Incontinentia pigmenti (Bloch-Sulzberger syndrome)
   Miliaria rubra
   Palmoplantar pustulosis
   Pustular psoriasis
   Viral blistering diseases

C Suprabasal
   Darier's disease
   Epidermolysis bullosa simplex
   Familial benign chronic pemphigus (Hailey-Hailey disease)
   Grover's disease
   Pemphigus vegetans
   Pemphigus vulgaris
   PUVA-induced bullae
   Solar keratosis, acantholytic type
   Warty dyskeratoma

(Fig. 2.1). In both diseases bullae may contain neutrophils and a few eosinophils. The epidermis, especially in late stages, is acanthotic. Differential diagnosis between the two forms is not possible by histology alone. A few acantholytic cells may also be found in bullous impetigo and in other blistering diseases featuring neutrophils within the bullae, as a result of their enzymatic activity. Subcorneal bullae with predominance of neutrophils are found in bullous impetigo, infantile acropustulosis, staphylococcal scalded skin syndrome, subcorneal pustular dermatosis and transient neonatal pustular melanosis. A few eosinophils are usually admixed with the predominant neutrophils in infantile acropustulosis, subcorneal pustular dermatosis and transient neonatal pustular melanosis. In this last, the epidermis shows signs of hyperkeratosis. In bullous impetigo, Gram–positive cocci can be demonstrated with the Gram stain. A predominance of eosinophils within the bullae is found in erythema toxicum neonatorum. In this disease, there also is a perifollicular infiltrate of eosinophils resembling that of eosinophilic folliculitis (Ofuji). Vesicles centred on the acrosyringium

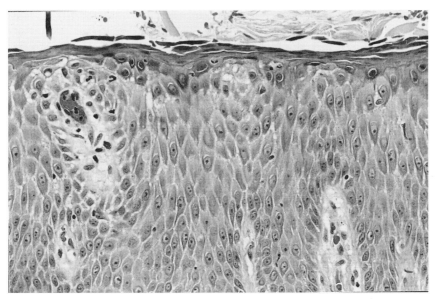

Fig. 2.1 Pemphigus erythematosus. The horny layer, in this case, is completely missing. Note acantholytic cells confined to the granular layer (H&E, original magnification ×250).

located directly below, or within, the stratum corneum are found in miliara crystallina. The affected sweat duct is ruptured.

Clinical features

Bullous impetigo occurs mainly in neonates or children and is associated with phage group II staphylococcal infection. Lesions are discrete and are predominantly located on the face, especially the nose and the perioral region, trunk and intertriginous sites. Bullae are clear or slightly turbid and arise on otherwise normal skin. Lesions in erythema toxicum neonatorum appear most frequently during the first 3–4 days of life, but may be present at birth. Morphologically there are erythematous macules, papules and pustules anywhere on the body (palms and soles can be spared). The disease is self-limiting. Blood eosinophilia may be present. Infantile acropustulosis usually affects black male children with onset between birth and 2 years of age. Vesicles and pustules are located mainly on the palms and soles but may also affect the wrists, ankles, face and scalp. They are intensely pruritic. Lesions resolve usually within 7–10 days, but recur after a few weeks. The disease resolves spontaneously by the time the patient reaches 2–3 years of age. There may be blood eosinophilia. In miliaria crystallina there are clear, small vesicles developing on otherwise normally appearing skin. Lesions are located mostly in intertriginous areas or on other parts of the body covered by clothes. They are caused by a superficial obstruction and subsequent rupture of the sweat ducts. Pemphigus erythematosus[4] affects elderly patients of both sexes. Predilection sites are the seborrheic areas of the face, scalp and trunk. Patients present with erythematous, hyperkeratotic, scaly plaques. Flaccid blisters may also be seen. In addition, there can be a butterfly erythema on the face resembling that of lupus erythematosus. Oral involvement is rare. The disease is usually associated with other autoimmune disorders (i.e. myasthenia gravis with thymoma, lupus erythematosus), but can also be induced by drugs (especially penicillamine). In pemphigus foliaceus[4] patients are mostly elderly, but children also may be affected. The disease presents most commonly with erosions, crusted patches and plaques arising on the face, scalp, upper chest and abdomen, but may involve the entire skin (exfoliative erythroderma). Involvement of mucous membranes is rare. Induction by penicillamine has been reported. An endemic variant is known in South America, mostly Brazil, as 'fogo savagem'. This variant occurs in children, adolescents and young adults. Staphylococcal scalded-skin syndrome is a disease of infants and young children, but it may occur in immunocompromised adults or in patients with renal impairment. Skin changes are caused by toxins produced by certain strains of *Staphylococcus aureus* (phage group II, mostly type 71). Erythematous and bullous lesions begin usually on the face, neck, axillae and groin, and subsequently become generalized. Mucous membranes are usually spared. Fever, when present, is low. In subcorneal pustular dermatosis superficial pustules develop on the trunk, particularly the intertriginous areas. Face and mucous membranes are never affected. A transient erythematous flare surrounds the pustules in the early phases. Patients are usually middle-aged. Women predominate over men. Some authors regard subcorneal pustular dermatosis as a variant of pustular psoriasis. In transient neonatal pustular melanosis lesions are usually present at birth. There are sterile vesicles and pustules located predominantly on the chin, forehead, neck, lower back and shins. Lesions usually disappear within 1–2 days leaving hyperpigmented macules.

Diagnostic tools other than histology

Tzanck's test reveals the presence of acantholytic cells in the two types of pemphigus, of eosinophils in infantile acropustulosis, and of neutrophils in bullous impetigo, infantile acropustulosis, staphylococcal scalded skin syndrome, subcorneal pustular dermatosis and transient neonatal pustular melanosis. Gram stain of a blister's content reveals Gram-positive cocci in bullous impetigo, but not in the other subcorneal blistering diseases. Organisms cannot be demonstrated within bullae of staphylococcal scalded-skin syndrome, but can usually be cultured at colonized sites of infection (umbilical stump, conjunctiva, external ear canal). Direct immunofluorescence shows intercellular deposits of IgG and/or C3 within the upper layers of the epidermis in pemphigus erythematosus and pemphigus foliaceus, but is negative in the other aforementioned disorders. Cases of subcorneal pustular dermatosis with a positive IgA intercellular deposits are currently classified as IgA pemphigus foliaceus. Indirect immunofluorescence shows circulating antiepithelial antibodies in pemphigus erythematosus and pemphigus foliaceus. Antinuclear antibodies and a positive lupus-band test on uninvolved skin can be observed in pemphigus erythematosus. A polypeptide associated with viral infections, thymosin alpha I, is markedly elevated in patients with the endemic variant of pemphigus foliaceus.

Blisters within the spinous layer

The diseases listed in Table 2.2B are characterized by blistering within the spinous layer. Blisters in this group may be caused by spongiosis, ballooning, or mechanical separation of the keratinocytes.

Histopathology – differential diagnostic features

Spongiosis is the mechanism of blister formation in allergic contact dermatitis, bullous mycotic infections, dyshidrotic dermatitis, hydroa vacciniformis, incontinentia pigmenti and miliaria rubra. Eosinophils are a prominent feature in incontinentia pigmenti, whereas a few neutrophils can be observed in bullous mycotic infections. In bullous mycotic infections, in addition, usually there is pronounced oedema of the superficial dermis, and the responsible microorganisms can be demonstrated with the PAS or Grocott stains. In miliaria rubra a hyperkeratotic plug can be seen overlying the spongiotic vesicle. Allergic contact dermatitis and dyshidrotic dermatitis may be indistinguishable histologically from one another. Ballooning is responsible for the formation of blisters in viral blistering diseases, bullous ichtyosis and friction blisters. In viral blistering diseases, in addition, one can observe large keratinocytes and giant cells, as well as a dense mixed-cell inflammatory infiltrate involving the entire dermis and sometimes the subcutaneous tissues. In bullous ichtyosis the epidermis is hyperkeratotic and the granular layer is thickened. Mechanic separation of the keratinocytes within the spinous layer is a feature of the Weber-Cockayne type of epidermolysis bullosa simplex. The inflammatory infiltrate in this form, if any, is very scarce. An intraepidermal pustule filled with neutrophils is found in palmoplantar pustulosis and pustular psoriasis. Differentiation between the two diseases is not possible on histological grounds alone, and some authors regard palmoplantar pustulosis as a variant of pustular psoriasis. Eosinophilic spongiosis can be observed in incontinentia pigmenti and allergic contact dermatitis (see Table 2.3). Necrotic keratinocytes are found in friction blisters and hydroa vacciniformis (see Table 2.4).

Clinical features

Allergic contact dermatitis occurs most frequently in young adults. It is rare in children and elderly patients. Predilection sites are the hand and feet, earlobes and scalp, but the entire body may be involved. Haematogenous

Table 2.3 Eosinophilic spongiosis in blistering and non-blistering diseases of the skin[22]

Arthropod bites (including scabies)
Bullous pemphigoid
Cicatricial pemphigoid
Dermatitis (contact, atopic, nummular, etc.)
Drug reactions
Epidermolysis bullosa
Factitial dermatitis
Herpes (pemphigoid) gestationis
Id reactions
Incontinentia pigmenti
Lichen planus
Mycosis fungoides
Pemphigus
Pityriasis rosea

Table 2.4 Necrotic keratinocytes in cutaneous blistering diseases

Bullous lichen planus
Bullous lupus erythematosus
Drug overdose-related bullae
Erythema multiforme/toxic epidermal necrolysis
Fixed drug eruption, bullous type
Friction blisters
Hydroa vacciniformis
Methyl bromide-induced bullae
Phototoxic dermatitis (phyto-photodermatitis)
Polymorphous light eruption (rare)
PUVA-induced bullae

spread can induce generalization of the cutaneous manifestations (erythroderma). In bullous ichthyosis, blisters on erythematous base appear usually within the first week of life. The blisters occur in crops and may be several cm in diameter. They are superficial and may rupture easily. Secondary infection is common. Bullous lesions localized mostly on the hands and feet are an infrequent complication of cutaneous mycotic infections. Lesions of dyshidrotic dermatitis are located solely on the palms, soles and lateral aspect of the fingers. Confluence of vesicles may give rise to large bullae. The Weber-Cockayne subtype of epidermolysis bullosa simplex[5-7] is the most frequent subtype of hereditary epidermolysis bullosa. Lesions are located on the acral sites, especially the feet (prolonged walks are a common cause of blistering). They usually heal with no scarring. The first symptoms occur during childhood or adolescence. Friction blisters develop at sites where the epidermis is thick (palms and soles, heels) after prolonged friction (prolonged walk, manual work). Hydroa vacciniformis is a seasonal disease of children, seen predominantly in boys during the summer months. Crusted patches, plaques and intact blisters on erythematous base arise on sun-exposed areas (nose and cheeks, neck, upper extremities). Incontinentia pigmenti usually appears at birth or within the first weeks of life. Females account for more than 90% of the patients. In the first stage there are erythematous and vesiculobullous lesions: they are located on the trunk and extremities, often arranged in a linear fashion along the Blaschko's lines. In the late stages verrucous and hyperpigmented lesions develop on areas previously affected by the eruption. Hypopigmentation may follow in a last, inconstant phase of the disease. Blood eosinophilia is present in about 70% of the patients, often lasting for months. The disorder is hereditary and affects the skin, hairs, nails, CNS, eyes, heart and skeletal system. The transmission may be X-linked. The incidence of miliaria rubra is greater in the first weeks of life, but the disease can be observed in infants, children and even adults. Pruritic, clustered papules and vesicles surrounded by erythema are observed mainly on the covered parts of the body. Palmoplantar pustulosis affects predominantly women aged between 40 and 60 years. Sterile pustules on erythematous ground are located on the palms and soles. Some cases possibly represent psoriasis pustulosa. Other are associated with bacterial infections localized on other parts of the body (so-called bacterid). There are two main variants of pustular psoriasis: a localized (palmoplantar) and a generalized form (syndrome of von Zumbusch). They occur usually in adults, but the generalized form may be observed in children. Multiple, partly confluent, erythematous, sterile pustules are located on the palms and soles (localized form) or the whole body (generalized form). In the generalized form there are also systemic symptoms such as fever, fatigue, severe malaise and inflammatory polyarthritis. There is leukocytosis in the peripheral blood. In viral blistering diseases lesions may be localized (i.e. herpes simplex, herpes zoster, milker's nodule, orf, hand-foot-mouth disease) or generalized (i.e. varicella). Clinical features vary according to the virus responsible.

Diagnostic tools other than histology

The Tzanck's test reveals large keratinocytes and giant cells in viral blistering diseases. In addition, a direct specimen identification/typing test or a PCR assay can show the presence of herpes simplex 1 or 2 viral DNA within intact blisters. Fresh preparations and tissue cultures allow identification of the responsible fungi in bullous mycotic infection. Direct and indirect immunofluorescence analyses in this group of diseases yield negative results. Electron microscopy helps in diagnosing and classifying cases of epidermolysis bullosa simplex and bullous ichthyosis. An abnormal phototest is usually found in patients with hydroa vacciniformis.

Suprabasal blisters

All diseases in this group (Table 2.2C) are characterized by suprabasal acantholysis, the only exceptions being epidermolysis bullosa simplex and PUVA-induced bullae. Some of them never present clinically with vesiculobullous lesions. However, I decided to include them because their histopathologic features may simulate those of a blistering disease.

Histopathology – differential diagnostic features

Acantholysis is confined mainly to the suprabasal layer in pemphigus vulgaris and pemphigus vegetans. Basal cells remain attached to the basement membrane while losing intercellular attachements, conferring the so-called 'tombstone' appearance to the specimen. The epidermis in pemphigus vegetans shows a prominent hyperplasia, but differentiation from pemphigus vulgaris, especially from older lesions of this disease, can be impossible. Although blistering in familial benign chronic pemphigus is also caused by suprabasal cell separation, acantholysis rapidly involves the entire thickness of the epidermis (so-called 'dilapidated brick wall' appearance). Mechanic separation of the keratinocytes is seen in epidermolysis bullosa simplex. In this disease, the split is so low within basal keratinocytes that the blister may appear subepidermal. However, PAS-stain shows the presence of the basement membrane on the bottom of the bulla. Detachment of the epidermis from the dermis owing necrosis of basal keratinocytes is found in PUVA-induced bullae. Dyskeratotic cells (corps ronds, grains) are observed in Darier's disease, Grover's disease, acantholytic solar keratosis and warty dyskeratoma. This last is characterized by a central pore showing features of viral infections at the margins (koilocytes). Epidermal changes (acantholysis, dyskeratosis) usually are more pronounced in Darier's than in Grover's disease, but differentiation at times may be impossible. Atypical keratinocytes above massive solar elastosis are a unique feature of acantholytic solar keratosis. Eosinophilic spongiosis may be encountered in pemphigus vulgaris and pemphigus vegetans (see Table 2.3).

Clinical features

Darier's disease is an autosomal dominant inherited disease presenting with papules and vesicles located on the seborrheic areas of the head, neck and trunk. Several forms of epidermolysis bullosa simplex[5–7] are recognized, in addition to the Weber-Cockayne subtype already described. The disease is inherited in an autosomal dominant manner. Intraepidermal separation is caused by a mutation in the genes encoding keratins 5 and 14. Lesions may be localized (acral regions) or generalized; symptoms appear first during childhood and usually improve considerably with age. Familial benign chronic pemphigus[8] is an autosomal dominant inherited disease with incomplete penetrance. Sporadic cases account for 25–30% of the total. The disease occurs in both sexes. First symptoms usually occur between 20 and 30 years of age. Predilection sites are the neck, axillae and intertriginous areas. Grover's disease presents with mildly pruritic papules and vesicles on the trunk in middle-aged adults. Occasionally, confluence of vesicles may give rise to large bullae. Pemphigus vulgaris[4,9] affects predominantly elderly patients of both sexes, but younger patients have been observed. Predilection sites are pressure points as well as the face and scalp, trunk, groin and axillae. Morphologically there are flaccid blisters and erythematous, crusted plaques. Secondary infection is frequent. Involvement of the oral mucosa with blisters, erosions and ulcers is common and may be the first manifestation of the disease in up to 50% of patients. Other mucosa may also be involved including anorectal mucosa, vulva, cervix, urethra, oesophagus, larynx and conjunctiva. Pemphigus vegetans[4] is a variant of pemphigus vulgaris characterized by vegetating lesions primarily affecting the flexures. Involvement of oral mucosa is common. There may be eosinophilia in the peripheral blood. PUVA-induced bullae occur on the acral regions as a rare complication of PUVA therapy, mostly 48–72 h after irradiation. They are caused by a phototoxic mechanism. Lesions of acantholytic solar keratosis clinically do not differ from common solar keratoses. They are confined to sun-exposed areas of elderly patients. Morphologically there are erythematous, slightly scaly, infiltrated patches. Warty dyskeratoma occurs usually as a solitary papule or small nodule, commonly located on the head and neck. Oral lesions have been reported.

Diagnostic tools other than histology

The Tzanck's test shows acantholytic cells in pemphigus vulgaris, pemphigus vegetans and familial benign chronic pemphigus. Direct immunofluorescence reveals intercellular deposits of IgG and, less frequently, IgA, IgM and C3 in pemphigus vulgaris and pemphigus vegetans, but is negative in familial benign chronic pemphigus. With indirect immunofluorescence antiepithelial antibodies directed against intercellular desmosomal cadherins are detectable in pemphigus vulgaris and pemphigus vegetans. Other suprabasal blistering diseases show a negative reaction. Electron microscopy and immunoelectron microscopy are helpful especially in classifying cases of epidermolysis bullosa simplex.

Subepidermal blistering diseases

With little or no inflammation

The diseases listed in Table 2.5A share the formation of a subepidermal blister with little or no accompanying dermal inflammatory infiltrate. In addition, cases of toxic epidermal necrolysis and bullous drug eruption may rarely present this pattern.

Histopathology – differential diagnostic features

Epidermal changes with necrosis of keratinocytes are found in acute radiodermitis, burns and drug overdose-related bullae. Preservance of the architecture of dermal papillae (festooning) can be observed in porphyrias, pseudoporphyrias and suction blisters, as well as in some cases of cell poor bullous pemphigoid (see Table 2.6) (Fig. 2.2). Hyaline deposits are found at the base of the blisters in bullous amyloidosis (Congo red- and

Table 2.5 Subepidermal blistering diseases

A With little or no inflammation
      Acute radiodermitis
      Angina bullosa haemorrhagica
      Blisters overlying scars
      Bullosis diabeticorum
      Bullous amyloidosis
      Bullous pemphigoid (cell-poor type)
      Bullous scleroderma
      Burns
      Drug overdose-related bullae
      Epidermolysis bullosa (junctional and dystrophic subtypes)
      Lymphatic bullae
      Porphyrias
      Pseudoporphyrias
      Suction blisters

B With predominant lymphocytic infiltrate
      Bullous leprosy
      Bullous leukemia cutis
      Bullous lichen planus – Lichen planus pemphigoides
      Bullous mycosis fungoides
      Erythema multiforme/toxic epidermal necrolysis
      Fixed drug eruption, bullous type
      Lichen sclerosus et atrophicus, bullous type
      Phototoxic dermatitis (phyto-photodermatitis)
      Polymorphous light eruption

C With predominant eosinophilic infiltrate
      Bullous drug eruptions
      Bullous pemphigoid
      Bullous reactions to arthropod bites
      Herpes (pemphigoid) gestationis

D With predominant neutrophilic infiltrate
      Bullous erysipela
      Bullous lupus erythematosus
      Bullous urticaria
      Bullous vasculitis
      Chronic bullous disease of children
      Cicatricial pemphigoid and Localized cicatricial pemphigoid
      Dermatitis herpetiformis (Duhring's disease)
      Epidermolysis bullosa acquisita
      Etretinate-induced bullae
      Linear IgA dermatosis
      Methyl bromide-induced bullae
      Sweet's syndrome (acute febrile neutrophilic dermatosis)

E With predominance of mast cells
      Bullous mastocytosis

Table 2.6 'Festooning' in cutaneous blistering diseases

Porphyrias
Pseudoporphyrias
Bullous pemphigoid
Epidermolysis bullosa acquisita
Suction blisters

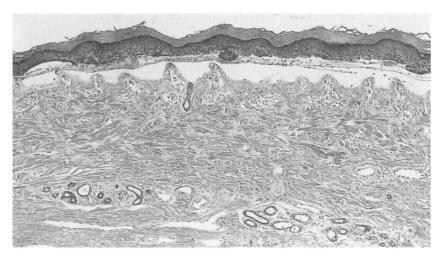

Fig. 2.2 Porphyria cutanea tarda. The architecture of dermal papillae is preserved (festooning). Note the absence of the inflammatory infiltrate (H&E, original magnification ×50).

thyoflavine-positive) and around blood vessels in the superficial dermis in porphyria cutanea tarda (PAS-positive). Sclerosis of the dermis is a feature of bullous scleroderma, whereas fibrosis is encountered in the dermis of blisters overlying scars. Massive haemorrhage is seen in angina bullosa haemorrhagica, and to a lesser extent in cryotherapy-induced and suction blisters. Differentiation of epidermolysis bullosa from cell-poor bullous pemphigoid may be impossible by light microscopy alone.

Clinical features

Acute radiodermitis with blistering occurs after a short time of latence within fields irradiated with > 8 Gy. Angina bullosa haemorrhagica presents with blood blisters on the oral mucosa in middle-aged or elderly patients. Development of a blister within a scar is uncommon; usually it happens within a few days after the surgical procedure. Bullae in patients with diabetes mellitus occur mainly on the hands and feet. They are a rare complication of the disease. Bullous amyloidosis is a rare variant of cutaneous manifestations of primary systemic amyloidosis. Bullae are usually localized on the area of minor trauma (hands and feet), but may be widespread. Other signs of cutaneous amyloidosis are present. Clinical aspects of cell-poor bullous pemphigoid[10] do not differ from that of bullous pemphigoid, except for the lack of erythematous changes at the base of the blisters. Bullous scleroderma[11] is a rare variant of localized cutaneous scleroderma (morphea). Lower extremities are the most common site of involvement. Tense, clear bullae develop following second-degree thermal burns, and sometimes following electrodesiccation therapy or cryotherapy. Bullae can occur following drug overdose. They arise at sites of pressure, possibly as a result of local ischaemia. Drugs implicated are amitryptidine, barbiturates, benzodiazepines, carbamezapine, heroin, imipramine, methadone and morphine. Lesions with similar clinico-pathological features have been observed also in carbon monoxide intoxication. Clinical aspects of junctional and dystrophic epidermolysis bullosa[5-7] vary according to the subtype. The disease is inherited in a recessive (junctional epidermolysis bullosa as well as four subtypes of dystrophic epidermolysis bullosa) or dominant manner (two subtypes of dystrophic epidermolysis bullosa). Clinical manifestations may be evident at birth or appear within the first years of life. In the junctional type there is a mutation in the genes encoding different chains of laminin 5, whereas in the dystrophic type the mutation is localized in an anchoring fibril collagen gene (COL7A1). Blisters may be localized to the acral regions, or generalized. They develop after minor trauma. Severe forms are lethal, usually within the first 2 years of life. Lymphatic bullae are a very rare complication of severe lymphoedema. They occur mainly on the extremities. Porphyrias are a group of inherited or acquired diseases characterized by altered haem biosynthesis resulting in accumulation of porphyrins or porphyrin precursors. Blisters can occur in the majority of the forms, but are usually observed in congenital erythropoietic porphyria, erythropoietic protoporphyria, porphyria cutanea tarda and variegate porphyria. The most common form is porphyria cutanea tarda. Blisters arise on sun-exposed areas (especially face and hands) following minor trauma. Cutaneous lesions with clinico-pathological features similar to those observed in the porphyrias (pseudoporphyrias) can be induced by drugs (furosemide, nalidixic acid, naproxen and tetracycline among others) or may be observed in patients receiving haemodialysis (bullous dermatosis of haemodialysis). This last occurs in 1–16% of patients receiving haemodialysis. Elevated levels of porphyrins can be found in the serum of patients with pseudoporphyrias; porphyrins in the stool and urine are normal or elevated. Subepidermal bullae may develop following suction of the skin. They usually represent a manifestation of dermatitis artefacta.

Diagnostic tools other than histology

Analysis of salt-split (NaCl-split) normal human skin with mapping for laminin, collagen IV, and bullous pemphigoid antigens allows identification of an epidermal, combined or dermal pattern. Bullous pemphigoid reveals an epidermal or combined pattern (epidermolysis bullosa acquisita, by contrast, shows a dermal pattern). Direct immunofluorescence shows IgG and C3 deposits around the vessels in the superficial dermis and in the basement membrane zone of lesions of porphyria cutanea tarda. Similar findings can also be observed in the pseudoporphyrias. Analysis of porphyrin levels in serum, urine and stool allows the diagnosis of porphyrias and pseudoporphyrias. The serum level of the responsible drug(s) are above normal limits in drug overdose-related bullae.

With predominance of lymphocytes

Subepidermal bullae with inflammatory infiltrates predominantly consti-
tuted by lymphocytes are featured by the diseases listed in Table 2.5B. In
addition, rare cases of bullous lupus erythematosus and bullous mycotic
infections also show this pattern.

Histopathology – differential diagnostic features

Necrotic keratinocytes within the basal layer (Civatte bodies) are a common feature of bullous lichen planus, erythema multiforme, fixed drug
eruption, phototoxic dermatitis and rarely of polymorphous light eruption
(see Table 2.4). Epidermotropism of atypical lymphocytes (sometimes with
formation of so-called Pautrier's microabscesses) is found only in mycosis
fungoides, but a few, solitary, non-atypical epidermotropic lymphocytes
may also be observed in most diseases belonging to this group. Mild spongiosis of the epidermis is usually seen in phototoxic dermatitis. Marked
oedema of the papillary dermis is associated with erythema multiforme,
phototoxic dermatitis and some cases of polymorphous light eruption.
Sclerosis and hyalinisation of the superficial and mid-dermis are a feature of
lichen sclerosus et atrophicus. The dermal inflammatory infiltrate shows a
granulomatous feature with prominent neural involvement in bullous leprosy. In this disease, acid-fast bacilli can be demonstrated with Fite or Ziehl-
Nielsen stains in a proportion of cases. Collection of small, monomorphous
lymphocytes within the subcutaneous tissues is seen only in bullous
leukaemia cutis.

Clinical features

Bullous leprosy is a very rare manifestation of borderline lepromatous leprosy. Typical, symmetrically distributed lesions of leprosy usually co-exist.
Bullous leukaemia cutis[12] may develop in patients with T-chronic lymphocytic leukaemia (CLL) or myeloid leukaemia, but mostly represent a manifestation of B-CLL. The occurrence is very rare (about 1.5% of patients
with B-CLL). Lesions may be generalized or localized to the extremities
and may be pruritic. Bullous lesions in patients with lichen planus may
appear on the top of pre-existing lesions (bullous lichen planus), or on normal skin (lichen planus pemphigoides)[13]. These last cases may rather represent examples of association of bullous pemphigoid with lichen planus.
Vesiculobullous lesions associated with a specific infiltrate may also develop
in patients with mycosis fungoides.[14] They can be localized on the hands
and feet ('dyshidrotic' mycosis fungoides) or arise on other areas of the
body. Typically, there is co-existence of 'classical' lesions of mycosis fungoides in other locations. Erythema multiforme presents with erythema,
papules and vesicles (hence the term 'multiforme') located on the upper
extremities (minor form) or generalized (major form). In this last type,
commonly there is involvement of the oral mucosa, as well as of the mucosa

of the eyes, nose, pharynx and trachea. Infectious diseases (i.e. herpes simplex, angina, rickettsiosis) usually precede the eruption by 1–3 weeks. Erythema multiforme can also be linked to drug ingestion or internal diseases (Crohn's disease, malignant tumors). Toxic epidermal necrolysis is now regarded as the most severe form of erythema multiforme, with lesions rapidly progressing to extensive shedding of the skin. Rapid loss of fluids and imbalance of electrolytes can be fatal. The bullous type of fixed drug eruption presents with solitary, rarely multiple brown-red blistering lesions. Predilection sites are the genital region, oral mucosa and extremities. Drugs most often involved are atropine, barbiturate, carisoprodol, diclofenac sodium, emetine, erythromycin, penicillin, pyrazolone, quinine and tetracycline. Bullous lichen sclerosus et atrophicus is a rare manifestation of lichen sclerosus. Lesions are commonly located on the genital area. Bullous lesions of phototoxic dermatitis develop after sun exposure following contact with certain plants, vegetables or perfumes containing furocumarine photosensitizer (i.e. 5-MOP and oil of bergamot among others). Berloque dermatitis, meadow grass dermatitis, dermatitis bullosa striata pratensis and phyto-photodermatitis are synonyms used in the literature. The eruption is usually seasonal. Lesions are localized in sun-exposed areas and often show a bizarre clinical configuration. They are intensely pruritic. Postinflammatory hyperpigmentation is a common sequela of the disease. Examples of plants and vegetables containing furocumarine photosensitizers are carrots, celery, figs and parsley among others. A subtype of polymorphous light eruption shows the formation of vesicular or bullous lesions. They are confined to sun-exposed areas and are intensely pruritic. The time of latence between sun exposure and onset of lesions varies from a few hours to 1–2 days.

Diagnostic tools other than histology

Immunohistochemistry shows an aberrant immunophenotype of B lymphocytes in bullous lesions of B-CLL (CD20+ / CD43+ / CD5+), as well as immunoglobulin light chain restriction (kappa or lambda). This last may be difficult to demonstrate in paraffin-embedded specimens. Analysis of the immunoglobulin gene rearrangement showed the presence of a monoclonal B-cell population in the majority of lesions studied.[12] In bullous mycosis fungoides immunohistochemistry usually reveals a 'normal' helper phenotype (CD3+ / CD4+ / CD8–). Gene rearrangement studies, however, may show the presence of a monoclonal population of T lymphocytes. Phototest shows a pathological reaction in patients affected by polymorphous light eruption. Exposition to the responsible drug (provocation test) may confirm the diagnosis of fixed bullous drug eruption.

With predominance of eosinophils

A subepidermal bulla with a predominantly eosinophilic infiltrate is present in all diseases listed in the Table 2.5C. With the exception of bullous reactions to arthropod bites, it may be extremely difficult to distinguish them from one another based solely on light microscopic findings.

Histopathology – differential diagnostic features

In contrast to the other diseases of this group, the inflammatory infiltrate in bullous reactions to arthropod bites involves not only the superficial but also the mid- and deep dermis. In this condition, eosinophils are typically arranged within collagen bundles. In bullous drug eruption the eosinophilic infiltrate is usually less pronounced than in bullous pemphigoid or herpes gestationis, but at times it may be impossible to distinguish it from that of the latter two. Differentiation of bullous pemphigoid from herpes gestationis is often not possible on histopathological grounds alone. A helpful feature, when present, is the observation of eosinophilic papillary microabscesses in herpes gestationis, and of neutrophilic papillary microabscesses in late lesions of bullous pemphigoid (see Table 2.7). In addition, lesions of bullous pemphigoid may rarely show festooning (see Table 2.6). Eosinophilic spongiosis can be observed in all of the disorders included in this group (see Table 2.3).

Clinical features

In bullous drug eruptions there are generalized erythematous macules and papules with blistering. Lesions may clinically resemble those of bullous pemphigoid. Bullous pemphigoid[10] affects mainly elderly patients without sex predilection (only a few cases of 'juvenile' bullous pemphigoid have been reported at present). Bullae are usually generalized, although in rare cases they may be localized. Oral involvement is found in up to 40% of the patients although in a less severe fashion than in pemphigus. Morphologically, lesions may be urticarial (especially in the prodromic phases of the disease), bullous, nodular-verrucous or vesicular (these last resembling dermatitis herpetiformis). Usually there is leukocytosis; blood eosinophilia and elevated serum IgE levels may also be observed. In some patient there is an association with other autoimmune diseases (rheumatoid arthritis and systemic lupus erythematosus among others). By contrast to

Table 2.7 Dermal papillary microabscesses in cutaneous blistering diseases

Neutrophils
  Chronic bullous disease of children
  Dermatitis herpetiformis Duhring
  Linear IgA dermatosis
  Cicatricial pemphigoid – Localized cicatricial pemphigoid
  Epidermolysis bullosa acquisita (rare)
  Bullous pemphigoid (late lesions, rare)
Eosinophils
  Herpes (pemphigoid) gestationis

what has been reported in the past, the association with internal cancer does not seem statistically significant. Bullous lesions may develop following arthropod bites. Lesions are solitary or grouped, and are very pruritic. Herpes gestationis[15,16] has clinical, histopathological and immunological features in common with bullous pemphigoid. However, it develops only in women who are pregnant, and therefore should be considered to be a distinctive expression of pregnancy. Lesions appear in the second trimester and usually disappear at or shortly after parturition. Recurrence in the following pregnancies is the rule.

Diagnostic tools other than histology

Direct immunofluorescence of skin lesions shows linear deposits of IgG and C3 or C3 alone along the basement membrane in bullous pemphigoid and herpes gestationis. With the salt-split test performed with patient's serum, circulating antibodies bind to the roof of the bulla in both of the aforementioned diseases (epidermal or combined pattern). Indirect immunofluorescence reveals the presence of antibodies against the 'bullous pemphigoid antigen' (located mainly in the hemidesmosomes) in the serum of patients with bullous pemphigoid, but may be negative in herpes gestationis patients.

With predominance of neutrophils

A subepidermal bulla with predominantly neutrophilic infiltrate is a feature of all diseases listed in Table 2.5D (Fig. 2.3).

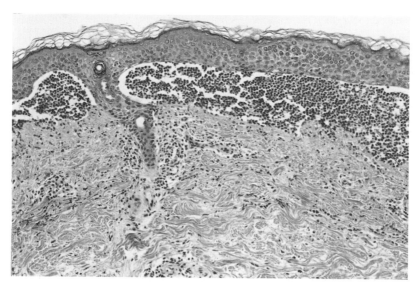

Fig. 2.3 Dermatitis herpetiformis. Subepidermal blisters filled with neutrophils (H&E, original magnification ×100).

Histopathology – differential diagnostic features

Necrotic keratinocytes are found in bullous lupus erythematosus and methyl bromide-induced bullae (see Table 2.4). In methyl bromide-induced bullae there is also oedema of the superficial dermis. Papillary microabscesses of neutrophils are a feature of chronic bullous disease of children, dermatitis herpetiformis, linear IgA dermatosis, cicatricial pemphigoid and rarely epidermolysis bullosa acquisita (see Table 2.7). Preservation of the architecture of dermal papillae (festooning) is commonly found in epidermolysis bullosa acquisita (see Table 2.6). The inflammatory infiltrate is usually arranged within the superficial and mid-dermis in most diseases of this group. However, in bullous erysipela and Sweet's syndrome the inflammatory infiltrate extends to the deep dermis and subcutaneous fat. Signs of vasculitis are a constant feature of bullous vasculitis, but vasculitic changes may rarely be found in other diseases belonging to this group. Differentiation of chronic bullous disease of childhood, dermatitis herpetiformis and linear IgA dermatosis is not possible on histopathological grounds alone.

Clinical features

In bullous erysipela, blisters develop on an erythematous ground. Patients are usually elderly. Lesions are located preferentially on the lower extremities. There are systemic symptoms such as fever and malaise, and the peripheral blood shows leukocytosis. Bullous lupus erythematosus[17] represents a very rare variant of systemic lupus erythematosus with localized or generalized skin manifestations. When localized, lesions are often limited to sun-exposed areas of the body, especially the acral regions. Bullous urticaria results from severe oedema of the superficial dermis. Typical lesions of urticaria co-exist. Bullae may rarely develop in severe, acute onset of vasculitis. Lesions are located preferentially on upper and lower extremities. Systemic symptoms may be present, especially in bullous vasculitis associated to septicaemia caused by *Vibrio vulnificus*. Chronic bullous disease of children[18] commences at ages ranging from 5–6 months to over 10 years. Females are affected more often than males. Preferential locations are the face, trunk, limbs, hands and feet, and genital area. In some patients lesions may be generalized. Involvement of mucous membranes is present in approximately 60% of the patients. Cicatricial pemphigoid[18] is a chronic disease with predilection for mucosal sites (especially oral mucosa). Involvement of the eyes commonly leads to blindness. Cutaneous blisters may be localized on palms and soles (cicatricial pemphigoid of Brownstein-Perry), or may be generalized. Dermatitis herpetiformis[18] occurs mainly in young adults. Male are affected twice as much as females. Intensely pruritic vesicles and small blisters are located on the extensor surfaces of the extremities and on the trunk. In a proportion of patients there is a gluten-sensitive enteropathy (sprue). Epidermolysis bullosa acquisita is caused by the production of autoantibodies directed against the type VII collagen. The disease can be associated with other pathological conditions (Crohn's disease, ulcerative colitis, diabetes mellitus and lupus erythematosus, among others). Lesions are often located on the extremities and develop after trauma. Involvement of the oral mucosa is frequent. Large, solitary bullae are a rare complication of therapy with etretinate. Linear IgA dermatosis[18–20] is a disease predominantly of middle-aged adults. Preferential locations are the trunk and limbs. There are itching or burning urticarial lesions, sometimes with a polycyclic configuration, eventually evolving in small blisters or large bullae. Involvement of mucous membranes is common. Lesions of the eyes may produce scarring. Tense bullae can develop after exposure to methyl-bromide used in fumigation. Sweet's syndrome affects predominantly women between 30 and 60 years of age. Blistering may occur as a result of severe oedema. Most common locations are the face and neck and the upper extremities. Some patients, however, present with generalized lesions. There are associated systemic symptoms such as fever, arthralgia and malaise. The peripheral blood shows leukocytosis with neutrophilia.

Diagnostic tools other than histology

Skin culture shows the presence of bacteria within lesions of bullous erysipela. Direct and indirect immunofluorescence represent the best tools for confirming the diagnosis of bullous lupus erythematosus, bullous vasculitis, chronic bullous disease of children, dermatitis herpetiformis and linear IgA dermatosis. Salt-split test on normal human skin can help the classification of unclear cases. However, immunofluorescence and salt-split skin tests may show similar results in chronic bullous disease of children, linear IgA dermatosis, and cicatricial pemphigoid of childhood, thus suggesting that these three diseases may represent variants of the same spectrum.[19] Gastrointestinal examination can enable the detection of the gluten-sensitive enteropathy (sprue) specific for dermatitis herpetiformis.

With predominance of mast cells

The only disease in this group is bullous mastocytosis (Table 2.5E). Usually it occurs in infants. Lesions are solitary (bullous mastocytoma), multiple (bullous urticaria pigmentosa), or diffuse (bullous mastocytosis). Any tendency towards blistering usually disappears within a few years. Histopathologically there is a subepidermal blister containing several mast cells. Mast cells are also present in the dermis outside the blister. Special stains (Giemsa, Leder) may help to identify the mast cells clearly.

Intradermal blistering diseases

Intradermal blisters are observed in bullous solar elastosis and penicillamine-induced bullae (Table 2.8). Histopathologically, severe actinic elastosis is a constant feature of bullous solar elastosis, whereas in penicillamine-induced

Table 2.8 Intradermal blistering diseases

Bullous solar elastosis
Penicillamine-induced bullae

bullae the dermis is markedly thinned, owing to decreased production of both collagen and elastic fibres.

Clinical aspects

Bullous solar elastosis[21] is a very rare complication of severe actinic damage. It occurs in elderly patients, especially on the forearms and dorsum of the hands. Penicillamine-induced bullae can occur after administration of high dosages of the drug used for Wilson's disease or cystinuria. There are wrinkled, atrophic lesions on trauma-prone areas (knees, elbows, feet, buttocks).

Key points for clinical practice

- Histological examination of cutaneous blistering diseases allows the identification of a 'pattern,' which is characteristic of a disease or, more frequently, a group of diseases.
- Matching histopathological with clinical features allows the number of diagnostic options to be narrowed considerably.
- Appropriate investigations (i.e. immunofluorescence, salt-split test, etc.) can allow specific diagnoses in unclear cases.

REFERENCES

1 Weedon D. The vesiculobullous reaction pattern. In: Weedon D, ed. The skin. 3rd edn. Churchill-Livingstone: Edinburgh, 1992: pp 127–163
2 Huilgol SC, Bhogal BS, Black MM, Immunofluorescence of the immunobullous disorders. Eur J Dermatol 1995; 5: 186–195
3 Pohla-Gubo G, Becher E, Romani N, Fritsch P, Hintner H. 'Salt-split' test on normal, non-sun-exposed skin of patients with autoimmune subepidermal bullous diseases. Dermatology 1994; 189: 123
4 Korman N. Pemphigus. J Am Acad Dermatol 1988; 18: 1219–1238
5 Eady RAJ, Dunnill MGS. Epidermolysis bullosa: hereditary skin fragility diseases as paradigms in cell biology. Arch Dermatol Res 1994; 287: 2–9
6 Bruckner-Tuderman L. Epidermolysis bullosa hereditaria. Hautarzt 1995; 46: 61–72
7 Fine JD, Bauer EA, Briggaman RA, et al Revised clinical and laboratory criteria for subtypes of inherited epidermolysis bullosa. A consensus report of the subcommittee on diagnosis and classification of the national epidermolysis bullosa registry. J Am Acad Dermatol 1991; 24: 119–135
8 Burge SM. Hailey-Hailey disease: an inherited disorder of cohesion. Eur J Dermatol 1995; 5: 277–282
9 Karpati S, Amagai M, Prussick R, Stanley JR. Pemphigus vulgaris antigen is a desmosomal desmoglein. Dermatology 1994; 189: 24–26

10   Korman N. Bullous pemphigoid. J Am Acad Dermatol 1987; 16: 907–924

11   Daoud MS, Su WPD, Leiferman KM, Perniciaro C. Bullous morphea: clinical, pathologic, and immunopathologic evaluation of thirteen cases. J Am Acad Dermatol 1994;
30: 937–943

12   Davis MDP, Perniciaro C, Dahl PR, Randle HW, McEvoy MT. Unusual vesiculobullous
lesions in patients with chronic lymphocytic leukemia: a comprehensive analysis of seven
new cases. J Cut Pathol 1995; 22: 57

13   Tamada Y, Yokochi K, Nitta Y, Ikeya T, Hara K, Owaribe K. Lichen planus pemphigoides:
identification of 180 kd hemidesmosome antigen. J Am Acad Dermatol 1995; 32:
883–887

14   Fränken J, Haneke E. Mycosis fungoides bullosa. Hautarzt 1995; 46: 186–189

15   Black MM. New observations on pemphigoid 'herpes' gestationis. Dermatology 1994;
189: 50–51

16   Wever S, Burger M, Langfritz K, et al Herpes gestationis. Klinische Spektrum und diag-
nostische Möglichkeiten. Hautarzt 1995; 46: 158–164

17   Yell JA, Allen J, Wojnarowska F, Kirtschig G, Burge SM. Bullous systemic lupus erythematosus: revised criteria for diagnosis. Br J Dermatol 1995; 132: 921–928

18   Wojnarowska F, Marsden RA, Bhogal B, Black MM. Chronic bullous disease of childhood, childhood cicatricial pemphigoid, and linear IgA disease of adults. J Am Acad
Dermatol 1988; 19: 792–805

19   Wojnarowska F, Allen J, Collier P. Linear IgA disease: a heterogeneous disease.
Dermatology 1994; 189: 52–56

20   Kuechle MK, Stegemeier E, Maynard B, Gibson LE, Leiferman KM, Peters MS. Drug-
induced linear IgA bullous dermatosis: report of six cases and review of the literature. J
Am Acad Dermatol 1994; 30: 187–192

21   Williams B, Barr R, Dutta B. Bullous solar elastosis. J Cut Pathol 1995; 22: 95

22   Ruiz E, Deng JS, Abell EA. Eosinophilic spongiosis: a clinical, histologic, and
immunopathologic study. J Am Acad Dermatol 1994; 30: 973–976

3

Mathematical modelling: a review of some recent books

D. W. K. Cotton

Fractal Physiology by Bassingthwaighte JB, Liebovitch LS, West BJ. Oxford University Press, 1994. £42.50

Understanding Nonlinear Dynamics by Kaplan D, Glass L. Springer Verlag, 1995. £23.50

The Algorithmic Beauty of Sea Shells by Meinhardt H. Springer Verlag, 1995. £34.00

Mathematical Biology by Murray JD. Springer Verlag, 1993. £29.50

Chaos Under Control by Peak D, Frame M. W H Freeman and Co., 1994. £19.50

Experimental biology in general and experimental pathology in particular employ a wide range of tools including intact animal models, tissue culture, isolated biochemical studies and mathematical modelling. Of course these are just a few examples of a rich investigative armamentarium and I have ordered them to suggest the progressive abstraction of techniques which can be applied. There are several types of limitations to these various approaches, both general limitations and limitations specific to the particular experimental modality. General criticisms include the objection that all models are incomplete and the very incompleteness may exclude the most interesting and important aspects of the situation being studied. Most experimental studies take this into account by using appropriate controls and good experimental design, including statistical evaluation of the problem as well as subsequent statistical evaluation of the results. The technique of isolating variables has been strikingly successful, but as this is progressively applied and the experimental system includes less and less of the total situation then the criticism that the experiment is too simplistic to yield useful information becomes more persuasive. For instance, if we wish to study malignant melanoma we can look at human patients; we can induce melanomas in experimental animals; we can study isolated melanoma cells in culture; we can study purified genetic and enzyme materials from melanomas; and we can model growth patterns mathematically. As we progress through this series we see that we can steadily gain control over the progressively reduced number of variables but at the cost of becoming progressively distanced from the original biological problem.

A glance at any current biosciences journal will reveal a world of genetic abstraction as separated from the oncology ward as any mathematical model could ever be, and we always have the opportunity of comparing our abstract models to the real world, so at least in this respect we are in advance of our colleagues who study cosmology or quantum mechanics.

The seminal English language work on mathematical modelling is *On Growth and Form* by D'Arcy Thompson written in 1917.[1] The insights provided by this book were considerable, but many of them were criticized as 'analytically unwieldy' (by no less an authority than Medawar!) and had to wait for the development of computers that could perform the experimental geometry manipulations that Thompson suggested in his most widely quoted chapter 'On the theory of transformations, or the comparison of related forms'. The concept of experimental geometry in its current manifestation is due to Benoit Mandelbrot in his extraordinary and idiosyncratic book *The Fractal Geometry of Nature*.[2] Subsequent to Mandelbrot's insights there has been an extraordinary explosion of interest in fractal geometry, and chaos, with many hundreds of attempts to apply this sort of mathematics to biological systems reported in the scientific literature, as well as hundreds of books of varying degrees of approachability for the non-mathematical but interested reader. There are many traps, for the unwary, lurking within mathematical models and perhaps the most seductive is the temptation to believe that the demonstration of similarity in *form* indicates an underlying similarity in *nature*. Structures such as the Mandelbrot figure have great beauty but it is pointless to seek examples of the Mandelbrot figure in nature, because it is a graph; it refers to a series of functions (called Julia sets) and one might just as well look for shapes like growth curves in a culture of cancer cells. Conversely, the graphical presentation of a wide range of mathematical functions can all produce the same pattern; does this mean that if that pattern appears in nature then it must be caused by all of those mathematical functions? Clearly not. Similarity is not identity, particularly when we are dealing with models where the majority of the features that make the phenomenon interesting have been excluded for the purposes of experimental study.

The mathematical manipulation known as the Fourier transform allows us to break down any complex waveform, such as a note on the guitar, into a series of oscillators, such as tuning forks, that defines that particular sound. In the opposite direction, it is possible to set up a series of electronic oscillators and select them for frequency, duration and volume such that they can generate any specific sound, such as the guitar note that we were just analysing. In practice the notes produced by such synthesizers are very convincing, in isolation, but different guitars and different guitarists produce a very wide range of variations that are exceedingly difficult to model completely. However, Fourier transform has a very important place in the analysis of complex waveforms, and synthesizers based on Fourier analysis are a multi-million pound industry. The point is that one needs to understand the limits of mathematical models and one needs to know how they may sensibly be employed, just as with any tool in science.

Fractal Physiology could hardly be bettered as an introduction and review of the application of the new mathematics to biological problems. The first section provides a brief overview of the subject area and the second section gets down to a definition of the kind of techniques used in fractal and chaos theory. Theoretical physicists and mathematicians often provide very specific mathematical explanations that other mathematicians are entirely satisfied with but which leave biologists feeling rather cheated. I am often disconcerted when, as I follow the evolution of some mathematical formula, the author suddenly says: 'differentiating this equation ...'; I think; 'Why? Where did that come from? What has happened?' like a child faced with a conjuring trick where not only does he not understand *how* it was done, he also has no idea *why* it was done. The second section of this book is mercifully free from this sleight of hand and the authors show there is nothing up their sleeves as they explain exactly the meaning and use of each transformation. The range of mathematics covered is very wide, how wide and how useful is revealed in the third section, which describes the application of this mathematics to physiological problems (actually, to a number of pathological processes too). The range of these problems is also impressive with sections on: ion channel kinetics; intra-organ flow dynamics; fractal growth; and the significance of chaos in physiology. This last section is very interesting as the intuitive temptation is to equate chaos with disease, but numerous studies have shown much more spontaneous (chaotic) variation in physiological than in pathological heartbeats, for example. One possible explanation is that chaotic systems are very dependent on initial conditions and tiny alterations in these values can start a system off on a totally new line, whereas stable systems are very hard to redirect and are thus less closely linked to short-term variations within the microenvironment of cells. Only a very boring experimental pathologist will fail to derive some inspiration from this book.

The basic requirement for this sort of study is some feeling for non-linear dynamics. Many simple physical systems exhibit linear dynamics where the reaction of a system is linearly proportional to the force employed. As a simple example, if the experimenter prods a cardboard box with a stick, the effect on the box will be directly proportional to the force employed. Once the inertial forces are overcome the box will move at a rate dependent on the force of prodding. If the experimenter prods a cat with a stick the specific results are unpredictable and dependent on a series of preconditions such as the state of alertness of the cat, its basic nature, its previous experience of being prodded and so on; what is produced is a series of non-linear dynamic responses. Interestingly, prodding a dead cat produces linear dynamic responses. *Understanding Nonlinear Dynamics* by Kaplan and Glass is a text that is said to have grown out of an undergraduate course taught to students in the biological sciences at McGill University in Canada. Consequently the exposition is lucid and the mathematics are kept simple and clear with a minimal assumption of prior mathematical knowledge. Nevertheless this is a thorough text and each section is illustrated by discussions of practical biological situations. Thus the section on Boolean networks and cellular automata is illustrated by descriptions including 'a lambda bacteriophage model', 'locomotion in salamanders' and 'spiral waves in chemistry and biology whilst the section on one-dimensional differential equations considers 'Gompertz growth of tumours' and 'heart rate response to sinusoid inputs' and the section on two-dimensional differential equations considers 'metastasis of malignant tumours'. I have spent some months working out the relationship between cobweb plots, time series, Verhulst process maps and the curious behaviour of the logistic equation used for describing growth in populations and in cell cultures, and here it all is very lucidly laid out in a fashion which I could have understood from the beginning.

It seems odd that short courses on statistics are now fairly general in medical curricula in this country but the mathematics of biological function is not even present as an option in most medical schools. Curiously the same prejudice does not apply in the other direction and there is a very interesting text for engineering students called *Invention and Evolution*, which considers the design solutions to problems that have been solved by evolution and uses these as models to illuminate engineering problems (the analogy between the Saltash bridge and *brontosaurus* is particularly appealing).[3] The mathematics required in Kaplan and Glass' book is fairly simple calculus but they recommend another book, for those who prefer a non-calculus approach, called *Chaos under Control* by Peak and Frame. This is a more popular book and has the expected advantages and disadvantages. It relates the new mathematics and the emerging science of complexity in a readable and entertaining form and even offers free software on the Internet as well as fascinating sections entitled 'Speculations'; but to do real research in this area it is the Kaplan and Glass book that will get you started.

Various techniques for dealing with large numbers are available; one can take means and effectively fit idealized curves, or one may employ statistics of greater complexity, but this has the disadvantage of smoothing out not only errors but also interesting actual fluctuations. Similar objections can be raised to the calculus approach. In respect of this mathematical smoothing it is instructive to consider the logistic equation so commonly used to model populations. It is easy to calculate the traditional sigmoid growth curve from the simple formula and it is easy to ignore the fluctuations that appear as the growth constant approaches 4, but the most interesting features of the curve and the most significant for an understanding of chaos in populations and cell cultures only appear when you take these variations seriously and do not just dismiss them as 'noise'. Even more interesting is the fact that we do not seem to observe such chaotic patterns in cell cultures or in many natural populations. But the mathematical model assumes a synchronized progeny from the original single cell, once we add a series of these curves together (analogous to a real population consisting of multiple clones with slightly different starting values) then we begin to see the re-emergence of the observed growth patterns.[4] This observation has clear significance for the treatment of human neoplasms because it suggests that synchronization of the cells before cytotoxic therapy might improve the kill rate of cancer cells. Conversely, it suggests a reason for the drug resistance of some tumours such as melanomas where the clonal diversity is known to be very high.

In 1952 that rather blurred genius Alan Turing published a speculative paper on morphogenesis showing how complex patterns could arise by the interaction of diffusing morphogens (what we would now call growth factors). Murray, in his extremely thorough work *Mathematical Biology* has shown in great detail how this can function in a consideration of the patterning of a wide variety of animal coverings. Murray's is the most complete and detailed book on the subject currently available; the mathematics is demanding but if you want references to the whole field, they are here. The book is a mine of mathematical models that have been found useful throughout all biological science and many of the models concern processes very similar to those studied by experimental pathologists, suggesting that the mathematics may also be similar.

The most startling and attractive demonstration of mathematical modelling of biological systems comes in a very pretty book called *The Algorithmic Beauty of Sea Shells* by Hans Meinhardt (algorithm derives from a misreading of the name of the Arabic mathematician al-Khowarizmi). This book demonstrates how the vastly complex, and apparently pointless, patterning of sea shells can be generated by very simple equations representing diffusing promoters and inhibitors of shell coloration (Turing's morphogens again). I say apparently pointless because many of these animals live most of their lives buried in the mud out of sight of predators and without the opportunity to impress prospective mates. Nevertheless they are highly patterned and this patterning can be reproduced by equations of relatively simple form that are very similar to those derived to explain the growth dynamics of simple animals such as *hydra*. Of course no one believes that the patterning of sea shells is a very important topic in itself but we can see that this is a non-trivial problem that begins to have some interest for students of human disease when we recall the striking appearance of the gyrate and figurate erythemas. These are highly patterned skin diseases whose form is sufficiently characteristic for them to acquire specific names (not really very unusual in dermatology).[5] When developing molluscs encounter some trauma their pattern may change for some time and only slowly revert to the normal patterning for that species, a condition very similar to that seen in Beau's disease of nails. Similarly, in the two shells of bivalve molluscs strikingly symmetrical patterns can appear, just as the lesions of lupus erythematosus, vitiligo and mitral malar flush are commonly bilaterally symmetrical. The software that comes with the book has instructions for changing the parameters of the equations and it is possible to sit and generate your own patterns. Given that we can now assay many growth factors and also use immunocytochemical markers to observe their distribution it should not be beyond the wit of experimental biologists to follow these in actual patients. Yet other interesting examples have recently appeared in Nature concerning the basis of skin colour in fish.[6,7]

Are there true and proven mathematical models which, in spite of their gross simplifications, still find an application within medicine? Fortunately there is the very convincing example of drug pharmacokinetics, which has the added advantage (for those interested in such things) of having been proven in the marketplace. No drug would now be offered on the market without such studies and Sir James Black has said that he could never have developed the thinking that led to beta-blockers and H_2 antagonists had he not approached partial antagonists from the basis of mathematical modelling. But is this a special case or are there general indications that mathematical modelling is of use in medicine? Read these books and their case studies of cardiac dysrhythmias, nerve impulse generation, vascular growth and tumour kinetics if you have any doubt. In our laboratory we have pursued a number of lines of enquiry using mathematical models in hip fracture[8] and in various types of measurement in pathology and the results are variable; some investigations show promise and others do not. The point is that mathematical modelling is like any other experimental tool and you have to use the right tool for the job; as it says at the beginning of chapter 2 of *Fractal Physiology*, if the only tool you have is a hammer, you tend to treat everything as if it were a nail (Abraham Maslow, 1966).

Reading these books has convinced me that mathematical modelling is a very important part of the future of biology, including pathology, and that the advent of the new mathematics of chaos, fractals and complexity is going to change that future. I think that pathologists ought to be involved in this, and more importantly we need to involve the next generation of medical students who are the people who will be doing the real work.

Acknowledgements

It is a pleasure to record my thanks to Professor James Underwood and Dr Simon Cross who are always ready to discuss, argue and enlighten me on these and all other matters and to the Faculty and participants at a recent Inserm Atelier in Paris, in particular Professor Jim Murray, who excited me about this subject all over again.

REFERENCES

1 Thompson D'A. On growth and form. Cambridge: Cambridge University Press, 1966
2 Mandelbrot BB. The fractal geometry of nature. New York: WH Freeman and Co, 1983
3 French MJ. Invention and evolution. Cambridge: Cambridge University Press, 1988
4 Cross SS, Cotton DWK. Chaos and antichaos in pathology. Hum Pathol 1994; 25: 630–637
5 Cross SS, McDonach JG, Stephenson TJ, Cotton DWK, Underwood JCE. Fractal and integer-dimensional geometric analysis of pigmented skin lesions. Am J Dermatopathol 1995; 17: 374–378
6 Kondo S, Rihito A. A reaction-diffusion wave on the skin of the marine angelfish Pomacanthus. Nature 1995; 376: 765–768
7 Meinhardt H. Dynamics of stripe formation. Nature 1995; 376: 722–733
8 Cotton DWK, Whitehead CL, Vyas S, Cooper C, Patterson EA. Are hip fractures caused by falling and breaking or breaking and falling? Photoelastic stress analysis. Forensic Sci Int 1994; 65: 105–112

4

Can we make sense of inflammatory skins?

D. W. K. Cotton

A preliminary disclaimer. I have almost as much trouble with inflammatory skins as anyone else and this article is, in part, my attempt to come to terms with the problem. The way that I have approached this is to go through a series of textbooks that I have found helpful over the years and try to combine their approaches into an algorithm that seems to work. A major problem with this kind of approach is that of suitable attribution. If several textbooks all comment on the same well known histological feature then I do not feel it necessary to reference one of them. If I use David Weedon's classification then I admit it and if I refer to some of Bernard Ackerman's 'Clues' then I place the word clue in italics and brackets at the appropriate place. Some judgement is required in all of this and I hope that the authors of these excellent texts will forgive inadvertent lapses. In general I have tried to protect myself by copying from many authors, so I can fairly say: 'almost none of this is my own work'.

The subject of inflammatory skins is one of the largest causes of frustration for junior pathologists (leaving aside their career prospects and personal lives) and even the occasional senior pathologist will admit to some areas of uncertainty, although only of a temporary or focal nature. The first heroic attempt to deal systematically with this subject was by A.B. Ackerman in the big golden book *Histologic Diagnosis of Inflammatory Skin Disease*[1] and he has followed this up in numerous other publications such as *The Lives of Lesions*[2] and the three volumes of *Clues to Diagnosis in Dermatopathology*;[3–5] all pathologists dealing with skin biopsies should have access to these books because they treat dermatopathology as a problem–oriented study, which is how it comes to us on the bench. Other essential books are *Pathology of the Skin: with Clinical Correlations*[6] by Philip McKee because he gives the gross pathology and the clinical correlations (what dermatologists call dermatology) and *The Skin*[7] edited by David Weedon because he approaches inflammatory skins as a series of reaction patterns. In Weedon's book the intention is that you should be able to identify the major reaction pattern type and then refine this to a specific diagnosis or at least a respectable differential.

A particularly sensitive area for pathologists is that they do not see the gross pathology, and the descriptions offered by the dermatologist or general practitioner who takes the biopsy is often less than rigorous. This can lead to some embarrassment when a perfectly reasonable histopathological interpretation is offered which is grossly at variance with the clinical picture and it is for this reason that Philip McKee's book[6] is valuable because it illustrates the clinical appearances as well as the histological. This means that the pathologist will be less tempted to suggest a focal lesion when the dermatologist has suggested a differential of diffuse widespread diseases. However, many cases remain clinically fairly distinct but histologically rather non-specific and here a knowledge of *Clues to Diagnosis in Dermatopathology* can make a large difference.[4]

The classifications of inflammatory skin disease into dominant reaction patterns as offered by both Weedon (Table 4.1) and Ackerman (Table 4.2), provide a helpful starting point even though mixed patterns do occur. Weedon describes six major and seven minor reaction patterns, Ackerman offers nine patterns that he subsequently divides further.

A comparison of Tables 4.1 and 4.2 shows that the two systems of classification both work; we can locate most disease in either system, but the reasons for doing so in either case are very different. The situation is not as bad as it seems because very broad categories in either system are usually immediately subdivided i.e. vesiculobullous in Table 4.1 is immediately divided into the familiar intraepidermal and subepidermal categories and superficial perivascular dermatitis in Table 4.2 is subdivided rapidly in order to separate psoriasis and lichen planus. In general, Weedon classifies the diseases on the basis of an archetype (his reaction patterns), which is morphological, whereas Ackerman classifies on the basis of the morphology without an intermediate recognition of an archetypal pattern. The Weedon method has the advantage of being like the way most pathologists think (this looks a bit like lichen planus but why are the lymphocytes so pleomorphic?) whereas Ackerman has science on his side in saying: 'let us not jump to conclusions, but just describe what is there'. Nevertheless, only the very beginner has no idea of what is going on; most of us can recognize the predominant pattern in much the way that Weedon describes and it is his first six categories that contain the majority of those inflammatory lesions with which we would like to get further than dermatitis or toxic erythema. The minor reaction patterns are not common and not difficult to classify into one group or another.

If you search a database such as *Index Medicus* using very general terms such as inflammatory skin disease, skin inflammation, etc., or even very specific terms such as lichen planus, lichenoid reaction or psoriasis, you will find hundreds of articles on these topics (especially if you use free text

Table 4.1 Morphological classification of inflammatory skin diseases according to Weedon

	Examples
Major patterns	
Lichenoid	Lichen planus
Psoriasiform	Psoriasis
Spongiotic	Contact dermatitis
Vesiculobullous	Pemphigus/bullous pemphigoid
Granulomatous	Sarcoidosis/tuberculoid
Vasculopathic	Hypersensitivity vasculitis
Minor patterns	
Epidermolytic hyperkeratosis	Bullous ichthyosiform erythroderma
Acantholytic dyskeratosis	Darier's
Cornoid lamellation	Porokeratosis
Papillomatosis	Basal cell papilloma
Angiofibromas	Fibrous papule of the nose
Eosinophilic cellulitis with flame figures	Well's syndrome
Transepidermal elimination	Perforating folliculitis

Table 4.2 Morphological classification of inflammatory skin disease according to Ackerman

Pattern	Examples
Superficial perivascular dermatitis	Psoriasis/lichen planus/contact dermatitis/porokeratosis (early)
Superficial and deep perivascular dermatitis	Lupus erythematosus
Vasculitis	Hypersensitivity vasculitis
Nodular and diffuse dermatitis	Sarcoidosis/tuberculoid
Intraepidermal vesicular and pustular dermatitis	Pemphigus/Darier's/bullous ichthyosiform erythroderma
Subepidermal vesicular dermatitis	Bullous pemphigoid
Folliculitis and perifolliculitis	Acne/lichen planopilaris
Fibrosing dermatitis	Scar/dermatofibroma/porokeratosis (late)
Panniculitis	Leukocytoclastic vasculitis/erythema nodosum

searches) but you will find almost no articles that are of help in diagnosis. There is much research into the molecular biology, immunology, growth factor levels and other interesting subjects but not much that is relevant to the practising pathologist with a tray of surgicals. Most of what there is appears in the *American Journal of Dermatopathology* and comes from Bernard Ackerman's laboratory. In some ways this is not surprising as it is unlikely that the complex technologies that are being applied to pathology, currently, would immediately yield diagnostic help. But our colleagues in radiology and microbiology are constantly publishing diagnostic articles. Whatever the cause it remains a fact that there is little new diagnostic information coming on the market, so the best that we can hope to do is to organize what we have in some helpful and accessible way using the numerous very good textbooks available.

Table 4.3 Pathology of major patterns of inflammatory skin reactions according to the Weedon classification

Pattern	Pathology
Lichenoid eroptions	Band-like lymphohistiocytic inflammatory infiltrate Basal cell damage (apoptotic Civatte bodies; liquefactive degeneration) Pigmentary incontinence Eventual atrophy of the epidermis
Psoriasiform	Epidermal hyperplasia Elongation of rete pegs Thickening, clubbing and fusing of rete pegs Thining of the suprapapillary plate 'Squirting dermal papillae' Inflammatory cells in the epidermis Parakeratotic hyperkeratosis Loss of the granular layer
Spongiotic pattern	Intercellular oedema of the epidermis Spongiotic vesicle formation Psoriasiform hyperkeratosis in older lesions
Vesiculobullous	Splits at various levels in the skin
Granulomatous	Pattern ranging from discrete granulomas to mixed reactions dominated by epithelioid macrophages
Vasculopathic	Pathological changes to vessels surrounded by inflammatory cells; there must also be evidence of vascular damage

The first stage is to get the groups of inflammatory skins down to manageable proportions and either of our classifications will do. On the whole I find myself starting with the Weedon classification. Table 4.3 summarizes the pathology of the major patterns of inflammatory skin reactions according to the Weedon classification.

One more category of inflammatory looking skins is those that eventually develop into lymphomas; can we distinguish these at an early phase? (Table 4.4) From the morphological point of view this does not seem to generally be possible. Even with the benefit of hindsight I cannot go back to the first lesions that were called non-specific inflammatory dermatosis and spot clues that would have led to a suspicion of early lymphoma. It is possible that a persistent lesion, for which no cause can be found and which is beginning to show abnormal cells and abnormal architecture, is a developing lymphoma. The problem is reflected in the current debate about the nature of this early disease: is it a benign inflammatory reaction that subsequently becomes neoplastic; is it a benign lymphoma that converts to a malignant lymphoma; or was it malignant from the start but only displayed its morphological correlates at a late stage? On the whole, a progression seems the most likely but whether this begins as a reactive process or a benign neoplasm remains unresolved as yet.

Table 4.4 Pathogenesis of some features important in diagnosis

Histological feature	Pathogenesis
Acanthosis	Basal cell damage resulting in sawtooth acanthosis–*lichenoid eruptions* Hard, sharp-edged acanthosis (virus taking over replicative cells to produce virions and transporting these to the surface for spread to new hosts)–*viral infections* Squirting papillae (polymorphs) between blunt acanthosis (epidermal defect in maturation)–*psoriasis* Squirting papillae (lymphocytes) between blunt acanthosis (epidermal stimulation)–*lichen simplex chronicus*
Apoptosis	Death programme triggered–*viral infection* Altered immune response–*graft versus host; T-cell lymphoma* Altered epidermal immune expression–*virus; lichen planus; drug reactions*
Epidermal hyperplasia	Thickening of the epidermis without marked acanthosis; there is no obvious outside damage as in lichen simplex chronicus and no basal damage as in lichenoid reactions so the stimulus may come from within the epidermis
Epithelioid macrophages	Activated macrophages with extensive rough endoplasmic reticulum and looking like epithelioid cells
Flame figures	Decoration of collagen fibrils with the eosinophilic granules from eosinophils; typical of Well's disease but common in situations with extensive eosinophil degranulation
Giant cells	More properly called polykaryons, those of macrophage lineage are derived from fused macrophage types and include Langhan's, foreign body and Touton. Viral and tumour giant cells may arise owing to nuclear division not followed by cytological division
Hypergranulosis	Increased keratohyaline granules in the upper layers of the epidermis occur in viral infections owing to admixture of virions into forming keratin; this brings the virions to the surface where they can infect other hosts
Leukocytoclastic vasculitis	A vasculitis in which the predominant cells are neutrophil polymorphs which are disintegrating (nuclear dust); this is usually associated with a drug reaction or with infection
Parakeratosis	Persistence of keratohyaline bodies into the keratin indicates incomplete keratin maturation usually as a result of rapid production, this often occurs with loss of the granular layer
Pigmentary incontinence	Basal layer damage results in damage to melanocytes with loss of pigment into the dermis where it is taken up by macrophages
Satellite cell necrosis	Single cell death in the epidermis in association with one or more lymphocytes, the implication being that the lymphocytes have triggered the apoptosis pathway
Spongiosis	Inter (and intra) cellular oedema putting stress on desmosomal prickles and resulting in rupture of these to produce intraepidermal pongiotic vesicles (no acanthocytes because desmosomal destruction is not circumferential)
Squirting dermal papillae	Dilatation and enlargement of vertical, papillary vessels responding to some presumed cytokine message from the epidermis; often accompanied by fibrosis (the picture is reminiscent of the features of solitary rectal ulcer/mucosal prolapse syndrome)
Transepidermal elimination	A mechanism by which the skin rids itself of abnormal substances; common in granulomatous diseases and some folliculitides
Vacuolar degeneration	A form of apoptosis in which vacuoles appear at the basal layer in association with lymphocytes (presumably killer cells of some type)
Vasculitis	Damage to blood vessels in association with inflammatory cells owing to a changed immune response to the vessels as a result of changed antigenicity, implantation of antigen or deposition of antigen/antibody complexes (the size of vessel involved may give a clue to the diagnosis)

Lichenoid reaction

As Weedon stresses, the fundamental pathological process in lichenoid reactions is damage to the basal layer. What we see in the well established lesion of lichen planus is a characteristic saw-tooth pattern of regeneration involving the rete ridges.

1. This attack on the basal layer kills basal cells, which can be seen as apoptotic bodies (Civatte bodies); apoptosis above the basal layer is very rare in lichen planus and clusters of necrotic keratinocytes within the epidermis suggest a lichenoid drug eruption.
2. Apoptosis without obvious lymphocyte association (satellite cell necrosis) is the commonest pattern, but satellite cell necrosis can predominate in graft versus host disease, regressing plane warts and erythema multiforme. Coincidentally melanocytes are also damaged and pigmentary incontinence is also seen. Whether the melanocytes are also killed by apoptosis or not remains unclear, but it should be easy enough to resolve because apoptotic basal cells will still contain cytokeratins and the remains of the melanocytes will not and should be positive for S100. That melanocytes are damaged in the process is attested to by the depigmentation often seen when lichen planus subsides.
3. Damage to the basal layer inevitably damages the integrity of the dermo-epidermal junction and small clefts (Max Joseph clefts) are usually seen, particularly in lichen planus where they can coalesce to form junctional bullae in lichen planus bullosa.
4. Another very characteristic feature of lichen planus that results from this basal layer damage is that the transition between the epidermis and the infiltrate is hard to see at low power because of the altered appearance of the lowest epidermal cells, which now look like keratinocytes and not basal cells.
5. At the top of the epidermis there is compact hyperkeratosis and wedge-shaped hypergranulosis that is common to all stages of lichen planus (*clue*).
6. Weedon points out that cell death in the basal layer is of two types: apoptosis and vaculor change; in some lichenoid conditions apoptosis is the main feature (lichen planus) whereas in others vacuolar damage predominates (lupus erythematosus, poikiloderma, drug reactions).

The common feature of lichenoid reaction patterns is a changed relationship between the epidermis and the lympho-histiocytic system: in regressing warts and tumours and lichenoid drug reactions this seems to be an alteration in the epidermis itself; while in lupus erythematosus, graft versus host disease and early mycosis fungoides the inflammatory cells are changed. In lichen planus itself the root cause is still obscure but there is no evidence that there is any initial altered immunity although some changes in immunity can be seen late in the process.

The pattern of a lichenoid infiltrate is characteristic: there is a band-like infiltrate with a flat base and the infiltrate is about 20 cells thick and consists largely of T lymphocytes (as do most lymphocytic skin infiltrates). Some interesting questions arise out of this; if the inflammatory cells are attracted by some soluble factor from the basal cells, why is the infiltrate so thick? Are the cells just 'queuing up' for the epidermis? Again, if the cells are attracted by something in or from the basal layer, why does the infiltrate not follow the contour of this? Is it just that the factors have all diffused to the same level in spite of the irregular acanthosis? Or are all of the inflammatory cells restricted to the papillary dermis as they seem to be?

The varieties of lupus erythematosus differ in degree and are difficult to distinguish histologically but they have in common a lichenoid infiltrate which attacks the basal layer of the epidermis. The infiltrate also attacks hair follicles causing their destruction with characteristic plugging. At low power the infiltrate has a 'lumpy bumpy' appearance in the dermis as it surrounds vessels and adnexae; such an appearance in the absence of a junctional lichenoid pattern suggests the enigmatic entity of Jessner's or sometimes polymorphous light eruption. LE is also light sensitive and although Civatte bodies are common on other body sites there are less common in lesions on the face. The junctional element of the eruption takes the form of mainly vacuolar degeneration and pigmentary incontinence is a feature. A late feature is a thickening of the basement membrane zone.

On the vulva, overlap conditions occur where it is not possible to confidently diagnose either lichen planus or lupus erythematosus, which indicates the possibility that these disease processes are not entirely distinct. Both lichen planus and lupus erythematosus may occur on the scalp causing scarring alopecia; other causes of baldness include pseudopelade of Brocq (infiltrate focused around the infundibulum), alopecia areata (all follicles in the same phase high in the dermis with a 'swarm of bees' lymphocytic infiltrate at their base) and trichotillomania (fragments of broken hair and disrupted follicles in the dermis).

Psoriasiform reaction

In these conditions the dominant effect is epidermal hyperplasia with rather regular, clubbed and fused rete ridges. There is no evidence that the rete pegs actually fuse but they give that appearance.

1. The suprapapillary plate is thinned and the papillae contain prominent vertical vessels from which inflammatory cells emerge into the epidermis. These appearances have given rise to the term 'squirting papillae', which may also be seen in lichen simplex chronicus where, however, the fibrosis is more marked and the infiltrate is more lymphocytic.
2. Biopsies of Reiter's syndrome are usually indistinguishable from pustular psoriasis.
3. Vertical and horizontal alternation of hyperkeratosis and parakeratosis is

characteristic of pityriasis rubra pilaris but may also be seen in evolving forms of psoriasis such as guttate psoriasis.

4. Lichen simplex chronicus has less regular acanthosis, the suprapapillary plates are thicker and the characteristic features are often superimposed on some other skin lesion.

5. Clear cell acanthoma can be mistaken for psoriasis but the lesions are solitary, small and well defined and the characteristic pale cell change is sharply demarcated.

6. Dermatophytes may also simulate psoriasis and the only firm distinction is to demonstrate hyphae (clues).

It is a moot point as to whether the vascular changes or the epidermal changes are the fundamental lesion in psoriasis, but certainly the vascular changes are seen first, although it is still possible that these occur in response to increased demands from the epidermis as it prepares to become hyperplastic. What is clear is that the epidermal hyperplasia is not a result of basal cell damage because there is no visible inflammatory involvement of the basal layer, although inflammatory cells do pass through into the epidermis proper. Even though there is an increased rate of mitosis in the epidermis of psoriasis there remains disagreement as to whether epidermal cells stay within the epidermis for a longer or shorter time (transit time) than normal. There is also no clear idea about the mechanisms that control epidermal growth and hyperplasia. However, it is known that the nucleotides from maturing keratinocytes are eventually recycled into the production of new cells and this must mean that cells in the superficial layers of the epidermis, which still have nuclei or remnants thereof, must be returning their DNA to some basal layer pool. This at least provides a theoretical possibility of a stratum corneum to basal layer signal. As psoriasis is characterized by the persistence of DNA into the stratum corneum (parakeratosis) it seems possible that this is the signal for epidermal hyperplasia. We know that in the case of lichen simplex chronicus it is the rubbing of the skin surface by the patient that causes the psoriasiform hyperplasia seen in that condition, together with squirting papillae, and that epidermal invasion by fungi have a similar effect.

Some common features leading to epidermal hyperplasia occurs in a great variety of diseases, which otherwise seem to have little in common. The dermal infiltrate can be radically different; psoriasis is characterized by neutrophil polymorph infiltration and lichen simplex chronicus is lymphohistiocytic unless complicated by secondary infection. Other diseases with a psoriasiform reaction may show an initial failure of maturation (Bowen's disease) or result from drug reactions or indicate internal malignancy (erythroderma). Clearly this is a heterogeneous group of diseases linked only by a histological similarity of epidermal hyperplasia with varied causes, effects and associations.

Spongiform reactions

Spongiosis is the presence of fluid between the epidermal cells, which holds them apart and makes the prickles of the drawn-out desmosomal intercellular bridges between cells very prominent. The archetypal lesion is that of an acute eczema even although the term 'eczema' lacks precision and is falling from favour (although if we were to dispense with all dermatological terms that lacked precision we would be left with a very small vocabulary). The origin of the intercellular fluid is unknown but because spongiosis is neither a feature of diseases with damage to the basal layer or those with squirting papillae nor of lesions with marked upper dermal oedema, such as erythema multiforme, it seems probable that the fluid comes from the epidermal cells themselves.

1. In contact hypersensitivity spongiosis is an early feature and is found low in the epidermis. As the stimulus is coming from the outside it seems reasonable to presume that spongiosis is not a direct effect from the allergen itself because we might then expect spongiosis to be most marked in the upper layers. The role of the Langerhan cells is to pick up allergen and display it to lymphocytes thus initiating the allergic response. It is therefore possible that the oedema fluid comes from epidermal cells and contains the allergen in sufficient concentration to attract the attention of the Langerhan cells.
2. Pemphigus folliaceus shows a similar appearance in the early stages and in this condition the early features are of intercellular oedema, with coating of the keratinocytes and desmosomes with IgG and C_3 and the eventual rupture of desmosomes. The clefts so formed then become confluent forming the typical intraepidermal bullae.

Even the spongiosis of eczema can become confluent and produce spongiotic vesicles, which feature gives rise to the term 'eczema' meaning 'to bubble up'. But the fully developed form of pemphigus is still classified as a vesiculobullous disease and eczema as a spongiotic disease. This illustrates two important and related points: first, inflammatory diseases of skin may fall into different categories at different phases of their development, a point very aptly dealt with by Bernard Ackerman in his book *The Lives of Lesions*;[2] and second; classifications based on morphology are always going to be misleading because similarity is not identity. I suppose that the most convincing demonstration of this is the fact that different drugs can induce the whole range of inflammatory skin reactions underlining the point that these are just *reactions*, even although in most cases we do not know what they are reactions to. When you consider that the features of inflammation were first described in skin it is remarkable that we understand the aetiopathogenesis of almost no skin disease except for some infections.

Weedon distinguishes three special types of spongiotic reaction pattern that differ from the classical form of eczematous spongiosis:

1. predominance of eosinophils may occur in allergic contact dermatitis and parasitic infestations and as a precursor lesion in pemphigus or an uncommon finding in bullous pemphigoid (eosinophilic spongiosis);
2. spongiosis may be specifically localized to the acrosyringium of eccrine sweat glands (miliarial spongiosis);
3. spongiosis may be specifically localized to the hair follicular infundibulum (follicular spongiosis).

These forms of spongiosis are readily distinguished as long as you think of them, but in the latter two cases the situation may be revealed only by careful serial (not step) sections.

In the great majority of spongiotic reaction the inflammatory infiltrate consists mainly of neutrophil polymorphs and the spongiosis is distributed randomly throughout the epidermis. And in general these diseases are the classic eczemas: irritant contact dermatitis; allergic contact dermatitis; nummular dermatitis; seborrhoeic dermatitis; atopic dermatitis; pompholyx; and spongiotic drug eruptions. Often the distinction between these is difficult to make histologically and one may have to rely on the clinical details for a likely cause. There are some features that may be of help:

1. strong concentrations of irritants may cause obvious damage to the surface of the epidermis with ballooning degeneration (a good sign in dermatitis artefacta);
2. mounds of parakeratosis containing plasma at the lips of follicular infundibula suggest seborrhoeic dermatitis (*clues*);
3. in the chronic lesion of atopic dermatitis there is an increase in mast cell numbers in the infiltrate and the epidermis may be thickened but without exaggeration of rete pegs.

Granulomatous

These are inflammatory reactions dominated by macrophages in some more or less organized pattern and frequently contain giant cells. Granulomas are quite varied in appearance and range from typical naked sarcoid-like structures to the very structured granulomas of tuberculosis and the so-called palisading granulomas associated with necrobiotic collagen. So great is the range that it is only the dominant presence of macrophages that holds the whole concept together. Much recent interest in granulomas has centred on the identification of various cytokines concerned in their formation and maintenance. However, interesting though this data is, it is not yet a help in diagnosis, nor is it ever likely to be unless there are any morphological correlates that arise from it Interleukin (II)-1 appears to initiate granuloma formation in synergy with tumour necrosis factor (TNF or cachexin), IL-2 is associated with increased size of granulomas and IL-5 may be an attractant to eosinophils in the granulomas associated with parasitic infections while IL-6 is believed to be important in tuberculosis granulomas. The relationship is complex and IL-4 and IL-10 are macrophage inhibitors; the complex balance between these and other cytokines are believed to be responsible for the differences in appearance of different granulomas as well as for the differing clinical pictures of diseases such as tuberculoid and lepromatous leprosy:

1. sarcoid granulomas have few lymphocytes (naked);
2. fibrin in the centre of naked granulomas strongly suggests sarcoid but is present in only about 25% of cases (*clues*);
3. in the Kviem test the marker injection site may show granulomatous change (dependent on the marker used and the individual's sensitivity).

Tuberculoid granulomas are highly structured and the fully formed lesion is very characteristic having caseous necrosis at the centre, epithelioid histiocytes with fused forms (mainly of Langhans cell type but also foreign body type), surrounded by a substantial rim of lymphocytes and plasma cells. The granulomas show a tendency to coalesce and are less well defined than sarcoid granulomas. They are also not restricted to tuberculosis and may be seen in various disorders including; tuberculids, leprosy, syphilis, leishmaniasis, rosacea and Crohn's. Tuberculosis in the skin may show no granulomas and may show almost any pattern of inflammation. Demonstration of the organisms is diagnostic but is far better performed by a microbiologist.

Necrobiotic granulomas form around altered collagen and are therefore seen in granuloma annulare, necrobiosis lipoidica, rheumatoid nodule and acute rheumatic fever nodules.

1. Necrobiotic collagen in granuloma annulare is rich in acidic mucins, in necrobiosis lipoidica it contains fat and in rheumatic nodules it contains fibrin.
2. The palisade around granuloma annulare is mainly lymphocytes and around necrobiosis lipoidica is mostly plasma cells (*clues*).
3. Necrobiosis lipoidica contains thickened bundles of collagen (*clues*).
4. The granulomas of granuloma annulare are small and oval, those of necrobiosis lipoidica are flat and horizontal and bigger, those of rheumatoid tend to be large, round and nodular.
5. Transepidermal elimination may occur in any granulomatous condition and the tracks of this may be apparent.

Suppurative granulomas contain neutrophil polymorphs in the centre of granulomatous structures and are an indication of infection with a variety of infectious agents such as chromomycosis, blastomycosis and cat scratch disease, and these should be sought for with appropriate stains and the help of the microbiologist.

Foreign body granulomas may arise owing to endogenous or exogenous materials; the common factor is that the body sees them as foreign.

Vesiculobulous

These conditions all have vesicles or bullae as their diagnostic feature. Diseases that also have a vesiculobullous phase but are classified under other headings include psoriasis, which may present as a sterile pustulosis, and eczema, which may be dominated by spongiotic vesicles. The diagnosis of vesiculobullous diseases is largely based upon the level in the skin at which the splits occur; another morphological feature whose aetiopathogenesis is obscure in many cases. Intraepidermal splits include the various forms of pemphigus, which are further subclassified on the basis of the level within the epidermis at which the split occurs.

Splits at or above the granular layer

Palmar or plantar holes of different sizes within the keratin suggest a fungal infection such as tinea nigra (*clue*), the presence of neutrophils in the stratum corneum is also a sign suggesting fungal infection. Superficial collections of neutrophils and organism can induce very superficial splits in the stratum corneum in impetigo and staphylococcal scalded-skin syndrome. Secondary infection may also occur in the initially sterile subcorneal pustular dermatoses.

Suprabasilar splits

All these conditions result from acantholysis and contain acanthocytes (rounded-up, single keratinocytes). These are very much less common in spongiotic vesicles, presumably owing to the fact that the cell separation in spongiosis is much more directly caused by physical forces than in the acantholytic diseases in which antibodies to both cell surface and desmosomes are commonly present. The acantholytic diseases include pemphigus vulgaris, pemphigus vegetans, familial benign chronic pemphigus (Hailey-Hailey disease), Darier's disease and Grover's disease. Incidental acantholysis can occur in solar keratosis and in squamous carcinoma as well as in physical and chemical damage.

As well as the standard features such as dilapidated brick wall appearance of Hailey-Hailey disease and the intercellular deposition of IgG in pemphigus the following points can be of help:

1. an apparent intraepidermal cleft can arise as the base of a junctional blister begins to re-epithelialise (bullous pemphigoid, dermatitis herpetiformis) but the base of such a blister does not bear adnexae; roofs of such blisters remain viable for a surprisingly long time in contrast to erythema multiforme;
2. Grover's disease is intensely pruritic and this condition is characterized by erosions, ulcerations and crusts superimposed on the basic acantholytic picture (*clue*);

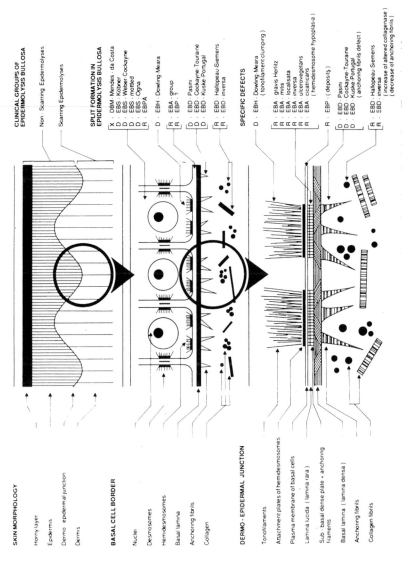

Fig. 4.1 The different sites at which splits occur in the various forms of epidermolysis bullosa (Reproduced from: *Diagnostic ultrastructure of non-neoplastic diseases.*[8])

3. numerous elongated acanthocytes in a pemphigus vulgaris-like setting suggest a physical or chemical cause (*clue*);
4. in chemical or physical blisters of this sort there is generally little inflammation until the roof is lost.

Subepidermal blisters

The structure of the basement membrane is complex but the way in which it holds the epidermis and dermis together is now being elucidated; for a review of this see Weedon. The basement membrane is known to contain a range of antigens, many of which take their names from specific disease entities and which are involved in the pathogenesis of these diseases. Consequently it is still the case that diagnosis is very dependent upon the demonstration of antibodies to many of these antigens. The components of the basement membrane cannot be distinguished by any of the standard light microscopic techniques and are thus not helpful in routine diagnosis, although an understanding of their biology is proving of great help in the understanding of the aetiopathology of many of them. It is still true that immunocytochemistry is less effective in the demonstration of extracellular antibodies than it is in the demonstration of intracellular ones. Consequently we remain dependent upon immunofluorescence for the diagnosis of most subepidermal bullous diseases. The various forms of epidermolysis bullosa can be distinguished by electron microscopy although the technique is often difficult; Fig. 4.1 is reproduced from *Diagnostic ultrastructure of non-neoplastic diseases*[8] and illustrates the different sites at which splits occur in the various forms of this complex disease group:

1. blisters with no inflammatory infiltrate suggest porphyria or (rarely these days) barbiturate poisoning;
2. clefts in the dermis occur in amyloidosis;
3. oedema in the upper dermis with single cell keratinocyte necrosis, which may become confluent as the blister develops, suggests erythema multiforme.

Vasculopathic pattern

This group includes all of those diseases with a predominant vasculitis or where the vasculitis is a significant component.

In any inflammatory disease the inflammatory cells have to get into the dermis by passing out of the bloodstream and through the vessel walls. Consequently it is not enough just to see vessels with inflammatory cells around them, one must see vascular damage. It is also important to bear in mind the distinction between thrombi causing vasculitis (such as primary vasculo-occlusive diseases like atrophie blanche and DIC) and vasculitis-causing thrombi (as in primary vasculitides). In the fully established or late lesion this may be difficult to distinguish but the primary event may be seen in isolation at the periphery of the lesion.

The urticarias result from marked vasodilatation and leakage of fluid and plasma proteins into the dermis (angio-oedema involves the deep dermis and mucous membranes and may co-exist). Urticaria, especially acute urticaria, is almost impossible to detect unless there is an inflammatory cell infiltrate because the other signs (spreading of collagen fibres) can all be reproduced by variations in fixation and section handling.

Summary

This covers the major groups of inflammatory skins; Weedon's minor categories are less of a problem and it is within the major categories that most difficulties occur. What makes inflammatory skins particularly problematic is that the inflammatory response is a stereotyped response to any trauma. Consequently there is a variable delay before the specific pattern has emerged and established itself. Added to this is the complex interplay of cytokine activities and the up-or down-regulation of receptors, all displayed upon the background of individual variability. Clearly there is no simple answer to this difficult diagnostic area, but it does seem that understanding the processes at work reduces the difficulties a little; the rest is experience and a subtle eye for even subtler signs.

REFERENCES

1. Ackerman AB. Histologic diagnosis of inflammatory skin disease. Lee and Febiger, 1978
2. Ackerman AB, Ragaz A. The lives of lesions. Masson Publishing USA. 1984
3. Ackerman AB, Jacoson, Vitale P. Clues to diagnosis in dermatopathology I. ASCP Press, 1991
4. Ackerman AB, Guo Y, Vitale P. Clues to diagnosis in dermatopathology II. ASCP Press, 1992
5. Ackerman AB, Guo Y, Vitale P, Vossaert K. Clues to diagnosis in dermatopathology III. ASCP Press, 1993
6. McKee PH. Pathology of the skin: with pathological correlations. J Lippincott, 1989
7. Weedon D. Systematic pathology 9. The skin. Churchill Livingstone, Edinburgh, 1992
8. Papadimitriou JM, Henderson DW, Spagnolo DV. Diagnostic ultrastructure of non-neoplastic diseases. Churchill Livingstone, Edinburgh, 1992

5

An update on chronic hepatitis

S. E. Davies

In the last decade there has been tremendous progress in the understanding of the hepatitis viruses, which has been reflected in the plethora of articles published on this subject. A spin-off from this has been increasing dissatisfaction with the existing terminology for the histopathological reporting of chronic hepatitis. These two areas of interest will be addressed in this chapter.

Chronic hepatitis – the terminology

What is chronic hepatitis?

The definition of chronic hepatitis is somewhat arbitrary, being defined as continuing disease without improvement in symptoms, enzymes or viral markers for 6 months. It must be appreciated that it is a clinicopathological syndrome, which has several causes. Many hepatic diseases can cause chronic inflammation within the liver and may enter the differential diagnosis but these are considered separate diseases; they include primary biliary cirrhosis and primary sclerosing cholangitis, metabolic abnormalities of alpha-1-antitrypsin deficiency and Wilson's disease, and some cases of alcohol injury.

Symptoms can be very variable or even absent. When present they are frequently mild and non-specific with general malaise being most common. Occasionally nausea, joint pain and abdominal pain are present. Specific features of liver disease including jaundice, darkened urine, itching and anorexia may be present with end-stage cirrhosis, acute exacerbation of chronic viral hepatitis or an acute onset of autoimmune hepatitis. The transaminases are frequently raised but may be normal and the levels do not reflect histological findings of inflammation. Alkaline phosphatase and gamma-glutamyl transpeptidase are minimally affected. Bilirubin, albumin and prothrombin time are relatively normal until late in the disease with development of end–stage cirrhosis.

The classification

Up until recently the classification of chronic hepatitis used the subdivisions chronic persistent hepatitis, chronic active hepatitis and chronic lobular hepatitis, (CPH, CAH and CLH, respectively), which originated in the late 1960s. These had been used on the grounds that they conveyed prognostic information. CAH implied a more severe lesion associated with progression to cirrhosis, and the presence of this type of lesion has been used as a standard indication for treatment.

However, since the availability of testing for hepatitis C virus (HCV) there has been an increasing dissatisfaction with this nomenclature on several grounds:[1–4]

1. CPH, CAH and CLH are not distinct and exclusive diseases. In any one individual e.g. a chronic carrier of hepatitis B virus (HBV) all these patterns may be seen at differing times in the natural history of the infection, being dependent upon the individual's immune status and state of viral replication;
2. chronic HCV infection can undoubtedly lead to the development of cirrhosis despite a common pattern in the early stages of CPH or borderline CPH/CAH;
3. similar histological patterns can be seen not only with chronic viral infections but also with autoimmune disease and adverse drug reactions (the metabolic causes of Wilson's disease and alpha–1–antitrypsin deficiency, although appearing similar may be differentiated histochemically);
4. the intra and interobserver concordance of histopathologists, even amongst experts, in assessing necrosis and inflammation can be quite poor;
5. piecemeal necrosis is the basis of the subdivisions rather than other forms of necrosis which may be of significance in determining outcome, in particular bridging necrosis;
6. there are limitations caused by sampling when small needle biopsies are performed.

The increasing consensus of opinion is to replace the classification of chronic hepatitis on purely histological criteria but to take into account the aetiology with clinical and serological factors.[5] This reflects a growing awareness that in patients with chronic hepatitis the cause of hepatitis is the most important factor in predicting clinicopathological outcome and determining what therapeutic regimens should be utilized. Classification based on the aetiology includes chronic viral hepatitis caused by HBV, HBV and hepatitis D virus (HDV), and HCV, autoimmune and drug-induced hepatitis. There remains some 10–25% of patients in whom no positive clinical or serological findings are identified and these are classified as cryptogenic. Hopefully this number will decline as further aetiological agents, presumably other viruses, are identified.

The most widely used scoring system for assessing CAH is the 'Histological Activity Index'.[6] Despite its popularity, not least with clinicians, it has inherent problems. The numerical scoring system gives a false sense of objectivity; the scoring is not linear, architectural abnormalities are the only consistently scored feature between pathologists[7] and the same value can be derived for markedly different histopathological appearances.

A modified scoring system has now been proposed by several individuals and an international panel of hepatopathologists[1,5,8–10] applying the ideas of grade and stage as already in existence with neoplasia. Put simply, the grade indicates the amount of necroinflammation and the stage the amount of architectural distortion. The necroinflammation incorporates both inflammatory infiltrate and cell loss and reflects its density/severity and the extent of tissue affected. An early simple proposal for alteration of terminology attempted to address the above criticisms.[1] The scores for grade and stage are separated and a similar value range given i.e. 0–4. Scores for necroinflammation assess both the portal/periportal activity and separate lobular activity. Such a system can record histopathological findings as verbal text or semiquantitavely, in addition to the aetiology when known. This simplified approach has met with approval although some advocate a scoring value of 1–4 for stage.[3] However, some suggestions are too simplistic,[11] with the scoring system suggested not allowing for differences in inflammation centred on portal tracts from that within the parenchyma.

Although semiquantitive textual descriptions of the presence, absence, distribution and extent of necroinflammatory activity and how this has affected the architecture should be practical for the majority of cases, scoring may still have a role to play, in particular, in clinical trials comparing the different treatment modalities utilized in various centres and also in assessing sequential biopsies from individuals. A more complex system involving nine categories still has the disadvantage of utilizing the terms CPH and CAH.[9] A leading paper representing a consensus view separates stage and grade but is quite complex;[10] separate categories exist for the assessment of portal inflammation, periportal or periseptal hepatitis, confluent necrosis and focal necrosis and inflammation, the values ranging from 0–4 or 0–6, possible discriminatory values being between 0 and 18. Staging has a score from 0–6 from normal to cirrhosis, reflecting both the degree of fibrosis in portal areas and how many portal areas are involved. Bridging necrosis is reserved for bridges linking portal tracts and terminal hepatic venules, conveyed by the term porto-central, and assessed under confluent necrosis. Further recommendations include the recording but not the scoring of other features including bile duct damage, steatosis, dysplasia, hyperplasia, iron and copper deposition and inclusions. Although complex this is an all-embracing model, which can be customized as individual need arises. The earlier proposed systems have the considerable advantage of simplicity and, when necessary, a qualitative verbal assessment of grade and stage in comparing different biopsies from any one patient can be given. However, a more complex system may be desirable when greater discrimination is required e.g. in a comparative trial of patients with only mild disease who may otherwise all score the same value.

Sampling errors should always be considered; is the biopsy material too scanty or inadequate for assessment? This is particularly important if any scoring is being performed with the associated implication of an objective 'scientific' assessment.

Rather than these proposals being met with dread at yet another new classification, they should be viewed as a change in emphasis. Hopefully, the nomenclature should make our job of reporting liver biopsies somewhat easier and remind clinicians of how important good clinicopathological correlation is in making sense of such material. Despite the proposal of aetiology being part of the pathological diagnosis there is still a role for the histopathologist, not least in confirming that the presumed aetiology is causing the liver abnormalities. The assessment of fibrosis and the absence or presence of cirrhosis together with the degree and type of inflammation present is still important.

Viral hepatitis

Although many systemic viral infections may induce liver damage, albeit usually mild, the term viral hepatitis is reserved for those whose prime effect is on the liver (Table 5.1). They are not biologically related. Up until the last decade the classification included hepatitis A virus, hepatitis B virus and, by exclusion, non-A non-B hepatitis (NANB). This was some what unsatisfactory, not least because the natural history of this last group showed considerable heterogeneity. The two distinct viruses hepatitis C and

Table 5.1 The hepatitis viruses

Virus	Type	Spread	Acute liver failure?	Progression to chronicity?	Prevention/ treatment
HAV	RNA	Faeco-oral	Occasional	No	Vaccination
HBV	DNA	Parenteral, sexual/vertical	Sometimes	Yes: especially if vertical	Immunization, interferon ~ 50%
HCV	RNA	Parenteral, unknown	Very rare	Yes: the majority	Interferon ~ 25%
HDV	RNA	Parenteral	Yes: > HBV	Yes	Interferon
HEV	RNA	Faeco-oral	In pregency	No	Hygiene
?HFV	?RNA	??	? cause	No	?
HGV	RNA	Parenteral	Not yet known	Yes	Not yet known

hepatitis E have now been described, possible candidates for hepatitis F have been proposed and a recognition of hepatitis G is emerging.

Hepatitis A virus

Hepatitis A virus (HAV) is an RNA virus of the picorna virus family that is spread via the faeco-oral route. There is a high prevalence in the developing world with the majority of infections occurring in young children. In the developed world numbers of cases have fallen such that only around 20% of the population have protective antibodies; the remainder being at risk of infection during foreign travel, although numbers may be higher in institutions.[12]

There is a short incubation period and prodrome followed by malaise, jaundice and deranged liver function tests. Acute infection is diagnosed by the presence of IgM antibody. Subclinical infection is common in that individuals with IgG antibodies frequently do not give a history of jaundice. HAV rarely leads to acute liver failure although occasionally protracted and cholestatic courses may be seen.

Histology of the liver does not give clues to the aetiology. Classical features of acute hepatitis with lobular disarray, hepatocyte necrosis and cell dropout with mononuclear cell infiltrate are present. Plasma cells may be numerous and cholestasis is common. Occasionally, portal tracts show a dense inflammatory cell infiltrate and an interface hepatitis may be seen (Fig. 5.1).[13] This gives a histological picture characteristic of chronic hepatitis and care must be taken not to make such a diagnosis in the absence of

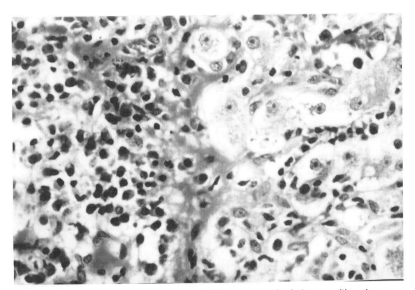

Fig. 5.1 The edge of a portal tract in acute HAV infection, left of picture, with a dense infiltrate of plasma cells and lymphocytes. These are seen infiltrating into and around hepatocytes in the adjacent parenchyma indistinguishable from the interface hepatitis seen with some cases of chronic hepatitis.

knowledge of the serology. Giant multinucleate hepatocytes may be present, albeit very rarely.

Preventive measures against infection are related primarily to education regarding improved hygiene in food handling and protection of water supplies from contamination. Gammaglobulins can be administered for passive immunisation but this is protective for a few months only. A vaccine for active immunization is now available.

Hepatitis E virus

Although biologically distinct, hepatitis E virus (HEV) has many similarities clinically to HAV, being responsible for many cases of enteric NANB hepatitis.[14,15] HEV is prevalent in developing countries and an important cause of epidemic hepatitis, having been found to be responsible for an epidemic affecting 30 000 people in India in the 1950s and over 100 000 people in China in the 1980s. Many sporadic cases are also seen. HEV has a short incubation period of 2–9 weeks and leads to the symptoms and signs of classical acute hepatitis with jaundice. Chronic disease is not seen although a minority of patients may have a prolonged viraemia with infective stools even after clinical recovery of their acute hepatitis. There is an overall low mortality of 0.5–4% but pregnant women are particularly susceptible with up to 20% mortality. Intrauterine infection can occur and has been implicated in subsequent abortion and perinatal mortality. To date, patients with acute HEV presenting in the UK have acquired their infection in the subcontinent as returning travellers or visitors.[14]

The virus is a non-enveloped single-stranded RNA virus.[16] Recombinant vaccines are being developed. HEV has been identified within the serum and hepatocytic cytoplasm in patients presenting with acute liver failure. The epidemics recorded have resulted from massive viral dose with gross contamination of water supplies. Somewhat unusual is that young adults, rather than children are primarily affected. Although antibodies appear to persist, the degree of protection is not yet known. Different strains may also account for later infection in life.

Histologically, acute HEV may be similar to acute HAV but with prominent cholestasis and portal inflammation,[17] although, to date, the data is somewhat scanty.

Hepatitis F and hepatitis G virus

Currently there is no universally recognized hepatitis F virus, partly because this has been used as a dustbin term. Some authors, particularly from the Far East have designated patients with either acute or chronic liver disease who have no serological markers of known hepatitis viruses as suffering from hepatitis F virus. This would seem inappropriate and against the trend of classification, not least because such a group of patients probably have several different viruses. Furthermore, in Japan, many patients presenting with acute liver failure have a mutant form of HBV, which can be demonstrated within the liver by polymerase chain reaction (PCR) despite negative serology.[18]

A single transmissible agent has been implicated in some cases of sporadic acute liver failure, being a 50–70 nm enveloped virus-like particle with similarities to toga viruses.[19] This was discovered within the cytoplasm of hepatocytes and in increased numbers after recurrence of severe hepatitis following liver transplantation. Although originally described in UK patients, similar particles have been described in patients from Thailand and Nepal. This agent has been termed 'candidate hepatitis F'.[20] It would seem unlikely that this single agent can account for all cases of acute liver failure of unknown pathogenesis and it has not been widely recognized as a unique and novel hepatitis virus.[21] Because of the lack of clarity surrounding hepatitis F, the most recent virus to be established has been called hepatitis G virus.

Another agent was identified after inoculation of serum from a patient with acute NANBNC hepatitis, (whose initials were GB), into primates. Passage studies in tamarins, utilizing oligonucleotide probes and PCR amplification, have revealed several genomically related agents that are hepatitic and they have been termed GBV-A, -B and -C.[22–24] Only the latter appears important in human infection and this is now recognized as hepatitis G virus (HGV). Although this is flavivirus-like it is not a genotype of HCV. Initial reports suggest HGV has a role in post-transfusion and community-acquired NANB hepatitis. About one-quarter of patients with acute HCV may also be HGV positive, although its pathogenicity is yet to be determined.[25]

A previous candidate for HGV was proposed when viral-type particles were identified ultrastructurally in patients with acute and chronic hepatitis that morphologically were distinguished by syncytial giant-cell hepatocytes. These particles were similar to paramyxovirus.[26] However, no further supporting evidence has come forward and this agent should not be confused with HGV as defined above. Although it may have been fitting for G to correspond to 'giant-cell' the presence of such hepatocytes is certainly not specific; found predominantly in the neonate they can also be present in several types of acute hepatitis and autoimmune chronic hepatitis.

Hepatitis B virus

The Virus and Pathogenesis

HBV is a small hepadnavirus consisting of a nucleocapsid core with a surrounding protein envelope. The envelope contains the surface antigen (HBsAg) and the core protein (HBcAg) surrounds the genome. This exists as incompletely double-stranded DNA with several overlapping reading frames, which code for the viral antigens. Cleavage of the large precore protein in the endoplasmic reticulum releases e antigen (HBeAg), which is associated with viral replication. A large P gene probably codes for the polymerase enzyme, and the protein encoded by the X gene is not fully determined although it is very common in chronic infection. Two further surface-related antigens have been demonstrated, both being larger than HBsAg and designated 'pre-S1' and 'pre-S2', the former being thought of importance in the attachment of the virus to the host cell. All of the viral antigens, apart from core antigen, may be demonstrable in the serum as are their respective antibodies. The presence of the various antigens and antibodies in the serum reflects the time from onset of infection and are different in acute and chronic infection. Viral replication is indicated by the presence of serum DNA and the specific DNA polymerase or alternatively by the presence of e and core antigens within hepatocytes. Antigens and HBV DNA can now be demonstrated within routinely fixed paraffin-embedded tissue.

The pathogenesis of liver injury and outcome of HBV infection in any individual is dependent upon the interplay of the properties of the infecting virus and the host immune response.

The immune reaction in chronic HBV infection consists of cytotoxic T lymphocytes that recognize and selectively lyse hepatocytes expressing HBcAg[27,28] and this can be modified by IgG antibodies against HBcAg. HBeAg is also expressed on the cell membrane. The core and e antigen are highly cross-reactive owing to substantial amino acid homology. It is now realized that T cells do not recognize large protein antigens but rather small peptide fragments, (of 18–16 amino acid residues), which are presented in a special groove on top of an human leukocyte antigen (HLA). T-helper cells produce cytokines in response to HBcAg and HBeAg in acute infection. In acute, self-limiting hepatitis there is a polyclonal response by cytotoxic T cells with specificity for multiple viral epitopes. There is some evidence that the presence of HBeAg epitopes leads to interference with the immune response and thus the immunotolerance seen in early chronic infection.

Interferon production in acute hepatitis is high and induces increased expression of HLA and associated processed viral antigens. The virus can affect production; the X protein stimulates interferon-β and the core protein inhibits production. There is some evidence that hepatocytes produce interferon-α. Production of interferon is impaired in those developing chronic infection. However, this is not the full story, otherwise all patients would respond to interferon therapy rather than only 50%. A terminal protein from the virus may inhibit the cellular response to interferon. The patient's HLA type may be important in determining outcome in that the expression of the viral epitope is in conjunction with this.

Molecular biological techniques have identified the highly variable nature of the HBV genome in populations, between different carriers and at different phases of the infection. However, there is no evidence that different viral genotypes account for the distinct clinical disease patterns. Individuals infected from the same source do not necessarily develop the same disease states indicating that the interaction between the viral genome and host remains paramount.

There are subtypes of HBsAg, (d, y, r, q, w1–4), which, whilst useful in epidemiological studies, are not associated with different natural history or pathogenicity. Several other mutants have now been described.[27,29] The first described is the 'precore mutant', which has a point mutation in the precore genome such that HBeAg is not expressed and there is antibody to the e antigen (HBeAb) in serum, despite there being ongoing replication and active liver disease. Initially the precore mutant was identified in fulminant hepatitis and rapidly progressive disease unresponsive to interferon but it has now been described in the full clinical spectrum of chronic disease including asymptomatic carriage. A mutant identified following vaccination is caused by an amino acid substitution in the major HBsAg protein, which alters its antigenicity. Antibodies induced against the wild, (naturally occurring), type cannot give protective immunity.

Other mutations will come to light with time. These may have considerable impact on vaccination programmes. Other mutations in the core and terminal regions might interfere with antigen expression and interferon production.[27] Whether clinical infection follows contraction of mutant forms into different individuals will depend on the individual's immune system. Recognition and rapid elimination may be possible.

Natural history

Chronic carriers show an early immunotolerant phase, particularly if infection is vertically transmitted, characterized by viral replication with HBeAg and HBV DNA in the serum and minimal liver damage. With time there is loss of tolerance with onset of active liver disease and persistent replication. The duration of this phase probably determines how much architectural distortion results. With elimination of virally infected cells there is seroconversion to HBeAb, cessation of replication and hepatic inflammation. There is spontaneous seroconversion of HBeAg positivity to HBeAb positivity in 10–20% of chronic carriers per year, frequently associated with clinicopathological exacerbation. Failure to eradicate replicating virus is associated with increased risk of progression to cirrhosis. Once cirrhosis has developed there is around 50% five-year survival.[30]

The virus is spread by close contact and parenteral routes. Transmission from infected mothers to babies is high, particularly if the mothers are e antigen positive, when the rate approaches 90%. Several studies of pregnant women have found that only 50% of the women who are surface antigen positive have classical risk factors.[31] Several countries, including the USA, are now advocating universal immunization, the most effective system being identification and immunization of high-risk cases at birth and the remaining population in late childhood. The UK does not currently have this policy. An alternative approach is performing antenatal screening on all pregnant women, combined active and passive immunization being offered to those found to be positive.

There are strong associations between HBV infection and hepatocellular carcinoma (HCC).[32] In geographical areas where HBV infection is endemic the prevalence of HCC is high and individuals developing HCC are usually chronically infected with HBV. Even in countries with low infection rates, 20–40% of HCC cases have HBV infection. Molecular studies show the presence of integrated HBV sequences in the vast majority of carcinomas in patients who are HBsAg positive and some with antibody to hepatitis B core and surface antigens (HBcAb and HBsAb, respectively). Some studies, but certainly not all, have found HBV DNA in carcinomas arising in cirrhotic patients who have no markers for current or previous HBV infection.

People most at risk of developing HCC are those who have become infected early in life, in particular during the perinatal period. Only around 50% of patients in high endemic areas have cirrhosis, and other factors, including aflatoxin, have been implicated. The tumours develop earlier than in patients with HCV infection, (see below), and may occur even in adolescence.

HBV markers may be present in up to 90% of patients with human immunodeficiency virus (HIV) infection.[33] Patients with HIV infection who become acutely infected with HBV are liable to become chronic carriers. However, liver damage is usually very mild with only slightly elevated liver enzymes and few necroinflammatory lesions.

Histopathology

No specific features of HBV are detected in acute infection. Acute hepatic changes of varying severity may be seen although those patients with severe disease are more likely to come to the attention of histopathologists. Viral antigens are not detected in the liver, apart from very occasionally in those with acute liver failure.

The full spectrum of chronic hepatitis may be seen in the livers of chronic carriers including the presence of cirrhosis, or alternatively minimal evidence of viral infection may be present. This reflects the relative expression of the virus and the immune status of the host. Hepatocellular carcinoma may be seen. Earlier reports identified the presence of dysplasia within hepatocytes with enlarged and bizzare hyperchromatic nuclei and these have been confirmed as showing aneuploidy. Such nuclei have a definite association with HBV infection and as this carries a risk of malignancy it has been postulated that dysplasia may represent preneoplastic change. However, this assertion is controversial and much emphasis is now being placed on foci of small hyperplastic hepatocytes as markers of premalignancy.

The presence of HBsAg within hepatocytes indicates chronic infection. The excess protein expands the endoplasmic reticulum, which is seen as a homogenous eosinophilic staining of the cytoplasm, the 'ground-glass' hepatocyte (Fig. 5.2, a and b). These cells stain positively with the orcein and aldehyde fuschin techniques. They can be identified specifically with immunocytochemistry. This technique can also identify HBcAg and HBeAg, the presence of which indicates ongoing viral replication. The

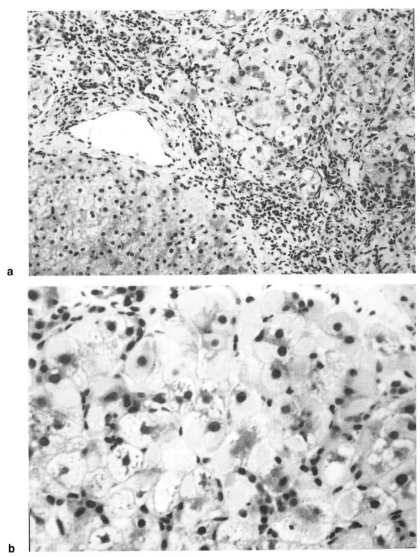

Fig. 5.2 (a) Chronic HBV infection with moderate activity and interface hepatitis; ground glass cells are discernible in the mid and upper right of the picture. They can be better visualized on higher power (**b**).

presence of cytoplasmic HBcAg correlates with the degree of necroinflammation. Persistent HBsAg can be seen even after the end of viral replication.

Treatment

Interferon-α response rates for chronic HBV are around 50% and a competent host immune response is required. Those who are immunologically tolerant owing to vertical transmission or immunosuppressed such as acquired immune deficiency syndrome (AIDS), renal transplant and dialysis patients, rarely respond. Interferon has antiviral and immunomodulatory effects.[34] Antiviral agents are aimed at inhibition of reverse transcriptase or DNA polymerase, but toxic side-effects may be experienced owing to interference with cellular and mitochondrial DNA synthesis in the host. Such agents include nucleotide analogues, which undergo phosphorylation and compete for integration into the genome, thus interfering with viral synthesis or transport.

The latest agent, lamivudine, has now undergone therapeutic trials.[35] In vitro studies have shown little toxicity on mitochondrial DNA synthesis. Lamivudine induces extensive lasting HBV suppression during treatment and occasional cases of eradication after cessation of therapy have been reported. The mechanism of action is unclear but a rise in liver enzymes precedes the decline in HBV DNA, as is frequently seen with successful interferon therapy, implying assistance in the host immune response.

Early cases of transplantation for HBV showed an unacceptably high morbidity and mortality, particularly in patients with active viral replication at the time of transplantation. A unique and novel histopathology, termed fibrosing cholestatic hepatitis, was described in some patients.[36] This was associated with universal fatality and appeared to have evolved following massive accumulation of viral proteins rather than by the normal immune mechanisms. Improved survival can be obtained with administration of immunoglobulin but this must be continued indefinitely. Trials utilizing antiviral agents and attempts at active immunization are ongoing.

Hepatitis D virus

The hepatitis D virus, (HDV), is a defective RNA virus that depends upon HBV for its replication and pathogenicity. It is a small RNA virus with similarities to plant virioids and is encapsulated in HBsAg. Infection is either at the same time as HBV or as superinfection of a chronic HBV carrier. It is associated with active disease biochemically and histologically. Co-infection has an increased risk of fulminant hepatitis. More rapid development of cirrhosis than with HBV alone has been repeatedly reported although some cases can show a long disease history. It is prevalent in drug addicts and in Mediterranean countries. Cirrhosis caused by HBV and HDV is associated with the development of HCC.

Serum markers alone do not distinguish acute and chronic infection. However, in chronic cases lobular inflammation may be pronounced. The presence of the delta antigen, (DAg), within hepatocytes is a more reliable indicator of ongoing infection than HDV antibody. The presence of HDV superinfection inhibits the replication of HBV and there is usually loss of HBV DNA in the serum and antigens may not be demonstrated within the liver. This effect on HBV may explain why patients transplanted for HBV and HDV liver disease have more favourable outcomes than those patients transplanted for HBV alone.[37]

Hepatitis C virus

The cloning of hepatitis C virus (HCV) and subsequent development of antibody testing was successful only in the late 1980s.[38] HCV is a 55 nm single-stranded RNA virus similar to flaviviruses, which include the yellow fever virus, with similarities also to pestiviruses. It has a genome of 9500 kb with genomic areas coding for structural core or capsid and envelope proteins, (C, E1 and E2) and non-structural proteins, (NS2, 3, 4 and 5). Initial diagnosis was based on detection of antibody to a large viral antigen using enzyme-linked immunosorbent assay (ELISA) but this proved unreliable in cases of acute infection and there were many examples of false positives, particularly in areas of low prevalence and in patients with hypergammaglobulinaemia.[39,40] Second generation testing with recombinant immunoblot assay (RIBA) directed against the structural nucleocapsid antigens is more reliable especially in early acute infection. Definite diagnosis of infection requires PCR using primers against the conserved non-coding region, the disadvantage being the expense and expertise needed to perform this reliably.

The genotype of HCV shows considerable heterogeneity indicating high mutation rates.[12,41] Strains differ between geographical regions, within individuals in the same region and within the same individual. Whilst some areas of the genome are conserved, the E2/NS1 region appears hypervariable. Diagnostic tests are aimed at identifying highly conserved domains, predominantly the 5′ non-coding region. There are 12 genotypes and at least 30 subtypes to date. The emergence of such mutants may explain the wide fluctuations in liver enzyme titres that are seen frequently in acute HCV and how, by escaping the host immune response, there might be a propensity for chronic infection. The specific genotypes also appear important with respect to response to interferon and rates of progression of disease to cirrhosis and hepatocellular carcinoma. Type 1 HCV is most common in Europe.

At present the pathogenesis is unclear, with contradictory data on the nature of the inflammatory infiltrate seen within the liver. Genetic susceptibility and other host factors have yet to be defined.

There appears to be some confusion and problems in trying to determine the significance of HCV infection. Who gets it, how do they get it and, more importantly, what is the natural history for those who have got it – these are all questions with incomplete answers.

Epidemiology

Difficulties in determining the prevalence of HCV have resulted from inclusion of false positives, (initial tests by ELISA being most unreliable),

failure to elucidate other risk factors, in particular a history of drug exposure, compounded by small sample size.

Without doubt HCV is the major cause for the majority of parenterally
acquired cases previously designated NANB hepatitis,[42] accounting for
60–90% of cases. Since the introduction of screening of donated blood for
anti-HCV antibodies in 1990, post-transfusion HCV infection is now less
than 1%.[43]

The majority of individuals who are found to be positive for anti-HCV
antibodies do not give a positive history of risk factors, particularly parenteral exposure.[43] Intravenous drug users are an at-risk group, up to 70% in
Australasia being positive.[39] The prevalence of community-acquired HCV
has been difficult to determine but 20% of cases of acute viral hepatitis in
the USA are thought to be caused by HCV. Despite the decrease in the
numbers of post-transfusion infections the numbers of cases identified
annually in the USA, approximately 150 000, has not declined. Risk factors
can be identified in around 60% of patients, usually percutaneous, intravenous drug and sexual/household exposure. Low socio-economic group
also appears to be a risk factor. The prevalence is highest in haemophiliacs
and long-term, (over 10 years), drug users, of whom more than 90% are
anti-HCV positive. Western-based hospital health-care workers have a
seropositivity prevalence of around 1% presumably owing to needle-stick
injuries, inapparant parenteral and possible mucus membrane transmission.
Haemodialysis patients show considerable geographical variation but may
have a prevalence as high as 20%.

With supplementary testing to exclude a high proportion of false positives, the incidence in UK blood donors is very low, being less than 0.01%,[44]
in North America and western Europe blood donors the seropositivity rate
is 0.3%, the highest rate being recorded in South America at 2%. Blood
donors cannot be considered as representative of the general population,
not least because they have been screened for high-risk behaviour and
other viral markers. The largest population study to date, involving over 10
000 individuals and performed in the USA found a prevalence of anti-
HCV positivity of 1.4%.[43]

Evidence for non–parenteral transmission comes from several small studies of the rate of infection in sexual partners of patients with anti-HCV, an
average of 5% of these being positive. The prevalence in other household
occupants is somewhat less, being 3.6%. Perinatal transmission rates have
been reported, varying from 0–13%, but does not appear to be a problem.

Natural history

The natural history of chronic HCV infection is still not established clearly.
It is unclear whether the majority of people infected have relentlessly progressive chronic liver disease with cirrhosis and its sequelae or a relatively
benign condition with long-term carriage in which morbidity and mortality are predominantly caused by co-existent disease.

Initial reports attempting to address these issues were confusing with some outright contradictory conclusions. One study of post-transfusion cases showed development of chronic liver disease in two-thirds, half of whom developed cirrhosis within 8 years.[45] Another, also of post-transfusion cases showed only a 3% mortality caused by liver disease after 18 years but most of which could be explained by alcohol.[46]

Subclinical disease is usual with less than 10% of acute infections causing an icteric illness.[42] HCV has only very rarely been implicated in acute liver failure in European or North American patients.[20,21] Approximately two-thirds of people acutely infected go on to develop chronic infection as indicated by persistent abnormal liver function tests after 6 months, regardless of whether the infection was parenterally or community acquired. However, transaminase values vary with time and may be normal for prolonged periods and the majority of carriers may be asymptomatic. Despite this the histopathology demonstrates active disease in over 50% of cases.[47]

Since the early 1980s an association between HCC and chronic NANB hepatitis has been identified. Testing for HCV showed that 60–80% of patients with an HCC not HBV related were anti-HCV antibody positive.[48] In Japan there has been a doubling in the number of cases of HCC from the mid-1960s to early 1980s and HCV now accounts for relatively more of these than does HBV. The time course appears to be that of a 20–30 year period. Many cases of chronic HCV infection were transfusion acquired, during the operations for pulmonary tuberculosis, which were widespread after World War II. The vast majority of cases arise within a cirrhotic liver.

The reported differences in patient outcome have been quite extreme. This partly reflects whether the sample population originates from a specialized referral centre and therefore is at the extreme of any disease spectrum; high morbidity being due to the co-existent disease associated with the transfusions, and there was the prolonged follow-up necessary to establish the natural history of HCV. The evolving picture is one of serious consequences in the minority of people.[49] However, extremely long follow-up may be necessary to determine more fully the natural history.

HCV and other hepatotrophic agents

A proportion of patients with alcoholic liver disease are consistently positive for anti-HCV antibodies, studies giving values of 25–65%.[50] Although originally this was thought to be false positivity similar to that seen in autoimmune hepatitis, HCV RNA positivity has been reported in 11–46% of patients with alcoholic liver disease, which is consistently higher than rates of HCV infection in alcoholics without liver disease. An obvious compounding factor in assessing the significance of this is that many of these patients are also intravenous drug users, such that in one study this could have accounted for 90% of patients' anti-HCV seropositivity. With exclusion of such patients, and also those with other risk factors including previous blood transfusion, there is still an excess of patients with alcoholic liver disease who are affected with HCV, the overall consensus being one-quarter to one-third.

Alcohol appears synergistic with HCV in that there is greater predisposition to severe liver disease than with either agent alone, this occurring at a younger age. A greater proportion of patients with alcoholic cirrhosis, around 40%, are anti-HCV positive compared with 20% of those with steatohepatitis and 2% of alcoholics with normal livers.[51] These patients may show more portal and lobular chronic inflammation. An increased risk of HCC in alcoholic cirrhosis with HCV infection has also been reported. Less commonly, a picture of chronic hepatitis more in keeping with a viral aetiology is present and may show considerable interface hepatitis.

In the context of HIV disease the outcome appears dependent partly on immune status,[52] particularly in haemophiliac patients with a high viral load. In early infections the significance of HCV infection seems much the same as in non-HIV patients but with declining immunity there is a risk of rapidly progressive devlopment of cirrhosis but with little inflammatory activity.

Up to one-fifth of patients with chronic HBV infection also have chronic HCV infection. A high percentage of carriers who only have antibodies against HBcAg but in whom PCR testing is positive for HBV also have anti-HCV antibodies.[53] There appears to be an increased risk of developing HCC when co-infected with both viruses.[54]

Extrahepatic manifestations

Several non-hepatic manifestations of HCV have been described, with immunological abnormalities having a high prevalence.[50,55] These appear to be of different types depending upon the putative mechanisms of injury, including immune-complex mediated and autoimmune with anti-tissue antibodies, and also in rare diseases, which have known associations with chronic liver disease. These manifestations are not dependent upon the serotype of HCV and have been seen with the strains prevalent in Europe and North America.

HCV infection appears to be the main cause of essential mixed cryoglobulinaemia–90% of patients have HCV RNA in their serum. Between one-third and one-half of patients with chronic HCV infection have demonstrable cryoglobulin. There is a high prevalence of rheumatoid factor positivity in 70% of patients and this may be important in the pathogenesis of the cryoglobulinaemia.

Various autoantibodies have been identified in up to one-half of individuals with chronic HCV including anti-nuclear, anti-smooth muscle and anti-LKM 1 antibodies. There is an association with autoimmune thyroiditis, with the presence of antibodies and hypo- and hyperfunction. Anti-mitochondrial antibodies have not been found. A lymphocytic infiltrate in labial salivary glands may be present in 50% of patients although a full-blown sialadenitis as seen in Sjoegren's syndrome is present in less than half of these and rarely causes symptomatic dryness.

A relationship between porphyria cutanea tarda, iron overload and chronic liver disease is well recognized. Early European studies have shown between two-thirds and three-quarters of patients with the sporadic form of the disease to be anti-HCV positive. They respond less well to venesection than HCV-negative patients. Chronic liver disease is also associated with lichen planus and HCV infection accounts for around half of these cases. Very rarely chronic corneal keratitis, a Mooren ulcer, has been described in HCV-infected patients.

HCV infection has been implicated in glomerulonephritis, of membranoproliferative type, although HCV antigens or RNA have not been demonstrated in the deposits within affected glomeruli. Proteinuria has been reduced in some patients by the use of interferon therapy. It is not yet fully established whether HCV infection plays a role in the pathogenesis of polyarteritis nodosum vasculitis, as is seen with HBV infection, or in the cutaneous manifestations of a vasculitic process.

Initial anti-HCV seropositivity by ELISA testing in patients with rheumatoid arthritis was found to be caused by hypergammaglobulinaemia rather than a true association. Lack of confirmatory tests refuted other possible associations, including pulmonary fibrosis. There are rare occurrences of aplastic anaemia complicating viral hepatitis but HCV infection has not been demonstrated convincingly as a causative agent.

The presence of a pericapillary lymphocytic infiltrate in salivary glands may be caused by immune complex deposition or by direct infection of the gland with HCV. Some studies utilizing PCR have identified HCV-RNA within the salivary gland and also the thyroid and seminal vesicle. HCV has been identified within peripheral blood but, as yet, there is contradictory data regarding the presence or absence of HCV in body fluids and secretions including saliva, semen, faeces and urine.[56]

Histopathology

The histopathology of HCV infection within the liver has emerged as more distinctive than descriptions of chronic NANB hepatitis but it is not diagnostic.[56] Several comparative studies of HCV infection with HBV infection and autoimmune hepatitis (AIH) have been performed in addition to detailed analysis of HCV and retrospectively of NANB hepatitis.[57–59]

There is usually a portal infiltrate of chronic inflammatory cells with distinctive lymphoid aggregates, occasionally germinal centre formation, and frequently centred upon bile ducts (Figs 5.3 and 5.4). This is quite distinctive being present in 50–80% of cases, as although lymphoid aggregates may be seen in HBV and autoimmune disease, follicles and germinal centres are not seen. Studies report frequencies of bile duct damage ranging from 25–90%. Part of this discrepancy reflects the individual criteria used to evaluate 'damage'. Although cytological disturbance of the biliary epithelium

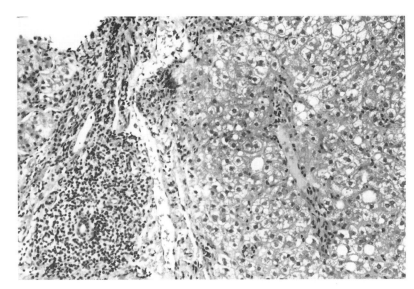

Fig. 5.3 A typical low power view of chronic HCV infection; the portal tract contains a moderate chronic inflammatory cell infiltrate including a lymphoid follicle, there is minimal disruption of the limiting plate, scattered parenchymal necroinflammatory foci are present with mild macrovesicular steatosis.

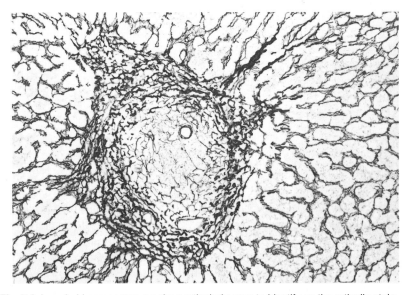

Fig. 5.4 Lymphoid aggragates may be particularly easy to identify on the reticulin stain. Chronic HCV infection.

may be seen together with infiltration by lymphocytes obscuring the ducts, chronic ductopenia as seen in primary biliary cirrhosis has not been identified.[60] There appears to be a positive relationship between level of inflammation and duct lesions.

The majority of patients show only focal and/or mild necroinflammation in periportal areas, the classical site for piecemeal (or more appropriately interface) necrosis typically being far less florid than that seen in cases of AIH (Fig. 5.3). Despite the absence of what has been considered aggressive lesions cirrhosis had developed in the majority of patients in one study.[57] Great difficulty has been encountered in trying to ascertain the category of chronic hepatitis in over one-quarter of patients.[59] There is a suggestion of more inflammation being present in cases of post-transfusion hepatitis, perhaps reflecting greater viral load.

A mild degree of macrovesicular steatosis is present in approximately two-thirds of patients, it being unusual to have severe fatty change (Fig. 5.3). Acidophilic bodies may be present in three-quarters of patients. Lobular infiltrate with prominence of Küpffer cells and lymphocytes in sinusoids may be prominent. Such changes may make differentiation from an acute hepatitis difficult, the presence of confluent necrosis in acinar zones 3 being a pointer to acute infection.[56] Occasional Mallory's body-like material has been seen in some cases[4,56] and granulomas have been reported in a small percentage of cases both within portal areas and acini, in cirrhotic and non-cirrhotic livers.[61–63]

In summary, the presence of lymphoid aggregates, mild necroinflammation, fatty change and lobular activity are highly characteristic of HCV infection although not found in every individual case. Once cirrhosis has developed, the amount of inflammation, including lymphoid aggregates, is diminished and there may be a decrease in fatty change giving a truly cryptogenic picture.[57]

Treatment

There are an estimated 3.5 million people in the USA who are positive for HCV of whom 8000–10 000 die annually and a further 1000 have liver transplantation performed.[64] In the UK there are approximately 200 000 infected people with HCV.[49] Who should be treated?

Any treatment should be focused on those individuals who are most risk of serious sequelae but, at present, the predictors of progression are not clearly understood. Reserving treatment for those who have already developed cirrhosis is inappropriate as failure rate in these patients is high.[65] Although 50% of patients who are positive for anti-HCV and, by PCR, have liver function tests within the normal range their livers are not normal. Histology shows necroinflammatory lesions, albeit predominantly mild. Therefore they cannot safely be considered as healthy carriers.[47] High levels of HCV RNA show a correlation with histological activity.[49]

The goal of any treatment should be the elimination of the virus but this obviously depends on sophisticated molecular techniques, although alternative stategies are possible if these are unavailable.[65] In clinical practice changes in alanine aminotransferase (ALT) may be adequate for assessment of response to treatment. Comparison between therapeutic trials may be difficult; older trials on the treatment of NANB hepatitis were by necessity focused on normalization of liver enzymes or improvement in histological activity.

Interferon therapy has been shown to decrease viral load, normalize transaminase levels and improve liver histology in some patients.[66] Early trials demonstrated 50% of patients as having an initial response but only 25% had a sustained remission as defined by normalization of ALT for longer than 6 months following cessation of treatment. This could have reflected patient selection in that only those individuals with abnormal liver function tests were candidates for treatment. However, similar values of 50% initial response but only 25–30% sustained response have been observed measuring serum HCV RNA. Sustained response is most likely in those who show a rapid decrease in liver enzymes and HCV RNA levels within the first month of starting therapy. Increased dose of interferon does not alter the response rate. However, extension of treatment time from 6 months to 12–18 months increased the number of sustained responses.[64] Factors which have emerged as associated with risk of poor response include increasing age, cirrhosis, long disease duration, high viraemic load and the type 1b genotype.[12,49,65] Higher serum ferritin and hepatic iron content have been noted in non-responders as compared with responders but of more significance is the presence of stainable iron within sinusoidal Kupffer cells and portal macrophages.[67]

The synthetic nucleotide analogue ribavirin has been tried as an antiviral agent in a few trials. Although improvement in biochemical markers may occur, in the majority of patients cessation of therapy is followed by a return to pretreatment values, and a significant decrease in HCV RNA has not yet been observed.[12]

Orthotopic liver transplantation has been performed successfully in a number of patients with end-stage liver disease, some of whom had complicating hepatocellular carcinoma. Recurrence in the graft and in the serum is nearly universal as judged by HCV RNA testing performed by PCR.[68] Although numbers are small it is apparent that in some cases there is more rapidly progressive liver disease with development of cirrhosis after 3–5 years.

Assessment of patients for treatment should probably be performed in specialist hepatology centres with consideration to possible infected partners, appraisal of carriers' general health for the suitability of treatment and clear endpoints decided upon with access to molecular biological techniques. Because of the protracted natural history of the disease much longer follow-up is necessary to determine if the risk of cirrhosis and hepatocellular carcinoma are reduced in those responsive to treatment.

Autoimmune hepatitis

Recent proposals from an international group of hepatologists recommend replacing the term Autoimmune Chronic Active Hepatitis with the term Autoimmune Hepatitis (AIH).[69] This has been deemed to be more appropriate because the term autoimmune itself implies chronicity and it is not necessary to fulfil the clinical criteria of symptoms or abnormal liver function persisting for more than 6 months. Because so many of these cases are responsive to steroids it would seem inappropriate, if not unethical, to delay starting treatment until this particular diagnostic criteria were met. Further, there may be absence of an interface hepatitis that warrants the diagnosis of CAH, either because of treatment or because of spontaneous fluctuations in disease activity. This nomenclature is in step with current trends on classifying chronic hepatitis as discussed above.

AIH is characterized by the presence of circulating autoantibodies, and as an autoimmune disease is more prevalent in females although also affects males and may be associated with other autoimmune manifestations. The pathogenesis is unknown; the antibodies present within the serum do not appear to be pathogenic. Possibly there is a genetic predisposition and initial triggering by viral infection. Problems in diagnosis may be encountered in that inducement of autoantibodies may occur following viral hepatitis and even drug-induced injury and that there may be complicating factors of high alcohol intake, drugs or even viruses present. Helpful clues to the diagnosis is the presence of autoantibodies and also hyperglobulinaemia, which is almost universally present. This particular form of liver injury is responsive to steroid therapy in 60–80% of patients although many require long-term maintenance.[70] Azathioprine can be used to lower the side-effects of steroids.

The diagnosis of AIH is based on a 3–10-fold increase in serum aminotransferases, high titres of anti-nuclear smooth muscle or liver-kidney microsomal antibodies, and an absence of other aetiological agents. The significance of the titres of antibodies is dependent upon age, being > 1:80 for adults but only 1:20 for children. However, problems may arise not least because there can be a great range in sympotology from near-fulminant presentations to asymptomatic and ill-defined onsets reflected in enzyme elevations, which may be minimal or massive. Up to 20% of patients lack seropositivity for antibodies at presentation. Children usually show lower titres of antibodies and there is an overlap with primary sclerosing cholangitis, which may need resolving with cholangiography.[71]

A diagnosis of 'probable AIH' (rather than definite) can be made when there is mild disease, lack of conventional autoantibodies or complicating aetiological factors. Such cases warrant a trial of steroid therapy.[69] The evaluation of response to treatment includes symptom control, normalization of liver enzymes and lack of necroinflammatory activity on liver histology.

The histopathology of AIH may show variation, although severe necroinflammation is seen frequently at presentation. Plasma cells are often

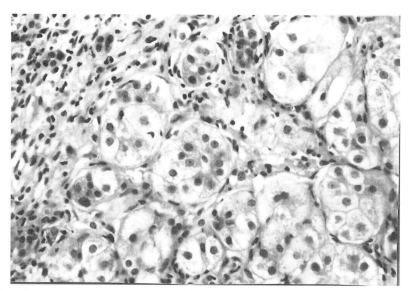

Fig. 5.5 Rosetting of periportal hepatocytes can be particularly prominent in interface hepatitis associated with autoimmune hepatitis.

prominent within the infiltrate together with interface hepatitis associated with obvious rosetting of hepatocytes (Fig. 5.5). Lobular activity may be florid with even cholestasis present. Multinucleate hepatocytes may be present in up to 30% of cases.[58]

Subtypes

Different subgroups of AIH can be identified depending on their autoantibody profile.[70] Classically described autoimmune chronic active hepatitis – also previously known as lupoid hepatitis, active chronic hepatitis and plasma cell hepatitis – is type 1. This is characterized by serum anti-nuclear (ANA) and/or smooth muscle actin (SMA) antibodies. Other antibodies may be present; soluble liver antigens (SLA) in up to 10% of patients, liver specific asialoglycoprotein receptor (also known as hepatic lectin; ASGP-R), neutrophil cytoplasm (ANCA) and others.[69,70]

Patients with type 2 AIH have anti-liver/kidney microsomal (ALKM-1) antibodies and are frequently children. This antibody reacts against cytochrome p450IIDb. Commonly, anti-liver cytosol (ALC) antibody is also present and, in some cases, may be the only identifying antibody. ALKM-1 has also been identified in about 5% of adults who are positive for HCV[50] and this infection seems to account for half of this type of AIH, being separately classified as type 2b. This may be related to the fact that part of the viral core region has an epitope identical to cytochrome p450IIDb. Chronic hepatitis D viral infection has been associated with AKLM-3 production and AKLM-2 with hepatitis induced by the drug ticrynafen.

Although this array of antibodies is of considerable interest there is still no direct link to pathogenesis or of differing aetiologies. At present it is probably unnecessary to subdivide them for diagnostic reasons as different therapeutic regimens are not considered and some subgroups are very small. More practically, the availability of testing other than for ANA, SMA and LKM1 is far from routinely available.

Overlap

A small subgroup of patients with anti-nuclear and smooth muscle antibodies normally consistant with AIH show histological features far more in keeping with primary biliary cirrhosis.[72] This includes heavy portal infiltrate centred on bile ducts which become attenuated. Portal granulomas are not seen but mild to moderate interface hepatitis is present. The aspartate aminotransferase (AST), ALT and alkaline phosphatase levels are all raised. Anti-mitochondrial antibodies, including the highly specific marker of PBC, anti-M2, are negative. This clinicopathological entity has been recognized as an autoimmune syndrome[73] and various names proposed including autoimmune cholangiopathy[74] The importance in recognizing this condition is the favourable response, biochemically and histologically, to steroid therapy.

Another small minority of patients who are anti-mitochondrial antibody positive have, on histological examination of their liver, very florid interface hepatitis and minimal evidence of biliary damage. These also represent an overlap syndrome and, again, may show steroid responsiveness. A similar small group of patients with a mixed hepatitic and cholangitic histology have positive findings for AIH and primary sclerosing cholangitis.[75]

Drug associated chronic hepatitis

Although adverse drug reactions may be manifest by any pattern of hepatopathology, including neoplasia, a picture of chronic hepatitis is rare.[76] The diagnosis may be difficult to establish and full clinical history including the use of non-proprietary compounds necessary. No specific tests are available but prompt resolution of clinical, biochemical and histological parameters are usual after withdrawal of the offending drug.

Histologically, portal inflammation with interface necrosis, fibrosis and even cirrhosis can be seen.[76,77] Occasionally eosinophils are present within the infiltrate and granulomas may also be present; on other occasions features typical of AIH including numerous plasma cells are seen. Progressive lesions are not seen after cessation of the drug. Oxyphenisatin, a laxative and now withdrawn from the market was an early recognized agent and associated with long-term use. Other drugs implicated include alpha-methyl dopa, nitrofurantoin, dantrolene, isoniazid, propylthiouracil, etretinate and sulphonamides.

Key points for clinical practice

- Modern molecular biological techniques have greatly advanced the understanding of the hepatitis viruses.
- Of great importance has been the identification of HCV as the main agent responsible for most cases of NANB hepatitis.
- HEV has been found to be responsible for endemic NANB disease in the developing world.
- Other causes of chronic NANB hepatitis are being identified, including HGV, although causes of acute liver failure remain more elusive.
- The natural history of HCV infection is only slowly emerging; acute infection leads to chronic infection in the majority with a definite but low risk of cirrhosis and hepatocellular carcinoma, albeit after a considerable time.
- Mutant forms of hepatitis B virus are emerging, which may have relevance to treatment and vaccination.
- The reporting of liver histology in patients with chronic hepatitis has been recently reassessed and change is recommended. The bottom line diagnosis should include aetiology, the grade of necroinflammatory activity and the stage of architectural distortion. Scoring systems may be appropriate in certain circumstances. Without the full clinical and serological information the histopathology may, on occasion, show features suggestive of the aetiological agent.

Acknowledgements

I wish to thank Professor P J Scheuer for helpful criticism and discussion in the preparation of this manuscript, and to Mr F Moll for technical assistance.

REFERENCES

1 Scheuer PJ. Classification of chronic viral hepatitis: a need for reassessment. J Hepatol 1991; 13: 372–374
2 Gerber MA. Chronic hepatitis C: the beginning of the end of a time-honored nomenclature? Hepatology 1992; 15: 733–734
3 Ludwig J. The nomenclature of chronic active hepatitis: an obituary. Gastroenterology 1993; 105: 274–278
4 Schmid M, Flury R, Buhler H, et al Chronic viral hepatitis B and C: an argument against the conventional classification of chronic hepatitis. Virchows Archiv 1994; 425: 221–228
5 Desmet VJ, Gerber M, Hoofnagle JH, et al Classification of chronic hepatitis: diagnosis, grading and staging. Hepatology 1994; 19: 1513–1520
6 Knodell RG, Ishak KG, Black WC, et al Formulation and application of a numerical scoring system for assessing histological activity in asymptomatic chronic active hepatitis. Hepatology 1981; 1: 431–435
7 Metavir study group. Intraobserver and interobserver variations in liver biopsy interpretation in patients with chronic hepatitis C. Hepatology 1994; 20: 15–20

8　Sheuer PJ. The nomenclature of chronic hepatitis: time for a change. J Hepatol 1995; 22: 112–114

9　Bianchi L, Gudat F. Chronic hepatitis. In: MacSween RNM, Anthony PP, Scheuer PJ, Burt AD, Portmann BC, eds. Pathology of the liver. Edinburgh: Churchill Livingstone, 1994: pp 349–395

10　Ishak K, Baptista A, Bianchi L, et al Histological grading and staging of chronic hepatitis. J Hepatol 1995; 22: 696–699

11　Hytiroglou P, Thung SN, Gerber MA. Histological classification and quantitation of the severity of chronic hepatitis: keep it simple. Semin Liver Dis 1995; 15: 414–421

12　Dusheiko GM. Rolling review – the pathogenesis, diagnosis and management of viral hepatitis. Aliment Pharmacol Ther 1994; 8: 229–253

13　Teixeira MR Jr, Weller IVD, Murray A, et al The pathology of hepatitis A in man. Liver 1982; 2: 53–60

14　Scharschmidt BF. Hepatitis E: a virus in waiting. Lancet 1995; 346: 519–520

15　Skidmore S. Hepatitis E. Br Med J 1995; 310: 414–415

16　Reyes GR, Purdy MA, Kim JP. Isolation of a cDNA from the virus responsible for enterically transmitted non-A, non-B hepatitis. Science 1990; 24: 1335–1339

17　Scheuer PJ. Acute hepatitis. In: DGD Wight, ed. Systemic Pathology Vol 11 Liver, biliary tract and exocrine pancreas. Edinburgh: Churchill Livingstone 1994; pp 53–70

18　Uchida T, Shimojima S, Gotoh K, et al Pathology of livers infected with 'silent' hepatitis B virus mutant. Liver 1994; 14: 251–256

19　Fagan EA, Ellis DS, Tovey GM, et al Toga virus-like particles in acute liver failure attributed to sporadic non-A non-B hepatitis and recurrence after liver transplantation. J Med Virol 1992; 38: 71–77

20　Fagan EA. Acute liver failure of unknown pathogenesis: the hidden agenda. Hepatology 1994; 19: 1307–1312

21　Lee WM. Acute liver failure. Am J Med 1994; 96: 3S–9S

22　Simons JN, Leary TP, Dawson GJ, et al Isolation of novel virus-like sequences associated with human hepatitis. Nature Med 1995; 1: 564–569

23　Schlauder GG, Dawson GJ, Simons JN, et al Molecular and serologic analysis in the transmission of the GB hepatitis agents. J Med Virol 1995; 46: 81–90

24　Simons JN, Pilot-Matias TJ, Leary TP, et al Identification of two flavivirus-like genomes in the GB hepatitis agent. Proc Natl Acad Sci 1995; 92: 3401–3405

25　Linnen J, Wages Jr J, Zhang-Keck Z-Y, et al Molecular cloning and disease association of hepatitis G virus: a transfusion transmissable agent. Science 1996; 271: 505–506

26　Phillips MJ, Blendis LM, Poucell S, et al Syncitial giant-cell hepatitis: sporadic hepatitis with distinctive pathological features, a severe clinical course, and paramyxoviral features. N Engl J Med 1991; 324: 455–460

27　Naoumov NV, Eddleston ALWF. Host immune response and variations in the virus genome: pathogenesis of liver damage caused by hepatitis B virus. Gut 1994; 35: 1013–1017

28　Lau JYN, Wright TL. Molecular virology and pathogenesis of hepatitis B. Lancet 1993; 342: 1335–1340

29　Foster GR, Thomas HC. Recent advances in the molecular biology of hepatitis B virus: mutant virus and the host response. Gut 1993; 34: 1–3

30　Wright TL, Lau JYN. Clinical aspects of hepatitis B virus infection. Lancet 1993; 342: 1340–1344

31　Boxall EH. Antenatal screening for carriers of hepatitis B virus. Br Med J 1995; 311: 1178–1179

32　Tabor E. Strongly supported features of the association between hepatitis B virus and hepatocellular carcinoma. In: Tabor E, Di Bisceglie AM, Purcell RH, eds. Etiology, pathology, and treatment of hepatocellular carcinoma in North America. Houston: Gulf publishing, 1991: pp 107–118

33　McNair ANB, Main J, Thomas HC. Interactions of the human immunodeficiency virus and the hepatotropic viruses. Semin Liver Dis 1992; 12: 188–196

34   Perrillo RP. The management of chronic hepatitis B. Am J Med 1994; 96: 34S–40S

35   Dienstag JL, Perrillo RP, Schiff ER, et al A preliminary trial of lamivudine for chronic hepatitis B infection. N Engl J Med 1995; 333: 1657–1661

36   Davies SE, Portmann BC, O'Grady JG, et al Hepatic histological findings after transplantation for chronic hepatitis B virus infection including a unique pattern of fibrosing cholestatic hepatitis. Hepatology 1991; 13: 150–157

37   Davies SE, Lau JYN, O'Grady JG, et al Evidence that hepatitis D virus needs hepatitis B virus to cause hepatocellular damage. Am J Clin Pathol 1992; 98: 554–558

38   Choo QL, Kuo G, Weiner AJ, et al Isolation of a cDNA clone derived from a blood-borne non-A non-B viral hepatitis genome. Science 1989; 244: 359–362

39   Mansell CJ, Locarnini SA. Epidemiology of hepatitis C in the east. Semin Liver Dis 1995; 15: 15–32

40   McFarlane IG, Smith HM, Johnson PJ, et al Hepatitis C virus antibodies in chronic active hepatitis: pathogenetic factor or false-positive result? Lancet 1990; 335: 754–757

41   Bukh J, Miller RH, Purcell RH. Genetic heterogeneity of hepatitis C virus: quasispecies and genotypes Semin Liver Dis 1995; 15: 41–63

42   Alter HJ, Purcell RH, Shih JW, et al Detection of antibody to hepatitis C virus in prospectively followed transfusion recipients with acute and chronic non-A non-B hepatitis. N Engl J Med 1989; 321: 1494–1500

43   Alter MJ. Epidemiology of hepatitis C in the west. Semin Liver Dis 1995; 15: 5–13

44   Dow BC, Coote I, Munro H, et al Confirmation of hepatitis C virus antibody in blood donors. J Med Virol 1993; 41: 215–220

45   Tremolada F, Casarin C, Alberti A, et al Long-term follow-up of non-A non-B (type C) post-transfusion hepatitis. J Hepatol 1992; 16: 273–281

46   Seeff LB, Buskell-Bales Z, Wright EC, et al Long-term mortality after transfusion-associated non-A non-B hepatitis. N Engl J Med 1992; 327: 1906–1911

47   Alberti A, Morsica G, Chemello L, et al Hepatitis C viraemia and liver disease in symptom-free individuals with anti-HCV. Lancet 1992; 340: 697–698

48   Okuda K. Hepatitis C virus and hepatocellular carcinoma. In: Tabor E, Di Bisceglie AM, Purcell RH, eds. Etiology, pathology, and treatment of hepatocellular carcinoma in North America. Houston, Gulf publishing, 1991: pp 119–126

49   Booth JCL, Brown JL, Thomas HC. The management of chronic hepatitis C virus infection. Gut 1995; 37: 449–454

50   Koff RS, Dienstag JL. Extrahepatic manifestations of hepatitis C and the association with alcoholic liver disease. Semin Liver Dis 1995; 15: 101–109

51   Pares A, Barrera JM, Caballeria J, et al Hepatitis C virus in chronic alcoholic patients: association with severity of liver injury. Hepatology 1990; 12: 1295–1299

52   Dhillon AP. Histopathology of hepatitis C and haemophilia. Haemophilia 1995; 1: 19–24

53   Jilg W, Sieger E, Zachoval R, Schatzl H. Individuals with antibodies against hepatitis B core antigen as the only serological marker for hepatitis B infection: high percentage of carriers of hepatitis B and C virus. J Hepatol 1995; 23: 14–20

54   Benvegnu L, Fattovich G, Noventa F, et al Concurrent hepatitis B and C virus infection and risk of hepatocellular carcinoma in cirrhosis – a prospective study. Cancer 1994; 74: 2442–2448

55   Pawlotsky J-M, Ben Yahia M, Andre C, et al Immunological disorders in C virus chronic active hepatitis; a prospective case-control study. Hepatology 1994; 19: 841–848

56   Dhillon AP, Dusheiko GM. Pathology of hepatitis C virus infection. Histopathology 1995; 26: 297–309

57   Scheuer PJ, Ashrafzadeh P, Sherlock S, et al The pathology of hepatitis C. Hepatology 1992; 15: 567–571

58   Bach N, Thung SN, Schaffner F. The histological features of chronic hepatitis C and autoimmune chronic hepatitis: a comparative analysis. Hepatology 1992; 15: 572–577

59   Gerber MA, Krawczynski K, Alter MJ et al Histopathology of community acquired chronic hepatitis C Modern Pathol 1992; 5: 483–486

60   Kaji K, Nakanuma Y, Sasaki M, et al Hepatic bile duct injuries in chronic hepatitis C:

histopathologic and immunohistochemical studies. Modern Pathol 1994; 7: 937–945

61 Okuno T, Arai K, Matsumoto M, Shindo M. Epithelioid granulomas in chronic hepatitis C: a transient pathological feature. J Gastroenterol Hepatol 1995; 10: 532–537

62 Emile JF, Sebagh M, Feray C, et al The presence of epithelioid granulomas in hepatitis C virus-related cirrhosis. Hum Pathol 1993; 24: 1095–1097

63 Attah EB. The presence of epithelioid granulomas in hepatitis c virus-related cirrhosis. Hum Pathol 195; 26: 463–464

64 Terrault N, Wright T. Interferon and hepatitis C. N Engl J Med 1995; 332: 1509–1511

65 Dusheiko GM, Khakoo S, Soni P, Grellier L. A rational approach to the management of hepatitis C infection. Br Med J 1996; 312: 357–364

66 Davis G. Interferon treatment of chronic hepatitis C. Am J Med 1994; 96: 41S–46S

67 Barton AL, Banner BF, Cable EE, Bonkovsky HL. Distribution of iron in the liver predicts the response of chronic hepatitis C infection to interferon therapy. Am J Clin Pathol 1995; 103: 419–424

68 Sallie R, Cohen AT, Tibbs CJ, et al Recurrence of hepatitis C following orthotopic liver transplantation: a polymerase chain reaction and histological study. J Hepatol 1994; 21: 536–542

69 Johnson PJ, McFarlane IG. Meeting Report: international autoimmune hepatitis group. Hepatology 1993; 18: 998–1005

70 Krawitt El. Autoimmune hepatitis: classification, heterogeneity and treatment. Am J Med 1994; 96: 23S–26S

71 Mieli-Vergani G, Lobo-Yeo A, McFarlane BM, et al Different immune mechanisms leading to autoimmunity in primary sclerosing cholangitis and autoimmune chronic active hepatitis of childhood. Hepatology 1989; 9: 198–203

72 Brunner G, Klinge O. A cholangitis with anti-nuclear antibodies (immunocholangitis) resembling chronic non-suppurative destructive cholangitis. Deutsche Med Wochenschr 1987; 112: 1454–1458

73 Goodman ZD, McNally PR, Davis DR, Ishak KG. Autoimmune cholangitis: a variant of primary biliary cirrhosis. Clinicopathologic and serologic correlations in 200 cases. Dig Dis Sci 1995; 40: 1232–1242

74 Ben-Ari Z, Dhillon AP, Sherlock S. Autoimmune cholangiopathy: part of the spectrum of autoimmune chronic active hepatitis. Hepatology 1993; 18: 10–15

75 Wurbs D, Klein R, Terracciano LM, et al A 28-year-old woman with a combined hepatitic/cholestatic syndrome. Hepatology 1995; 22: 1598–1605

76 Davies SE, Portmann BC. Drugs and toxins. In: DGD Wight, ed. Systemic Pathology Vol 11 Liver, biliary tract and exocrine pancreas. Edinburgh: Churchill Livingstone, 1994: pp 201–236

77 Zimmerman HJ, Ishak KG. Hepatic injury due to drugs and toxins. In: MacSween RNM, Anthony PP, Scheuer PJ, Burt AD Portmann BC, eds. Pathology of the liver. Edinburgh: Churchill Livingstone, 1994: pp 568–593

6

Trophoblastic disease

H. Fox

The term 'gestational trophoblastic disease' is, by convention, restricted to hydatidiform moles, choriocarcinoma and placental site trophoblastic tumour. These are all defined in purely morphological terms but any classification of trophoblastic disease also includes one non-morphological component, namely 'persistent trophoblastic disease'; this term is applied to a biochemical abnormality, i.e. an elevated level of human chorionic gonadotrophin (hCG) following a molar pregnancy, and this diagnosis not only lacks any specific morphological connotation but becomes invalid if a morphological diagnosis is achieved.

The term 'gestational trophoblastic neoplasia' is sometimes used as an alternative to gestational trophoblastic disease and indeed many seem to feel, often at a subliminal level, that these various conditions represent a neoplastic spectrum, with moles at the benign end of this spectrum, choriocarcinoma at the malignant extreme and invasive hydatidiform mole being equivalent to a neoplasm of borderline malignancy. This is a totally misleading approach for there is nothing to suggest that a hydatidiform mole, of any type, is a form of neoplasia; it is, without question, a specific form of abortion. A choriocarcinoma is usually considered to be neoplastic but, as will be discussed later, even this may be no more than an unusual type of abortus in some cases and the only undoubtedly neoplastic entity within this group of conditions is the placental site trophoblastic tumour.

Hydatidiform moles

During the last few decades molar disease has been divided into complete and partial hydatidiform moles, the distinction between these two entities being based originally on their differing morphological features.[1,2]

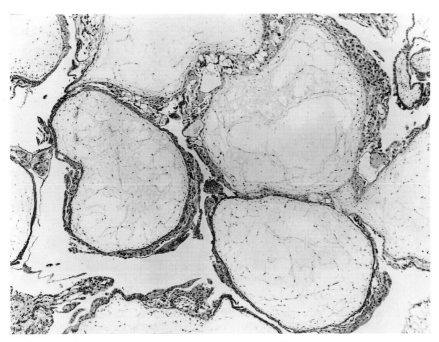

Fig. 6.1 Histological appearances of a complete hydatidiform mole. There is marked villous swelling, central cistern formation and an abnormal pattern of trophoblastic growth. (Reproduced with permission from: Elston CW. Gestational trophoblastic disease. In: Fox H, ed. Haines and Taylor, Obstetrical and gynaecological pathology, 3rd edn. Edinburgh: Churchill Livingstone, 1987.)

Morphology

Classically, a complete mole is characterized by diffuse vesicular change which involves, to a greater or lesser degree, the entire villous population, thus producing the classical 'bunch of grapes' appearance; the mass of villous tissue is increased markedly, to an extent that an in situ mole can fill or even distend the uterus, no remnant of a normal placental shape is discernible and neither a fetus nor a gestational sac is present. Histological examination confirms that all the villi are avascular, swollen and oedematous, some very markedly so but others only minimally (Fig. 6.1); central cistern formation is common. It is usually maintained that trophoblastic hyperplasia is a characteristic feature of a complete mole but, in reality, the degree of trophoblastic proliferation in such lesions is often no greater, and sometimes less, than that seen in the normal first trimester placenta. It is the pattern, rather than the degree, of trophoblastic proliferation that is abnormal in a complete mole; whilst in a normal pregnancy trophoblast proliferates along one side or at one pole of a villus, in a complete mole the villous trophoblastic proliferation is either circumferential or multifocal. A moderate degree of nuclear atypia is commonly present in molar trophoblast although

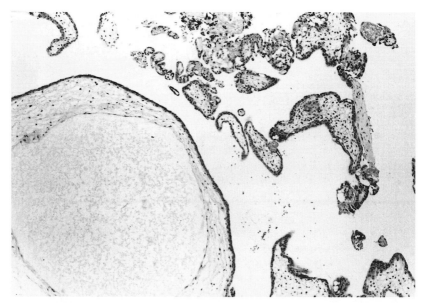

Fig. 6.2 Histological appearances of a partial hydatidiform mole. One villus is markedly vesicular whilst adjacent villi are of normal size. (Reproduced with permission from: Fox H. Obstetrical pathology. In: Anderson MC, ed. Systemic pathology, 3rd edn. Volume 6 Female reproductive tract. Edinburgh: Churchill Livingstone, 1991.)

this is often no more marked than that seen in the trophoblast of placentas from normal first trimester pregnancies. Because of the use of ultrasound, anembryonic gestations and hence molar pregnancies are now being diagnosed at an earlier stage of gestation than in the past. In these early lesions the classical gross appearances of a complete mole will not be apparent and only a proportion of the villi may show vesicular change; indeed in very early complete moles there may be no vesicular change and it is suggested that in such cases the presence of branching villi with small sprouts and a polypoid or lobulated appearance on cross-section are typical.[3] Stromal blood vessels and fetal red cells may be present in these very early moles and even in the absence of overt vessels endothelial cells may be visualized with a stain for Factor VIII.

A partial mole differs in numerous respects from a complete mole: it is commonly associated with a fetus, retains a placental shape and does not have a greatly increased villous mass. Only a proportion of the villi show macroscopically visible vesicular change, these being scattered within normal placental tissue. Histologically the presence of both oedematous swollen villi and vascularized villi of normal size, albeit often with an unusually fibrotic or cellular stroma, is confirmed (Fig. 6.2). The vesicular villi commonly have a very irregular, scalloped outline, this resulting in the 'Norwegian fjord' appearance: cutting of some of these deep indentations in cross-section results in the presence of so-called 'trophoblastic inclusions' within the villous stroma. There is abnormal trophoblastic proliferation, this, as with complete moles, usually being either circumferential or multi-focal; the degree of trophoblastic proliferation is usually not only less than that seen in complete moles but is less than that encountered in normal first trimester placentas. The villous trophoblast frequently has a somewhat vac-uolated, or 'lacy', appearance. It is often maintained that partial moles are characterized by 'syncytiotrophoblastic hyperplasia' but it is, of course, quite impossible for the villous syncytiotrophoblast to be hyperplastic for this is a post-mitotic, terminally differentiated tissue, which is incapable of DNA synthesis and cell division. In some partial moles an angiomatoid appear-ance is seen.

It should be noted that the use of the word 'partial' to describe a mole does not mean that one portion of the placenta is normal and another por-tion molar. This latter situation is encountered if a complete mole, or very much less frequently a partial mole, is part of a dizygotic twin pregnancy and associated with a normal twin;[4] in such pregnancies one placenta is molar and the other non-molar whilst in a true partial mole there is an intermingling of molar and non-molar villi with the molar villi distributed throughout the entire placenta.

Cytogenetics

It has been recognized for some time that complete moles are androgenetic, i.e. all their nuclear DNA is paternally derived: furthermore, approximately 95% of complete moles have a 46XX chromosomal constitution, the remainder having a 46XY karyotype. Banding studies have shown that the vast majority of 46XX complete moles are derived from a single sperm (monospermic or homozygous moles) whilst all 46XY moles and a small minority of 46XX moles are derived from two sperms (dispermic or het-erozygous moles).[5] A hypothetical model has been proposed to explain these findings, namely that homozygous moles are caused by fertilization of a 'dead' ovum (i.e. one containing no viable genomic material) by a single haploid sperm, which then undergoes endoreduplication of its genetic material without cell division, and that heterozygous moles result from entry into a 'dead' ovum of two haploid sperms, which then fuse and repli-cate. It has to be stressed that this concept is purely theoretical and that the mechanism of the loss of the maternal genome is unknown: there may be a primary loss of the genome or maternal chromosomes may be excluded in the cell divisions following fertilization. That fertilization has actually occurred in molar gestations is certain, for the mitochondrial DNA is of maternal origin.

Partial moles contain both paternal and maternal genomic material and the vast majority are chromosomally triploid, usually 69XXY but some-times 69XXX or 69XYY. It is, of course, known that not all triploid gesta-tions are associated with molar change in the placenta and it is now clear that if the extra chromosomal load is of paternal origin a partial mole will result, whilst if the extra chromosomal content is contributed from the mother a non-molar placenta will develop.[6] It is thought that paternally derived triploidy is usually the result of two haploid sperms fertilizing a haploid ovum but that a few cases may be caused by fertilization of a haploid ovum by a diploid 46XX sperm.

This relatively simple subdivision into androgenetic diploid complete moles and biparentally derived triploid partial moles is not, however, the whole story. Cytogenetic studies have yielded a few instances of triploid and tetraploid complete moles and of diploid and tetraploid partial moles.[7] Furthermore, flow cytometric studies, whilst in general confirming that most complete moles are diploid and most partial moles triploid, have nevertheless rather consistently revealed small subpopulations of diploid partial moles and triploid complete moles.[8] To complicate the matter still further there have been very occasional instances of androgenetic partial moles and biparentally derived complete moles,[7] entities for which there is, at the moment, no very plausible explanation.

It should be noted that these anomalies have been detected in moles for which a rigorous morphological diagnosis had been made. Triploid complete moles may well be caused by three haploid sperms entering a 'dead' ovum but many of the reported diploid partial moles have, in reality, been examples of a complete mole with an accompanying concomitant non-molar twin pregnancy; nevertheless, a distinct entity of diploid partial mole does exist which, it has been suggested, merits consideration as a separate third type of molar pregnancy, such cases possibly being a result of uniparental disomy or of malfunction in the maintenance of imprinting.[9]

Studies of mice models[10] have indicated that paternal genes play a dominant role in placental development whilst maternal genes have a major role in fetal development, this being the result of genomic imprinting. This concept would be in accord with the cytogenetic findings in complete moles which, with their double content of paternal alleles might express a double dose of genes such as *IGF2*, which is genomically imprinted to the paternal copy. However, the maternally imprinted gene *H19* is also expressed in complete moles[11] and this suggests that imprinting is lost, possibly because the imprinting process may require a biparental genome.

Histological diagnosis

Pathologists can usually diagnose well established complete hydatidiform moles with some degree of accuracy although whether this applies also to very early complete moles must be in some doubt. Their ability to distinguish between a partial hydatidiform mole and a hydropic abortion is, however, rather poor, there being considerable interobserver variation.[12] In making this distinction emphasis has to be placed on the circumferential or multifocal, rather than polar, pattern of trophoblastic proliferation that characterizes a mole: in truly doubtful cases flow or static cytometry is of considerable value in establishing the correct diagnosis.[8,13]

Postmolar disease

In the UK about 8% of patients who have had a complete mole will develop persistent trophoblastic disease: the figure in the USA is rather higher because of the use of different diagnostic criteria. The actual cause of persistent trophoblastic disease is generally unknown: there may have been incomplete removal of the mole but it is equally possible that many of these cases are invasive hydatidiform moles with residual invasive molar tissue within the myometrium or its vasculature; it is also possible that some are early cases of choriocarcinoma. It is thought that the risk of development of a clinically overt choriocarcinoma following a complete mole is less than 5%.

The incidence of persistent trophoblastic disease following a partial mole has been much disputed but there is now no doubt that it occurs although the magnitude of the risk is very much lower than is that for complete moles. The eventual risk of choriocarcinoma in patients with partial moles is also unknown: choriocarcinomas have been reported following partial moles but this, in itself, does not necessarily mean that this condition increases the risk of a choriocarcinoma for this can follow a normal pregnancy.

Prognostic factors

As it is widely agreed that all women who have had a molar pregnancy should enter a follow-up surveillance programme, there is therefore no practical point in attempting to define those cases at most risk of developing post-molar disease. Nevertheless, from a purely theoretical viewpoint it is of interest to consider if a high-risk group can be defined. It was at one time considered that the risk of eventual post-molar disease was related directly to the degree of trophoblastic proliferation in the mole but this has proved not to be the case[14] and grading of moles in terms of their degree of trophoblastic proliferation has now been abandoned. Attempts to identify those cases at greatest risk for post-molar disease by the use of cell proliferation markers, the expression of proto-oncogenes such as c-erb-B2 and flow cytometry[15–17] have failed but it has been maintained that heterozygous (dispermic) moles have a much higher risk of subsequent post-molar complications than do homozygous (monospermic) moles:[18] doubts have, however, been cast upon this claim by the failure to find any association between the presence of a Y chromosome, detected by the polymerase chain reaction or by chromosome in situ hybridization, in a mole and an excess incidence of post-molar disease.[19,20]

Invasive hydatidiform mole

An invasive hydatidiform mole is one that penetrates into the myometrium or invades the uterine vasculature (Fig. 6.3). A deeply invasive mole usually becomes clinically evident several weeks after apparently

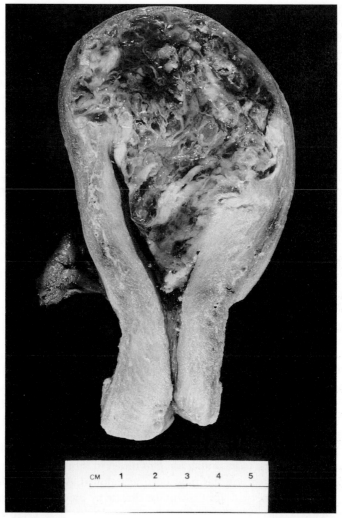

Fig. 6.3 Invasive hydatidiform mole. The uterus is occupied by a hydatidiform mole that is invading deeply into the myometrium. At one point the mole infiltrates almost to the serosa. (Courtesy of Professor D O'B Hourihane, Dublin, and reproduced with permission from: Fox H, Buckley CH. Pathology of gestational trophoblastic disease. In: Blackledge GRP, Jordan JA, Shingleton HM, eds. Textbook of gynecologic oncology. London: Saunders, 1991.)

complete evacuation of a mole from the uterus, the patient usually presenting with hemorrhage. If a hysterectomy is performed at this stage the appearances range from at one extreme, only a small haemorrhagic focus in the myometrium to, at the other end of the spectrum, a large deeply cavitating haemorrhagic lesion of the uterine wall (Fig. 6.4), which mimics a choriocarcinoma: rarely, a mole penetrates the full thickness of the myometrium, this leading either to uterine perforation or to extension of the mole into adjacent structures, such as the broad ligament. The histological distinction from a choriocarcinoma is dependent upon the finding of molar villi within the uterine wall, these more commonly being seen in the myometrial vascular channels than between the myometrial fibres: the molar villi show a very variable degree of trophoblastic proliferation and sometimes this is far from being a conspicuous feature.

Invasive moles have, in the past, caused death from uterine bleeding or perforation but their mortality rate is now virtually zero because of the success achieved in their treatment by a limited course of chemotherapy. In fact the diagnosis of an invasive mole, which can only be made with certainty on a hysterectomy specimen, is now almost obsolete because nearly all invasive moles are subsumed into the category of persistent trophoblastic disease.

It has to be stressed that the invasive capacity of some moles is not an indication that they are neoplastic. Normal trophoblast has the ability to invade both the myometrium and the uterine vessels whilst villi from a normal placenta can invade deeply into, or even through, the uterine wall to give rise to a placenta increta or a placenta percreta, both of which are the exact non-molar equivalents of an invasive mole.

Molar tissue can be transported via the bloodstream to extrauterine sites, particularly to the vagina and lungs: the transported molar trophoblast can then grow in these sites to form nodules that are either clinically or radiologically detectable. The development of 'metastatic' lesions implies that molar trophoblast has entered the uterine vessels and hence their presence is taken as *de facto* evidence of the presence of an invasive mole; the 'metastatic' nodules are not, however, usually associated with evidence of molar invasion of the myometrial tissues.

The 'metastatic' nodules commonly appear several weeks after evacuation of a mole from the uterus but may occur concurrently with a mole or can be the presenting symptom of such a lesion. Vaginal lesions form haemorrhagic submucous nodules; histologically, these often contain villous structures, a finding that rules out a diagnosis of choriocarcinoma. Even if villi are not present in a post-molar vaginal lesion and the mass is formed of biphasic trophoblast, a diagnosis of choriocarcinoma is not warranted if the trophoblast is not invading normal tissues: following a non-molar pregnancy the diagnosis of a lesion such as this would be choriocarcinoma even in the absence of tissue invasion. Pulmonary lesions can cause haemoptysis but are usually an asymptomatic radiological finding: histological examination of these will also usually reveal the presence of villi. These extrauterine lesions may resolve spontaneously but are commonly treated with limited chemotherapy, which achieves excellent results.

The fact that molar trophoblast is transported to extrauterine sites is not an indication of neoplastic behaviour. Trophoblast enters the maternal bloodstream in every normal pregnancy[21] and is transported to sites such as the lung;[22] this transported trophoblast only gives rise to detectable lesions if it is molar in nature.

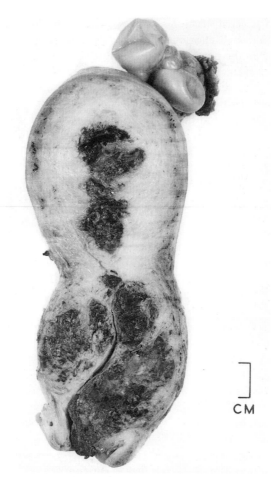

CM

Fig. 6.4 Uterus containing a choriocarcinoma. This is forming multiple haemorrhagic nodules, those in the cervix probably being metastases. (Reproduced with permission from: Elston CW. Trophoblastic tumours of the placenta. In: Fox H. Pathology of the placenta. London: Saunders, 1978.)

Choriocarcinoma

Approximately 50% of choriocarcinomas follow a molar pregnancy, 30% occur after an abortion and 20% follow an apparently normal gestation. The time interval between the antecedent pregnancy and the clinical presentation of a choriocarcinoma is very variable, ranging from a few weeks or months to 15 years.

Morphology

Within the uterus a choriocarcinoma forms single or multiple haemorrhagic nodules, which are often accompanied by local metastasis to the

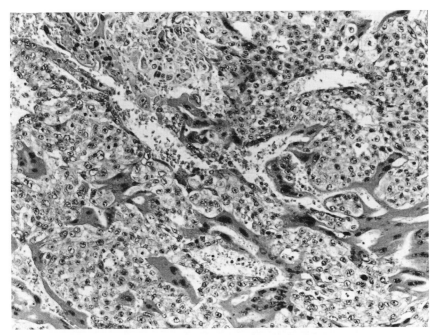

Fig. 6.5 Histological appearances of a choriocarcinoma. This shows a bimorphic pattern of cytotrophoblast and syncytiotrophoblast, which are showing a regular and orderly relationship with each other. (Reproduced with permission from: Elston CW. Gestational trophoblastic disease. In: Fox H, ed. Haines and Taylor, Obstetrical and gynaecological pathology, 3rd edn. Edinburgh: Churchill Livingstone, 1987.)

cervix and vagina (Fig. 6.4). The neoplastic masses consist of a central area of haemorrhagic necrosis and, usually, although not invariably, a peripheral rim of viable tumour tissue. The central, sometimes complete, necrosis of the neoplastic tissue is a reflection of the fact that a choriocarcinoma has no intrinsic blood supply, relying for oxygenation on its ability to invade the uterine blood vessels: it is therefore only the growing edge of the tumour that is oxygenated adequately, the remainder undergoing ischaemic necrosis.

Histologically, a choriocarcinoma typically has a biphasic structure that recapitulates, often to a striking degree, that of the trophoblast of the normal implanting blastocyst, central sheets or cores of cytotrophoblast being 'capped' by a peripheral rim of syncytiotrophoblast (Fig. 6.5). The trophoblastic cells in a choriocarcinoma commonly show no greater degree of atypia and mitotic activity than is seen in an implanting blastocyst. Villi are never present in an extraplacental choriocarcinoma and, indeed, the presence of villous structures negates a diagnosis of choriocarcinoma. Although a biphasic structure is characteristic of choriocarcinoma, a monophasic variant, composed solely of cytotrophoblast, has been described anecdotally.

Because of the need to obtain an oxygen supply, a choriocarcinoma is avariciously invasive of vascular channels in the myometrium, vessels which, it should be noted, are also invaded by trophoblast during the process of normal implantation. The tumour cells tend to form solid plugs within the myometrial vasculature and, although there is often extravascular extension, the malignant trophoblast tends to infiltrate between the muscle fibres with very little tissue destruction. The propensity for vascular invasion is the basis for the predominantly haematogenous dissemination of a choriocarcinoma to sites such as the lungs, brain, liver, kidney and gastrointestinal tract: large tumour emboli may impact within the pulmonary arteries. Lymph node deposits of a choriocarcinoma are usually tertiary metastases from a large extrauterine lesion.

Origin

There are many puzzling aspects of choriocarcinoma such as their status as an allograft (which they must be because of their content of paternal anti-gens), their increased frequency in women of blood groups A with group O spouses and in group O women with group A spouses[23] and their rather strange, almost bizarre, epidemiological risk factors, which include dieting, a family history of dizygotic twins, more than one marriage and infrequent sexual intercourse:[24] by far the most perplexing problem they pose is, how-ever, their origin. As already discussed, choriocarcinomas may follow either a normal or a molar pregnancy, more commonly the latter, and there is a considerable gap in our knowledge as to the relationship between the pre-vious pregnancy and the subsequent choriocarcinoma. Is the neoplasm actually derived from the trophoblast of the prior pregnancy and, if so, what has been happening to this trophoblast during the intervening months or years? The application of genetic techniques, such as the study of cytoge-netic polymorphism,[25] DNA restriction fragment-length polymorphism assays[26,27] or the study of tandem repeat regions amplified by the polymerase chain reaction[28,29] has shown that some, but by no means all, choriocarcino-mas are androgenetic. It has been presumed that the androgenetic tumours were derived from a previous molar gestation and this has indeed been proven to be so in several cases by showing complete genetic identity between the mole and the choriocarcinoma, this despite the fact that in two such cases there had been a full-term normal delivery intervening between the molar pregnancy and the development of the choriocarcinoma.[28–30] In one of these cases the time interval between the mole and the choriocarci-noma was 10 years[30] and it is difficult to understand how tissue from the mole remained in the uterus for that length of time, and throughout a later normal pregnancy, to then subsequently undergo a neoplastic resurgence; this typifies the questions posed by this enigmatic lesion.

Some points are, however, becoming clearer; it seems increasingly probable that many, possibly most or even all, choriocarcinomas that follow an apparently normal pregnancy are, in reality, metastases from an undetected small intraplacental choriocarcinoma. Only a small number of intraplacental choriocarcinomas have been described and in nearly all the choriocarcinoma was very small and easily overlooked unless the placenta was examined meticulously: in most cases the placenta had been subjected to such examination because metastases had developed in the mother during pregnancy and only in only two cases had the tumour been detected in the absence of such complications.[31,32] One case[33] is of particular interest insofar as a patient developed an apparently primary choriocarcinoma soon after a normal pregnancy: re-examination of the placenta at that time revealed a tiny intraplacental choriocarcinoma.

Intraplacental choriocarcinomas are histologically identical to extraplacental choriocarcinomas but are often separated from the normal villous population by villi with a surrounding mantle of choriocarcinoma-like trophoblast that has replaced the normal trophoblast: this therefore confirms the long held opinion, based largely on the ability of choriocarcinomas to secrete hCG, that a choriocarcinoma is a lesion of villous trophoblast despite the invariable absence of villi from extraplacental tumours. It is not yet known if all choriocarcinomas following a normal pregnancy are biparental rather than androgenetic but if this were proven to be so it would strengthen the case for such lesions being metastases rather than primary neoplasms.

If choriocarcinomas following a normal pregnancy are in reality metastases from an intraplacental choriocarcinoma, are those which follow a molar gestation similarly derived from an intramolar choriocarcinoma? This is certainly a possibility, for one such lesion has been described[34] although it was not associated with subsequent disease. The prolonged time interval, in many cases, between a molar pregnancy and the development of an overt choriocarcinoma does, however, suggest that by no means all post-molar choriocarcinomas are derived from intramolar lesions and it is certainly conceivable that some such choriocarcinomas are new pregnancies, the choriocarcinoma *ab initio* that has long been considered as a possibility.[35] Some choriocarcinomas, which have not obviously followed a normal pregnancy, have been biparental or even of purely maternal origin and there seems no good reason why a pregnancy, of any genetic type, should not evolve directly into a choriocarcinoma: there is an excellent precedent for the belief that a pregnancy can appear to be neoplastic, namely the now generally agreed concept that a teratoma is a parthogenetic pregnancy. This raises the question, however, as to whether such pregnancies should be considered as truly neoplastic or simply as aberrant gestations. Choriocarcinomas invade vessels and spread to distant sites but so does normal trophoblast; histologically they resemble acutely the trophoblast of the normal implanting blastocyst and their response to methotrexate, whilst being quite different to that of virtually every other neoplasm, is not unlike that of a normal, but ectopic, early gestation. This is, of course, pure speculation but nevertheless the possibility that some choriocarcinomas are simply abnormal pregnancies should not be dismissed too lightly.

Placental site trophoblastic tumour

This is an uncommon tumour that is derived from the extravillous trophoblast of the placental bed (sometimes referred to as 'intermediate trophoblast'). In the vast majority of cases the neoplasm develops after a
normal pregnancy, only 5% occurring after a molar gestation.[36] Patients present at anything from a few weeks to 18 months after the antecedent pregnancy with a complaint of irregular vaginal bleeding or, perhaps more
commonly, amenorrhoea: a small proportion of patients develop a
nephrotic syndrome that appears to be caused by chronic intravascular
coagulation initiated by factors released from the tumour.[37] The uterus is
commonly enlarged but a pregnancy test is positive in only one-third of
patients, this reflecting the fact that the principal secretory product of
extravillous trophoblast is human placental lactogen (hPL) rather than hCG.

The tumours tend to form tan, white or yellow masses within the
myometrium and often protrude into the endometrial cavity, sometimes
forming a polypoidal mass. Histologically, the tumour replicates, in an anar-
chic form, the appearances seen in the normal placental bed. The tumour is
formed principally of mononuclear cytotrophoblastic cells with an irregular
and inconsistent admixture of multinucleated cells, the latter resembling the
multinucleated cells of the placental bed rather than true syncytiotrophoblast. The tumour cells infiltrate between, and dissect, the myometrial
fibres as cords and sheets with a striking absence of necrosis and haemorrhage (Fig. 6.6). Invasion of vessels by tumour cells is common but the massive intravascular growth that characterizes a choriocarcinoma is not seen
and some vessels within the tumour are surrounded, but not invaded, by
neoplastic cells. Non-infiltrated vessels often show fibrinoid necrosis of
their wall, whilst a pseudodecidual change, and sometimes an Arias-Stella
reaction, may be apparent in the adjacent endometrium.

About 15–20% of placental site trophoblastic tumours behave in a malignant fashion[37] and either recur locally or spread to distant sites such as the
liver, lung and central nervous system. Assessment of the degree of malignancy of any individual neoplasm is, however, difficult for although those
which have run a malignant course have usually had a high mitotic count
this is not an invariable rule[38,39] and a low mitotic count should not necessarily engender a sense of security; both deep myometrial invasion and a
high proportion of cells with clear cytoplasm tend to be associated with an
aggressive course. Flow cytometry of placental site trophoblastic tumours
has been performed only rarely but most of the tumours appear, irrespective
of their clinical behaviour, to be diploid;[40] there has been one triploid neoplasm which, very surprisingly, followed a normal term pregnancy.

A placental site trophoblastic tumour can pose diagnostic problems in
curettage material, the major difficulty being in distinguishing such a neoplasm from an exaggerated, but otherwise normal, placental site reaction.
The shorter the time interval between the preceding gestation and the
curettage the more likely is the diagnosis to be that of placental site reaction

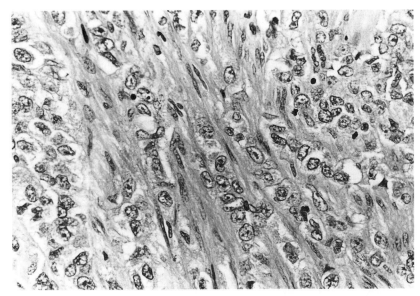

Fig. 6.6 Histological appearances of a placental trophoblastic site tumour. Cords and sheets of mononuclear are infiltrating between, and compressing, the myometrial fibres. (Reproduced with permission from: Fox H. Obstetrical pathology. In: Anderson MC, ed. Systemic pathology, 3rd edn. Volume 5 Female reproductive tract. Edinburgh: Churchill Livingstone, 1991.)

but this is not an inviolate rule for I have seen a highly malignant placental site tumour that became apparent only 10 days after a normal delivery. Other findings suggestive of a placental site trophoblastic tumour are the presence of an intrauterine mass and the finding of mitotic figures.

It is of note that the placental site trophoblastic tumour responds very poorly to the cytotoxic drug therapy which is so successful in choriocarcinoma;[37] indeed the response to any form of chemotherapy is unsatisfactory and surgery is the basis of treatment.

Key points for clinical practice

- Hydatidiform moles, of all types, are a form of abortion.
- Partial hydatidiform mole can be complicated by persistent trophoblastic disease and by choriocarcinoma: patients with such moles should be followed-up.
- Normal trophoblast is invasive and metastatic: invasive moles share these qualities, which are not an indication of malignancy or neoplasia.
- Choriocarcinoma can be derived from a hydatidiform mole despite an intervening normal pregnancy.
- Choriocarcinoma following a normal pregnancy may be a metastasis from an unnoticed intraplacental choriocarcinoma.

- Some choriocarcinomas may be new pregnancies.
- About 15–20% of placental site trophoblastic tumours behave in a malignant fashion.
- Features suggesting that a placental site trophoblastic tumour may behave in an aggressive fashion are a high mitotic count, deep myometrial invasion and many cells with clear cytoplasm. Tumours may, however, be malignant in the absence of any of these features.

References

1 Szulman AE, Surti U. The syndromes of hydatidiform mole. I. cytogenetic and morphologic correlations. Am J Obstet Gynecol 1978; 131: 665–671

2 Szulman AE, Surti U. The syndromes of hydatidiform mole. II. Morphologic evolution of the complete and partial mole. Am J Obstet Gynecol 1978; 132: 20–27

3 Paradinas FJ. The histological diagnosis of hydatidiform moles. Curr Diag Pathol 1994; 1: 24–31

4 Steller MA, Genest DR, Bernstein MR, Lage JM, Goldstein DP, Berkowitz RS. Clinical features of multiple conception with partial or complete molar pregnancy and coexisting fetuses. J Reprod Med 1994; 39: 147–154

5 Roberts DJ, Mutter GL. Advances in the molecular biology of gestational trophoblastic disease. J Reprod Med 1994; 39: 201–208

6 Jacobs PA, Szulman AE, Funkmouska J, Maatsura JS, Wilson CC. Human triploidy: relationship between paternal origin of the additional haploid complement and development of partial hydatidiform mole. Ann Hum Genet 1982 46: 223–231

7 Vejerslev LO, Fisher RA, Surti U, Walke N. Hydatidiform mole: cytogenetically unusual cases and their implications for the present classification. Am J Obstet Gynecol 1987 157: 180–184

8 Lage JM, Popek EJ. The role of DNA flow cytometry in evaluation of partial and complete hydatidiform moles and hydropic abortions. Semin Diag Pathol 1993 10: 267–274

9 Sunde L, Vejerslev LO, Jensen MP, Pedersen S, Hertz JM, Bolund L. Genetic analysis of repeated, biparental, diploid, hydatidiform moles. Cancer Genet Cytogenet 1994; 66: 16–22

10 Barton SC, Surani MAH, Norris ML. Role of paternal and maternal genomes in mouse develoment. Nature 1984; 311: 374–376

11 Ariel I, Lustig O, Oyer CE, et al Relaxing of imprinting in trophoblastic disease. Gynecol Oncol 1994; 53: 212–219

12 Howat AJ, Beck S, Fox H, et al Can histopathologists reliably diagnose molar pregnancy? J Clin Pathol 1993; 46: 599–602

13 Topalovsky M, Hankin RC, Michael C, Hunter SV, Edwards AM, Chen JC. Ploidy analysis of products of conception by image and flow cytometry with cytogenetic correlation. Am J Clin Pathol 1995; 103: 409–414

14 Genest DG, Laborde O, Berkowitz RS, et al A clinical–pathologic study of 153 cases of complete hydatidiform mole (1980–1990): histologic grade lacks prognostic significance. Obstet Gynecol 1991; 77: 111–115

15 Cheung AN, Ngan HY, Collins RJ, Wong YL. Assessment of cell proliferation in hydatidiform mole using monoclonal antibody MIB1 to Ki-67 antigen. J Clin Pathol 1994; 47: 601–604

16 Cameron B, Gown AM, Tamimi HK. Expression of c-erb-B-2 oncogene product in persistent gestational trophoblastic disease. Am J Obstet Gynecol 1994; 170: 1616–1621

17 Hemming JD, Quirke P, Womack C, Wells M, Elston CW, Pennington GW. Flow cytometry in persistent trophoblastic disease. Placenta 1988; 9: 615–621

18 Wake N, Fujino T, Hoshi S, et al The propensity to malignancy of dispermic heterozygous moles. Placenta 1987; 8: 318–326

19 Mutter GL, Pomponio RJ, Berkowitz RS, Genest DR. Sex chromosome composition of complete hydatidiform mole: relationship to metastasis. Am J Obstet Gynecol 1993; 168: 1547–1551

20 Cheung AN, Sit AS, Chung LP, et al Detection of heterozygous XY complete hydatidiform mole by chromosome in situ hybridization. Gynecol Oncol 1994; 55: 386–392

21 Mueller UW, Hawes CS, Wright AE, et al Isolation of fetal trophoblast cells from peripheral blood of pregnant women. Lancet 1990; 336: 197–200

22 Attwood HD, Park WW. Embolism to the lungs by trophoblast. J Obstet Gynaecol Br Cwlth 1961; 68: 611–617

23 Bagshawe KD. Recent observations related to chemotherapy and immunology of gestatonal choriocarcinoma. Adv Cancer Res 1973; 18: 231–263

24 Buckley JD, Henderson BE, Morrow CP, et al Case-control study of gestational choriocarcinoma. Cancer Res 1988; 48: 1004–1010

25 Chaganti RSK, Koduru PRK, Chakraborty R, Jones WB. Genetic origin of a trophoblastic choriocarcinoma. Cancer Res 1990; 50: 6330–6333

26 Azuma C, Saji F, Nobunaga T, et al Studies of the pathogenesis of choriocarcinoma by analysis of restriction fragment length polymorphisms. Cancer Res 1990; 50: 488–491.

27 Osada H, Kawata M, Yamada M, Okumura K, Takamizawa H. Genetic identification of pregnancies responsible for choriocarcinoma after multiple pregnancies by restriction fragment length polymorphism analysis. Am J Obstet Gynecol 1991; 165: 682–688.

28 Suzuki T, Goto S, Nawa A, Kurauchi D, Saito M, Tomoda Y. Identification of the pregnancy responsible for gestational trophoblastic disease by DNA analysis. Obstet Gynecol 1993; 82: 629–634

29 Fisher RA, Soteriou BA, Meredith FJ, Paradinas FJ, Newlands ES. Previous hydatidiform mole identified as the causative pregnancy of choriocarcinoma following birth of normal twins. Int J Gynecol Cancer 1995; 5: 54–70

30 Fisher RA, Newlands ES, Jeffreys AJ, et al Gestational and non-gestational trophoblastic tumours distinguished by DNA analysis. Cancer 1992; 69: 839–845.

31 Driscoll SG. Choriocarcinoma: an 'incidental finding' within a term placenta. Obstet Gynecol 1963; 21: 96–102.

32 Fox H, Laurini RN. Intraplacental choriocarcinoma: a report of two cases. J Clin Pathol 1988; 41: 1085–1088

33 Hallam LA, McLaren KM, El-Jabbour JN, Helm CW, Smart GE. Intraplacental choriocarcinoma: a case report. Placenta 1990; 11: 247–251.

34 Heifetz SA, Csaja J. In situ choriocarcinoma arising in partial hydatidiform mole: implications for risk of persistent trophoblastic disease. Pediatr Pathol 1992; 12: 601–611

35 Acosta-Sison H. Can the implanting trophoblast of the fertilized ovum develop immediately into choriocarcinoma? Am J Obstet Gynecol 1955; 69: 442–444.

36 Lage JM, Young RH. Pathology of trophoblastic disease. In: Clement PB, Young RH, eds. Tumors and tumorlike lesions of the uterine corpus and cervix. New York: Churchill Livingstone, 1993: 419–475

37 Young RH, Kurman RJ, Scully RE. Proliferations and tumors of the placental site. Semin Diag Pathol 1988; 5: 223–237

38 Eckstein RP, Paradinas FJ, Bagshawe KD. Placental site trophoblastic tumour (trophoblastic pseudotumour): a study of four cases requiring hysterectomy, including one fatal case. Histopathology 1982 6: 221–226.

39 Alvero R, Remmenga S, O'Connor D, Burnhill D, Park R. Metastatic placental site trophoblast tumor. Gynecol Oncol 1990; 37: 445–449.

40 How J, Scurry J, Grant P, et al Placental site trophoblastic tumor: report of three cases and review of the literature. Int J Gynecol Cancer 1995; 5: 241–249.

7

Role of the stroma in neoplastic growth and progression

E.-N. Lalani   G. W. H. Stamp

Much of the research effort in the last few years has been directed into the analysis of the genetic events which underlie the generation of the transformed epithelial phenotype. This has to some extent overshadowed understanding of the biology of tumour stroma, which is not only the framework imparting the distinctive morphological appearances that are the basis of classification and grading and the conduit for nutritional support, but functional activities of the stromal cells exert major influences over the proliferative capacity, differentiation and invasive/metastatic potential of the malignant cell population.

This selective review concentrates on recent advances in the biology of tumour stroma and the desmoplastic response. Stromal cell populations are non-neoplastic and are less prone to become refractory to conventional drugs and biotherapies, unlike tumour cells with accumulating genetic damage during progression.

The composition of tumour stroma

The stroma surrounding or included within the boundaries of a neoplasm is a complex mixture of cell types enmeshed in a matrix of modified or newly synthesized extracellular components. The cellular complement comprises:

1. fibroblasts;
2. endothelial cells;
3. smooth muscle cells and myofibroblasts;
4. macrophages and inflammatory cells; and
5. entrapped cells (dependent on anatomical location).

This diversity of cell types in the tumour microenvironment results in complex cascades of events that modify the growth and development of tumours to a highly variable degree, and their differing contributions may account for many of the variations in biological behaviour of tumours which display similar genetic aberrations in the neoplastic component. Our account will concentrate on the non-specialized (at least morphologically) cellular populations of the desmoplastic response, a cellular proliferation of stromal fibroblasts and indeterminate cells, which is usually maximal in the centre of neoplasms.[1] These non-endothelial stromal populations interact via synthesis of and/or binding to matrix components, secretion of soluble factors and cell–cell contacts. The extracellular matrix is the key factor in normal and neoplastic structure, being a composite of insoluble fibres and soluble polymers. The principal fibres are collagens and the soluble molecules include proteoglycans and glycoproteins. The latter have the potential to bind or activate growth factors and cytokines. It is frequently evident on morphological examination that the extracellular matrix (ECM) is different in carcinomas arising from different anatomical sites, to such a degree that it may become the dominant feature of the neoplasm, and form the basis of many conventional histological classifications. These differences are the sum of many different factors, which include stromal cellularity, matrix composition and epithelial cell distribution and cytoarchitecture. Continuing evolution and modulation of ECM during the growth of a neoplasm is accompanied by changes in matrix composition, which may then result in modulation of neoplastic cells and stromal cells in the vicinity. We are only beginning to appreciate the complexity of network interactions, or the interdependent gene expression termed 'dynamic reciprocity'.[2,3]

Stromal fibroblasts and neoplasia

The exact molecular signalling mechanisms that occur between epithelial and mesenchymal cells and the dependency of such interactions on soluble factors, cell–cell communication or neosynthesis of ECM components is unclear.[2-6] Embryogenesis, wound healing and neoplasia are similar in many respects, the role of mesenchymal cells in the first two situations not being in doubt.[7,8] During morphogenesis the mesenchyme directs epithelial cell differentiation and growth, for example in the lung, kidney, skin, salivary gland and mammary gland.[9] Substituting a mesenchymal element from a different site results in incomplete epithelial differentiation or may even induce a switch to the lineage appropriate to the mesenchymal origin.[10]

It has been claimed that site-specific fibroblasts may differentially regulate tumour cells from that site and may explain experimental observations where tumour cell lines from mammary gland or colon metastasize when implanted in orthotopic sites.[11-13] In other experiments, there is evidence that fibroblasts in tumour environments secrete factors that enhance tumorigenicity of xenografted cell lines, especially when combined with matrix components.[14] Normal fibroblasts exert a differentiating effect on MCF-7 mammary carcinoma cells that is not observed with tumour-derived fibroblasts[15] although such effects can be variable depending on the lineages involved.[16] There is some evidence that the ability to induce a desmoplastic stroma is inversely related to the invasive/metastatic capability but this may not be invariable.[17] There are many such examples of tumour–fibroblast interdependence, and these effects could be mediated via two predominant routes:

1. degradation and neosynthesis of stromal matrix modulating cell structure and function via specific cell-surface receptors;
2. secretion of positive and negative regulatory molecules including growth factors and cytokines.

It is more likely that each aspect is involved with direct and indirect consequences for both the epithelial and mesenchymal compartments, hence the need to evaluate both when analysing data derived from tumours, rather than isolated cells in vitro. However, the composition and modification of the ECM and the response of the neoplastic cell to the dynamic changes in the microenvironment will ultimately determine its morphology and function.

Fibroblasts – the orchestration of tumour growth via ECM

Experimental studies have indicated the role of ECM proteins, especially collagens, in controlling epithelial cell proliferation, differentiation and gene expression.[5,10,18] Other ECM components, including those of the basement membrane (BM) and the immature matrix, which characterizes embryogenesis, wound healing and neoplastic desmoplasia, also exert powerful effects on cellular shape, motility and function. ECM may affect the ability of cells to grow in vitro and in vivo. For example, simple preparations of interstitial collagen may neither support growth of some cell lines nor promote differentiation, but the purified ECM produced by the EHS murine sarcoma (matrigel), which contains more complex components including Type IV collagen and laminin, will promote differentiation in vitro and facilitate the growth of certain tumour cell lines in immunosuppressed mice.[19,20]

However, fibroblasts do not merely synthesize interstitial collagens or accommodate the developing vascular network. It is now clear that they have far more diverse and dynamic functions, amongst which neosynthesis of extracellular matrix components are foremost. These components include fibronectin (FN), vitronectin (VN) and tenascin (TN) as well as an embryonic-like trimeric Type 1 collagen. Additionally, in the stable differentiated environment, ECM proteins such as interstitial collagen and BM components, as well as abnormal accumulations of structured matrix such as elastin, predominate. These synthetic abilities differ among different tumour types and in different regions of the same tumour.

Structural components of the neoplastic ECM

Collagens

The collagens comprise a superfamily of at least 17 genetically distinct types of extracellular matrix proteins encoded by over 30 genes, which appear to function primarily as structural components. At least 19 different types of collagens have been identified.[21] They can be divided into subfamilies based on the nucleic acid and protein sequences, into fibrillary collagens (Type I–III, V, XI), facit collagens (Types IX, XII, XIV), BM (Type IV), short chain collagens (Types VIII, X) and others (VI, VII, XIII).[22] The collagens contain three alpha (α) polypeptide chains, with amino acid Gly–X–Y repeats where X and Y are often proline and hydroxyproline, forming right handed polyproline helices. The three α-chains in turn form a left handed, triple helical molecule called the collagenous (COL) domain. However, owing to their complex structures it is becoming increasingly difficult to define accurately what is a collagen and what is not. Therefore, at least three collagens appear to comprise the protein core of proteoglycans. The role of collagens in controlling epithelial cell proliferation, differentiation and gene expression have been well documented.[22-25]

Elastin

Human elastin is a non-glycosylated, hydrophobic, insoluble protein forming the central core of elastic fibres, the outer sheath of which comprises a microfibrillary network containing fibrillin and other proteins.[26] It is encoded by a gene found on chromosome 7 q11.2, consisting of 45 exons of approximately 45 kb.[27,28] The hydrophobic and cross-linked repeats of the molecule are encoded by distinct exons. Elastin is a common component of the matrix of several types of carcinoma but typifies invasive ductal carcinomas of the breast or pancreas, where it accumulates in the 'oldest' regions of the tumour, maximally around pre-existing structures such as ducts, blood vessels, etc. There are cell surface receptors that bind preferentially to elastin and may promote migration, partly by promoting traction but little work has yet been done on the functional assessment of elastin receptor signalling in tumours.[29-31] However, elastin-rich ECM is often sparsely cellular and the cells low in proliferative activity, and abundant elastin may act as a growth inhibitor or migration inhibitor rather than a promoter. The association of basal and squamous cell carcinomas of the skin with elastosis may also be important in this respect as it may be relevant to the relative indolence of these tumours. The structure of the elastin fibrils and cellular elastin receptors may also be critical. In tubular and cribriform carcinomas of the breast, where BM components are sparse or absent and elastinis diffuse rather than aggregated the cells are highly differentiated and growth appears to be slow. Induction of elastin synthesis in stromal cells appears to be a specific property of certain neoplastic cells as it may be observed in the metastases in lymph node or liver of breast and pancreatic carcinoma, for example, but it is rarely observed in other tumour types. Elastin contains fibrillin, which is composed of microfibrils that possess a motif similar to that of (TGF)-β 1 transforming growth factor binding protein[32] and may be relevant in terms of the cellular response to matrix-associated cytokines that include the TGF-β family, and which may therefore act as a growth or migration inhibitor in such regions, which are often found to be sparsely cellular and low in proliferative activity.[30,31]

Fibronectin

Fibronectin (FN) is an ubiquitous extracellular glycoprotein that exists in soluble form in body fluids and insoluble form in ECM. It plays a role in many physiological processes including embryogenesis wound healing, haemostasis and thrombosis.[33,34] FN is secreted as a dimer, with a molecular mass of 220–250 kDa, and in common with many ECM components including laminin, thrombospondin and tenascin, it is a mosaic protein.[35] It is composed of three types of module.[35] These modules are arranged into functional domains that are resistant to proteolysis and contain binding sites for other ECM proteins including collagen and thrombospondin, cell surface receptors, which include the integrin superfamily, circulating blood proteins (e.g. fibrin and plasmin) glycosaminoglycans (heparan and chondroitin sulphate) and growth factors such as fibroblast growth factors (FGFs).

FN is known to have profound effects on cellular spreading, migration and proliferation, the extent of these changes differing among cells of variable lineages. A further layer of complexity arises because there are several potential splice variants of FN, which may be differentially expressed between tumours of differing histogenetic origins, and even heterogeneously within individual tumors. FN is synthesized early in the wound healing response and is abundant in early embryogenesis and morphogenesis, situations in which there is epithelial cell migration and spreading, functions that may be mediated by different cellular receptors, and may facilitate invasion and metastasis. Our knowledge of the structure and synthesis of FN has increased significantly but despite this many questions still remain to be addressed, including the recent suggestion that on proteolytic cleavage, FN reveals many cryptic active sites.[36,37] FN gene knock-out studies in mice by George and colleagues[38] found that FN knock-out produces lethality and major mesodermal defects whereas cell migration was only mildly affected.[38]

Tenascin

Tenascin (cytotactin, hexabrachion or J1) is expressed in similar situations to FN and is abundant in neoplastic stroma. It may also promote cellular migration in embryogenesis, wound healing and neoplasia.[39] It is a six subunit glycoprotein of high-molecular weight, the gene for which is on human chromosome 9 (q 32–34) with a coding region spanning ~ 80 kb and consisting of 27 exons. Whether FN and tenascin actively interfere with the establishment of the stable, immobile and differentiating phenotype is, as yet, unclear. The first deliberately engineered mutation of an ECM protein gene was the knock-out of the mouse tenascin-C gene.[40] These mice, suprisingly, developed to term and were overtly normal and fertile. This clearly suggests that the expression of tenascin-c is not essential for development and that there is a great deal of redundancy or compensation.

Tenascin may enhance adhesion in certain cell lines but under other conditions has antiadhesive properties, mapped to an alternatively spliced region in a FN-like domain and served to enhance migration on FN and Type IV collagen substrates.[41] It is maximal at the invasive edge of mammary carcinomas but is also abundant in the invasive but non-metastatic basal cell carcinomas of the skin.[42,43] Tenascin is transiently expressed in many developing organs coinciding with cellular migration during morphogenesis. Therefore, reappearance in tumours is of great interest.

Vitronectin

Vitronectin (VN) is a factor that promotes cell adhesion and spreading, and is also found in both plasma and tissues. In plasma it exists in two forms, a single chain and a heterodimer bound by disulphide bonds. The human VN gene is approximately 5 kb and comprises eight exons generating a 1.7 kb transcript. It is located in the centromeric region of chromosome 17q.[44] VN is a ligand for at least three integrins ($\alpha V\beta_1$, $\alpha V\beta_3$ and $\alpha V\beta_5$); it contains the RGD motif. Site-directed mutagenesis of the RGD sequence to either RGE or RAD resulted in complete loss of cell adhesion activity, confirming that, in VN, the RGD sequence is essential to VN-mediated cell adhesion.[45] VN also promotes cellular migration and is more abundant in the tumour stroma and in embryogenesis,[46] and VN receptors (members of the integrin superfamily) are up-regulated on invasive and metastatic tumour cells.[47] It has been demonstrated that activation of such receptors will enhance secretion of 72 kDa Type IV collagenase/MMP-2,[48] which is associated with the invasive/metastitic phenotype in carcinomas (see below). VN also binds to proteins of the complement and coagulation pathways and inhibits cytolysis.

Other components

Other components of the new (or immature) matrix include differing proportions of proteoglycans and glycoproteins whose roles are as yet unclear. Proteoglycans are a rather diverse family composed of protein cores with covalently bound glycosaminoglycan side-chains encoded by a number of distinct genes[49] and include heparan sulphate and chondroitin sulphate proteoglycans. The side-chains are composed of dissaccharide repeats of two different sugars, one of which is usually a hexuronate and the other a hexosamine. These molecules have a ubiquitous distribution and are found in the extracellular compartment, intercellularly and in intracellular storage granules. They may act either as primary adhesive components or serve to mask adhesive sites in other proteins. Unlike Type IV collagen and laminin they appear to be products primarily of epithelial cells in vivo. Thrombospondin (TSP) is a matrix component that has antiangiogenic effects and promotes aggregation of activated platelets, but also modulates cell growth and motility in fibroblasts, and may promote adhesion in epithelial cells.[2] Furthermore, TSP is able to bind to collagen, FN, laminin and plasminogen in its central regions. It is possible that part of its function may be to abrogate effects of angiogenesis-stimulating factors such as FGFs by binding to its heparin-like domains[50] although TSP may promote synthesis of FGF-1 in certain mesenchymal cells and it may also bind TGF-β (Sage and Bornstein 1991). Its role in tumour growth and progression is yet to be fully evaluated.[51] The effects of cellular binding to TSP compared with mature interstitial collagen or BM has not been investigated comprehensively but it is theoretically possible that cell surface binding could induce a number of genes active in invasion via second messenger systems or alteration in cytoskeletal structure by redistribution of the cell surface anchorage points.

As stromal ECM becomes increasingly remodelled within the vicinity of differentiating cells, formation of the BM commences. This is a highly organized structure comprising numerous components based on an interlacing network of Type IV collagen molecules forming a sheet, to which adhere various components and complex molecules of high-molecular weight such as laminin, entactin and HSPG. It used to be considered that the synthesis of these components was purely an epithelial (or specialized mesenchymal cell) function, and studies on isolated epithelial cells in culture demonstrated that they were able to synthesize such components. However, experiments in vivo (cross-species recombination, xenografting and in situ hybridization) and in vitro (culture of fibroblast populations) show that the BM is to a large extent a product of the mesenchymal cell.[52]

It is a consistent observation that loss of BM formation, either structurally or immunohistochemically, is one feature of less differentiated cells in neoplasia and contentiously said to be an indication of early invasive activity. If this is indeed a co-operative activity based on the epithelial-mesenchymal interaction, is this also a consequence of down-regulation of activity in stromal cells, perhaps favouring the synthesis of products such as FN and tenascin? The re-establishment of BM integrity is closely related to differentiation, and it is difficult to ascertain whether BM synthesis is a function of differentiation, secondarily up-regulating the expression of appropriate cell surface receptors of integrin and non-integrin types, or whether these are mutually reciprocal processes, i.e. does the presence of BM induce the expression of receptors which then mediate differentiation in an increasingly cyclical process, or are these all a reflection of an appropriately functioning cell directed to the achievement of its highest differentiated state?

Disturbance of the BM is not solely due to decreased formation, but also to active degradation of the structural Type IV collagen. This is specifically effected by members of the matrix metalloproteinase (MMP) family (see below) including a 72 kDa Type IV collagenase enzyme (MMP-2) but also by others including stromelysin-1 (MMP-3) and 92 kDa Type IV collagenase (MMP-9). The balance between formation, maturation and degradation of the BM is critical to cytoarchitectural organization and control of epithelial cell function in normal and neoplastic tissues.

Functional properties of the desmoplastic fibroblast

Enzymic degradation of ECM

It is vital that a neoplastic cell acquires the ability to break down normal structural components of the ECM such as BM, which while permitting focal cytoplasmic contacts is impermeable to epithelial cells. Liotta and Stetler-Stevensons (1991) proposed the three-step hypothesis that essentially involves 1 cell attachment; 2) ECM degradation; and 3) locomotion.[53]

It is the shift in the balance of protease action and antiprotease activity that may determine the outcome of the interaction.[54] Once the invasive cell has transgressed the BM, it then has to bind to other structural components of the ECM including interstitial collagen, which also has to be degraded, and interact with newly synthesized molecules such as FN, VN and tenascin. The end result of this process is to create a dynamically interactive and primitive environment reminiscent of embryogenesis and wound healing. The different ligands in the altered ECM dictate profound alterations in the cellular structure and function by redirecting cell surface receptors, in the direction of a less differentiated phenotype that characterizes the malignant cell. Re-establishment of the BM may theoretically reverse some or all of these changes provided the cell has retained the genetic information necessary to respond to it.

Specific protease activity in neoplasia

There are four major classes of endoproteinases involved in ECM degradation: serine, cysteine, aspartic and metallo proteinases. Of these, overexpression of certain MMPs has been shown to increase tumour cell invasion in vivo.[55] and this can be reversed by their specific inhibitors, the tissue inhibitors of metalloproteinases (TIMPs).[56] MMPs are members of a family of a common structural group of proteases, which contain a metallic ion, zinc, for catalytic activity and whose principal characteristics and substrate specificies are summarized in Table 7.1. In all of the metalloproteinases there are two highly conserved regions, the cysteine-switch, an interaction between two highly conserved regions, the first PRCG/(V/N)PD, immediately upstream from the propeptide cleavage site, and the zinc-binding

Table 7.1 Principal characteristics and substrate specifications of matrix metalloproteinases (MMPs)

Group Member		M_w (kDa)	Substrate specificity	Source
Collagenase				
Intersitial collagenase	(MMP-1)	55	collagens I,II,III,X; gelatin; proteoglycans	fibroblasts
Neurophil collagenase	(MMP-8)	75	as for MMP-1	neutrophils
Collagenase-3	(MMP-13)	?	collagenase I,II,III	
Stromelysins				
Stromelysin-1	(MMP-3)	57	proteoglycans; collagens II,IV,IX, X,XI; fibronectin; laminin	fibroblasts macrophages
Stromelysin-2	(MMP-10)	57	as MMP-3 but less activity	macrophages
Stromelysin-3	(MMP-11)	51	?	desmoplastic fibroblasts
PU-MMP				
Matrilysin/PUMP	(MMP-7)	28	As stromelysins; elastase	immature monocytes; mesangial; tumour cells; (not fully defined)
Mouse MMP				
Metalloelastase	MMP-12)	57	elastin, fibronectin	macrophages
Gelatinases/ Type IV collagenases				
Gelatinase A	(MMP-2)	72	denatured collagens collagens I,IV,V,VII, X,XI; elastin	most cell types
Gelatinase B	(MMP-9)	95	as gelatinase A	monocytes, macrophages, ?tumour cells
Transmembrane MMPs				
MT1-MMP	(MMP-14)	63	gelatinase A collagen III, fibronectin, laminin	plasma membranes
MT2-MMP	(MMP-15)	70	gelatinase A	plasma membranes
MT3-MMP	(MMP-16)	66	?	plasma membranes
MT4-MMP	(MMP-17)	70	?	plasma memb. and leucocytes

PU-MMP = Putative uterine metalloproteinase

regions (HEXXHXXGXXH), which co-ordinate the catalytic zinc ion.[57,58] Disruption of this interaction is an essential prerequisite for subsequent enzyme activation.[59] Together, MMPs have the capacity to degrade all of the major structural components of the ECM.

Some MMPs are expressed constitutively but others such as MMP-1 are secreted in response to microenvironment changes.[60] MMP activity can be regulated at various levels: gene transcription, mRNA stabilization, translation, processing and secretion, binding to cell membranes and/or ECM, activation, inhibition and degradation. One major control of MMP activity is exerted by the TIMPs, all four of which described so far having 12 conserved cysteine residues paired into six disulphide bonds giving rise to a three-loop structure with a C-terminal tail, differences in the latter which may determine binding affinities. TIMPs form 1:1 complexes with MMPs to inhibit activity and may also act to prevent autoactivator and transactivation. The complex interactions of TIMPs with MMPs have been recently reviewed in detail.[54] TIMP-2 is the specific inhibitor of MMP-2, which is usually expressed with the latter but may be differentially regulated by certain factors such as oestrogens, thus potentially altering the net enzymic activity at a particular site.[61]

Most of the MMPs except MMP-2 are activated in vivo by plasmin and/or pro-urokinase type plasminogen activator (uPA). In addition there is some evidence for activation or transactivation by MMPs, as stromelysin may activate both interstitial collagenase (MMP-1) and MMP-9[62,63] and MMP-1 is activated by MMP-3.[64] Stromelysins have fairly comprehensive substrate specificity, and can degrade HSGs and elastin. They can cleave the globular but not the fibrillar regions of Type IV collagen. Stromelysin-1 is also expressed in subsets of desmoplastic fibroblasts in experimental skin carcinomas.[65] Stromelysin-3 may be more important in neoplasia as it appears to be expressed in close proximity to invasive tumour cells and the degree of expression appears to correspond approximately to the level of invasive activity.[66,67]

MMP-1 appears to be induced in stromal cells by tumour-derived factors[68] which potentially include interleukin (IL)-1, tumour necrosis factor-α (TNF-α) bFGF and platelet-derived growth factor (PDGF),[69] and stromelysin-3 is synthesized by stromal cells in a similar fashion.[70] Matrix glycoprotein may also serve to protect stromal collagen fibrils from MMP-dependent degradation.[71]

MMP-2 and MMP-9 specifically degrade the BM by cleaving the triple helical portion of the Type IV collagen of BM at a pepsin-resistant triple helical domain into one-quarter and three-quarter fragments (but may also act on Type V collagen.[72] They have a large FN-like collagen-binding domain composed of three 58–59 amino acid repeats each encoded by a separate exon, and MMP-9 also contains a small Type V collagen-like domain. The FN-like domain of MMP-2 is required for the substrate specificity against Type IV collagen.[73] This enzyme is disproportionately up-regulated in malignant tumours compared with wound healing or benign tumours, and neoplastic cell lines expressing high levels of this enzyme have greater metastatic potential.[53,74-76] In the mouse, MMP-2 is highly expressed in mesenchymal cells during development,[77] with a completely different pattern to MMP-9. In addition, MMP-2 and MMP-9 have very different promoter regions, and their expression is differentially regulated by cytokines in certain cell lineages.[78] There is also an abundance of evidence that cellular binding to certain ECM substrates may lead to enhanced expression of proteases, including epithelial cell binding to Type 1 collagen.[79] melanoma cell binding to VN,[48] HT 1080 cells to FN[80] and macrophages to Type I collagen.[81]

Antibodies raised to both the profragments and to the other domains of MMP-2 appear to localize maximally to neoplastic cell cytoplasm, in tumour cells of mammary,[82] colon[83] thyroid,[84] ovarian[85] and lung carcinomas.[86] MMP-9 is often expressed in macrophages and possibly other leukocytes in tumours, and may be derived largely from areas of necrosis[87] but occasionally mRNA is localized in tumour cells themselves.[88] Additionally, in vitro data from cell lines reinforced the impression that the neoplastic cell was the origin of the enzyme in homogenates of tumours in vivo and similar conclusions were drawn from Northern analysis of extracted mRNAs from tumours.[89]

However, we and others showed that the desmoplastic stromal cell may potentially make an equivalent or greater contribution to the disruption of BMs, as they appear to transcribe the MMP-2 gene at high levels, judging from in situ hybridization experiments,[83] as well as its specific inhibitor TIMP-2. The same situation appears to be true for mammary carcinomas and the more indolent, non-metastasizing basal cell carcinomas of the skin.[90] In studies of human tumours, 92 kDa gelatinase mRNA localizes to a tumour-infiltrating population, probably macrophages rather than tumour cells, and in a completely different distribution to MMP-2.[91]

Interstitial collagenase and stromelysin-3 are also synthesized in the desmoplastic stromal fibroblasts in malignant tumors of colon and breast respectively,[70,92] and a membrane-associated factor appears to be responsible for the fibroblast stimulation of interstitial collagenase production.[68] The possibility that a neoplastic cell-derived cytokine or soluble factor was involved was also supported by the observation that fibroblasts on the tumour periphery and around foci of in situ carcinoma also expressed MMP-2 and TIMP-2 mRNAs, albeit at a relatively lower level.[90] MMP-2 mRNA and secreted enzyme is increased in fibroblasts co-cultured with human carcinoma cell lines or their conditioned media, implicating a soluble factor in this role.[93]

Several explanations could be offered for these apparently conflicting data, including artefactual localization of mRNA or protein. It could be that there is stabilization of mRNA in stromal cells, but this would seem an unlikely basis given the relative abundance of the mRNA in stromal fibroblastic cells. For an explanation of the immunolocalization to neoplastic cells, there is in vivo evidence for uptake of intact or degraded enzyme.[89] Similarly, uPA bound to PAI-1 is also rapidly internalized. Careful examination also revealed apparently genuine immunoreactivity for MMPs in the more inconspicuous cytoplasm of stromal non-endothelial fibroblastic cells.[83]

Experimental in vitro evidence provides a potential explanation for these contradictory findings. The active form of MMP-2 binds to cell membranes via the C-terminal, and activated enzyme was present at areas of invasion and cytoplasmic extremities in chick embryo fibroblasts (invadopodia).[94] The presence of activated MMP-2 at the tumour-stromal interface appears to be caused by physiological activation as no mutations in the active site have been demonstrated. We also showed that a synthetic inhibitor, which binds tightly to activated but not pro-MMP-2, also localizes to the neoplastic cell membrane.[95,96] Labelled activated enzyme was also demonstrated on the cell surface of certain mammary carcinoma cell lines indicating the presence of high affinity receptors that are presumably different to the cell surface activator.[97]

More recently, Sato and co-workers have identified and characterized a novel and uniquely transmembrane metalloproteinase (MT-MMP) that activates pro-MMP-2, which may explain its activation mechanism.[98] This, in a fashion similar to uPA, provides a mechanism whereby secreted MMP-2 is taken up on the cell membrane, and there, subsequently, becomes activated by MT-MMP. Inactivation and degradation may give rise to intracellular immunoreactivity. Such a hypothesis does not exclude the possibility that neoplastic cells may also synthesize pro-MMP-2 in certain circumstances, thus contributing to the imbalance with TIMP-2 in the pericellular stroma. Such a high level of complexity would permit directional control to the invasive cell and avoid the complete destruction of the immediate pericellular matrix, which would destablize the cell and prevent locomotion.[53] The expression of MT-MMP may occur in both tumour cells and in desmoplastic fibroblasts, and may correlate with vascular invasion.[99]

Protease degradation of ECM is also mediated by serine, cysteine and aspartyl proteases as well as MMPs. Oversecretion of members of each group has been documented in tumours including serine proteases such as trypsin, kallikrein, elastases and plasminogen activator,[100] cysteine proteases, e.g. cathepsin B,[101] the levels of which vary considerably in differing tissues, and aspartyl proteases, e.g. cathepsin D,[102] but in many if not all of these systems the enzyme is derived from an infiltrating population and direct involvement in tumour progression is debatable. Plasmin may degrade several components of ECM itself, but as well as autoactivating its proform it can activate some MMPs, and cathepsin B may activate uPA, so there is potential for more complex inter-relationships and cascades.[100] Plasminogen and uPA bind to co-localized specific cell surface receptors thus offering potential for highly controlled degradation at the epithelial-stromal interface and this activity is regulated by specific inhibitors.

Soluble factors and the tumour stroma

Transforming growth factor -β family

Prime among these are members of the transforming growth factor -β (TGF-β) family (which has at least 24 members showing high levels of conservation). TGF-βs have protean effects on epithelial and mesenchymal cells in vitro. Members of the TGF-β family have wide-ranging effects in controlling cellular differentiation and growth during embryogenesis, and while in general they appear to inhibit the growth and promote differentiation of epithelial cells and stimulate the growth of mesenchymal cells, the biological effects are dependent on many factors including the nature of the target cell and interaction with other growth factors and cytokines. One main mechanism appears to be via the regulation of the expression of molecules that mediate complex epithelial mesenchymal interactions.[103] TGF-β has been demonstrated to promote fibroblast proliferation, angiogenesis, synthesis of ECM components by mesenchymal fibroblasts and epithelial cells (such as tenascin, elastin, FN, collagens, laminin and also their cell-surface receptor molecules, including the integrin superfamily of heterodimeric ECM receptors), modulate macrophage and lymphocyte function, and variably affect tumour cell proliferation and differentiation. At high levels TGF-β may inhibit epithelial cell proliferation, but in low concentration the reverse effect may be seen. TGF-β may also directly or indirectly affect other stromal-modulating factors including up- or down-regulation of metalloproteinases[104] and other proteases, and synthesis of cytokines, although all of these effects are cell-type dependent.

Mature TGF-β_1 is a 25 kDa, 125 amino acid polypeptide homodimer, which is secreted as an inactive complex in association with the 40 kDa precursor (latency-associated protein) and a much larger binding protein. Activation results by cleavage of the N–terminal 50 amino acids, either by acidic microenvironment, proteases, binding to ECM or other as yet unknown mechanisms, and dissociates the complex to yield the active form. Activated TGF-β may then bind to one of at least three known receptors on the cell surface to mediate its effects. Types I and II TGF-β receptors are transmembrane serine/threonine kinases but the Type III receptor (betaglycan) may not have signalling activity[105] but could enhance presentation to the Type II receptor.[106] Adding to the complexity there are TGF-β_2 and TGF-β_3, which are differentially expressed in embryogenesis and neoplasia.[107] This simplified account of the mechanisms involved in this complex process involves synthesis, secretion, activation, ECM binding, and receptor expression, binding and signal transduction, so it is perhaps not surprising that observations on the topography of TGF-β expression are difficult to interpret because they may not reflect the biology of the system, which in a neoplastic environment may be aberrant in one or more of these steps. Resistance to TGF-β effects is not infrequently observed in neoplastic cells and may explain some aspects of tumour progression.[108,109]

Flanders and co-workers raised polyclonal antisera to the amino terminus of TGF-β_1, and two of these produced remarkably different patterns; one (LC 1 30) recognized intercellular TGF-β, the other (CC 1 30) recognized ECM-associated TGF-β. In basal cell carcinomas of the skin, we showed that intracellular TGF-β was confined mainly to stromal cells and occasional differentiating (?entrapped) keratinocytes, whereas the ECM-associated form was abundant in the stroma and would explain many of the biological features of basal cell carcinomas.[110] In situ hybridization studies show epithelial cells to be the primary source of TGF-β_1 mRNA, at least in ovarian and colorectal carcinomas, but active desmoplastic stroma in mammary and colorectal carcinomas has also been found to be rich in the ECM-associated form of TGF-β_1. Immunoreactive TGF-β has not been found in benign tumours e.g. of the thyroid gland, but is focally present, at least in the intracellular form, in a majority of thyroid carcinomas. It has been claimed that TGF-β immunoreactivity correlates with degree of differentiation of neoplastic cells but others have found that all active epithelia in the breast and prostate express intracellular TGF-β_1, and that there is little correlation with differentiation. Ultrastructural immunoelectron microscopy and immunohistochemical staining in prostate cancer suggests stromal cells are the source of TGF-β in desmoplastic stroma, which is a paradoxical observation reminiscent of the situation with MMP-2.[111,112]

The cellular growth response to TGF-β in vitro has been found to be dependent on both cell type and culture conditions, but there is in vitro evidence that maximal response is seen in well-differentiated cell lines. Furthermore, growth response may be different depending on local concentration of the growth factor.[109] This may be at least in part a consequence of alterations in the expression of ECM molecules and their receptors, which may enhance differentiation and inhibit proliferation. Such a mechanism is of central importance, up-regulating certain integrins in some cell types, down-regulating them in others[113] and also promoting the synthesis of ECM which may, in turn, act to generate specific spatiotemporal patterns of integrin distribution on the cell surface. ECM alterations per se might also further enhance the synthesis of TGF-β by certain epithelial cell types.[114] TGF-β_1 inhibitory elements are also found in some MMP gene promoters, which inhibit the transcription of some MMPs such as stromelysin.[115] TGF-β has been shown to upregulate MMP-2 in keratinocytes,[116] although the promoter of this gene lacks a TGF-β response element suggesting that this may be an indirect effect.[117] Furthermore, TGF-β may down-regulate MMP-1 gene expression by indirect mechanisms involving synthesis of Jun-B, which is a negative regulator of c-*jun*.[118]

Hepatocyte growth factor/scatter factor and trefoil peptides

Hepatocyte growth factor/scatter factor (HGF/SF) is an example of a substance which would in theory enhance the motile phenotype of neoplastic cells and promote invasion and metastasis, and is considered to be a product of mesenchymal cells[119] although mRNA for HGF/SF localizes to neoplastic cells in breast carcinoma and hyperplastic breast disease. In vitro, HGF/SF induces a dispersive effect on certain cell lines, which may be enhanced on certain substrates. HGF/SF also promotes proliferation of endothelial cells. However, the relevance of HGF/SF expression to tumour progression in vivo is still to be established. Other such factors are autocrine motility factor[120] and migration stimulatory factor[121] and the newly defined family of trefoil peptides, which have recently been shown to have similar dispersive effects.[122]

Tumour necrosis factor-α

Tumour necrosis factor-α (TNF-α) was originally considered to be primarily a product of tumour cells, and to have a number of biological activities and possibly systemic effects including cancer cachexia.[123] TNF-α receptors are predominantly expressed on the surface of neoplastic cells. Its production can induce tissue remodelling[124] and in ovarian cancers it may be able to promote tumorigenesis by increasing local vasculature,[125] having wide-ranging effects on endothelial cells including chemotaxis, proliferation, and angiogenesis.[125,126] TNF-α may alter adhesion events in the ascitic stage of the disease that contribute to implantation as demonstrated in previous studies on ovarian cancer xenografts.[127] TNF-α also acts directly as a growth factor for normal fibroblasts[128] that may contribute to the generation of tumour stroma.

TNF-α expression has been demonstrated in colorectal and ovarian carcinoma in vivo by Northern analysis of extracted mRNA, although in situ hybridization demonstrated that this expression appears to be confined to a minority of infiltrating macrophages and is not detectable in the neoplastic epithelial cells.[129,130] Critical examination revealed that even in epithelial areas much of the mRNA corresponded to an infiltrating mononuclear cell population. Recent data suggests that tumours themselves secrete chemotactic factors that attract macrophages into the tumour including members of the macrophage chemoattractant protein family[131] and IL-8. As already noted, tumour-associated macrophages may be the primary source of soluble factors, so misleading data may be obtained if only homogenates are examined or intratumoral subpopulations not defined.

TNF-α up-regulates gene expression of some metalloproteinases that are particularly associated with high invasive activity and metastatic potential, including stromelysin and MMP-2.[69] The role of TNF-α in cancer cachexia is still contentious although experiments in rat models have provided some evidence[132] that suggest a role in this complex wasting syndrome. TNF-α is capable of suppressing elastin synthesis by fibroblasts probably via jun/fos binding to an AP-1 site in the elastin gene promoter[133] and a similar mechanism operating in MMP-1 synthesis by fibroblasts.[134] TNF-α and IL-1 can also induce uPA synthesis in human endothelial cells,[135] and MMP and TIMP expression in endothelial cells.[136] IL-1b is able to enhance the amount of membrane-associated MMP-2 on human skin fibroblasts.[137] Cytokines such as TNF-α, IL-1α and interleukin-α (IFN-α) may also be relevant in modulating integrin expression.[130,138]

Other factors

There are many other factors that may affect the composition and function of the desmoplastic stroma. These include insulin-like growth factors[139] and FGF, which form a family including acidic and basic FGF as well as int 2 and hst 3, which appear to have certain tumorigenic properties when expressed in epithelial cells (possibly affecting secretion and binding to ECM). Basic FGF will induce expression of both uPA and PAI.[140] bFGF may also be a product of the non-neoplastic myoepithelial cell in the breast[141] and is present in BM extracts.[142] Association of bFGF with heparan sulphate appears to be necessary for activation of its receptor.[143] aFGF may enhance motility in fibroblasts and carcinoma cells and both aFGF and bFGF are overexpressed in pancreatic cells and synthesized by neoplastic cells and stromal fibroblasts.[144] PDGF may also be found in the tumour microenvironment of highly vascular tumors or may be synthesised de novo by desmoplastic fibroblasts and is also abundant in the epithelial-mesenchymal inductive environment of skin appendages and basal cell carcinomas.[145] It may also act by up-regulating stromelysin or interstitial collagenase.

Key points for clinical practice

- The consequences of stromal functional activity to tumour growth and progression should not be underestimated.
- Single parameter analysis (e.g. tumour homogenates, mRNA estimation, in vitro propagation of cell lines freed from stromal populations, or immunohistochemistry) may give misleading data when interpreted in isolation.
- The formation and structure of the extracellular environment dictates tumour growth and differentiation, via specific interactions at the cell surface. Manipulation of these factors may provide opportunities for regulating tumour growth.
- Early steps to regulate tumour growth now being taken with the development of synthetic MMP inhibitors or recombinant cytokine 'biotherapies', now a major growth area in modern oncology. Pathologists should be at the forefront in monitoring the localization and cytostatic/cytolytic effects of such agents.

REFERENCES

1 Hewitt RE, Powe DG, Carter GI, Turner DR. Desmoplasia and its relevance to colorectal tumour invasion. Int J Cancer 1993; 53: 62–69

2 Sage EH, Bornstein P. Extracellular proteins that modulate cell-matrix interactions. SPARC, tenascin, and thrombospondin. J Biol Chem 1991; 266: 14831–14834

3 Juliano RL, Haskill S. Signal transduction from the extracellular matrix. J Cell Biol 1993; 120: 577–585

4 Nathan C, Sporn M. Cytokines in context. J Cell Biol 1991; 113: 981–986

5 Howlett AR Bissell MJ. The influence of tissue microenvironment (stroma and extracellular matrix) on the development and function of mammary epithelium. Epithelial Cell Biol 1993; 2: 79–89

6 Slack JM. Embryonic induction. Mech Dev 1993; 41: 91–107

7 Adams JC Watt FM. Regulation of development and differentiation by the extracellular matrix. Development 1993; 117: 1183–1198

8 DeSimone DW. Adhesion and matrix in vertebrate development. Curr Opin Cell Biol 1994; 6: 747–751

9 Sakakura T. New aspects of stroma-parenchyma relations in mammary gland differentiation. Int Rev Cytol 1991; 125: 165–202

10 Bernfield, M, Banerjee S, Koda J, Rapraeger A. Remodelling of the basement membrane: morphogenesis and maturation. Basement membranes and cells movement. Ciba Foundation Symposium. London. London: Pitmans 1984: 179–196

11 Morikawa K, Walker SM, Nakajima M, Pathak S, Jessup JM, Fidler IJ. Influence of organ environment on the growth, selection, and metastasis of human colon carcinoma cells in nude mice. Cancer Res 1988; 48: 6863–6871

12 Price JE, Polyzos A, Zhang RD, Daniels LM. Tumorigenicity and metastasis of human breast carcinoma cell lines in nude mice. Cancer Res 1990; 50: 717–721

13 Fidler IJ, Wilmanns C, Staroselsky A, Radinsky R, Dong Z, Fan D. Modulation of tumor cell response to chemotherapy by the organ environment. Cancer Metastasis Rev 1994; 13: 209–222

14 Noel A, Nusgens B, Lapiere CH, Foidart JM. Interactions between tumoral MCF7 cells and fibroblasts on matrigel and purified laminin. Matrix 1993; 13: 267–273

15 Brouty Boye D, Mainguene C, Magnien V, Israel L, Beaupain R. Fibroblast-mediated differentiation in human breast carcinoma cells (MCF-7) grown as nodules in vitro. Int J Cancer 1994; 56: 731–735

16 Schuster U, Buttner R, Hofstadter F, Knuchel R. A heterologous in vitro coculture system to study interaction between human bladder cancer cells and fibroblasts. J Urol 1994; 151: 1707–1711

17 Nakanishi H, Oguri K, Takenaga K, Hosoda S, Okayama M. Differential fibrotic stromal responses of host tissue to low- and high-metastatic cloned Lewis lung carcinoma cells. Lab Invest 1994; 70: 324–332

18 Mackenzie I, Rittman G, Bohnert A, Breitkreutz D, Fusenig NE. Influence of connective tissues on the in vitro growth and differentiation of murine epidermis. Epithelial Cell Biol 1992; 2: 107–119

19 Fridman R, Kibbey MC, Royce LS, et al Enhanced tumor growth of both primary and established human and murine tumor cells in athymic mice after conjection with matrigel [see comments]. J Natl Cancer Inst 1991; 83: 769–774

20 Topley P, Jenkins DC, Jessup EA, Stables JN. Effect of reconstituted basement membrane components on the growth of a panel of human tumour cell lines in nude mice. Br J Cancer 1993; 67: 953–958

21 Olsen BR. New insights into the function of collagens from genetic analysis. Curr Opin Cell Biol 1995; 7: 720–727

22 Olsen BR, Ninomiya Y. Collagens. In: Kreis T, Vale R, eds. Guidebook to the extracellular matrix and adhesion proteins. Oxford: Oxford University Press, 1993: 32–47

23 McCarthy J, Turley EA. Effects of extracellular matrix components on cell locomotion. Crit Rev Oral Biol Med 1993; 4: 619–637

24 Rooney P, Kumar S. Inverse relationship between hyaluronan and collagens in development and angiogenesis. Differentiation 1993; 54: 1–9

25 Weber KT Sun Y, Katwa LC. Local regulation of extracellular matrix structure. Herz 1995; 20: 81–88

26 Mecham R.P. Elastin. In: Kries T, Vale R, eds Guidebook to the extracellular matrix and adhesion proteins. Oxford: Oxford University Press, 1993: 50–53

27 Fazio MJ, Mattei MG, Passage E et al Human elastin gene: new evidence for localization to the long arm of chromosome 7. Am J Hum Genet 1991; 48: 696–703

28 Foster K, Ferrell R, King Underwood L, et al Description of a dinucleotide repeat polymorphism in the human elastin gene and its use to confirm assignment of the gene to chromosome 7. Ann Hum Genet 1993; 57: 87–96

29 Parsons DF. Tumor cell interactions with stromal elastin and type I collagen: the consequences of specific adhesion and proteolysis. Tumour Biol 1993; 14: 137–143

30 Katchman SD, Hsu Wong S, Ledo I, Wu M, Uitto J. Transforming growth factor-beta up-regulates human elastin promoter activity in transgenic mice. Biochem Biophys Res Commun 1994; 203: 485–490

31 Reitamo S, Remitz A, Tamai K, Ledo I, Uitto J. Interleukin 10 up-regulates elastin gene expression in vivo and in vitro at the transcriptional level. Biochem J 1994; 302: 331–333

32 Rosenbloom J, Abrams WR, Mecham R. Extracellular matrix 4: the elastic fiber. FASEB J 1993; 7: 1208–1218

33 Colvin RB. Fibronectin in wound healing. In: Mosher DF, ed. Fibronectins. London: Academic Press, 1989; 213–254

34 Thiery J-P, Duband J-L, Dufour S, Savanger P, Imhof BA. Roles of fibronectins in embryogenesis. Fibronectins. In: Mosher DF, ed. London: Academic Press, 1989: 181–212

35 Potts JR, Campbell ID. Fibronectin structure and assembly. Curr Opin Cell Biol 1994; 6: 648–655

36 Fukai F, Iso T, Sekiguchi K, Miyatake N, Tsugita A, Katayama T. An amino-terminal fibronectin fragment stimulates the differentiation of ST-13 preadipocytes. Biochemistry 1993; 32: 5746–5751

37 Barkalow FJ, Schwarzbauer JE. Interactions between fibronectin and chondroitin sulfate are modulated by molecular context. J Biol Chem 1994; 269: 3957–3962

38 George EL, Georges Labouesse EN, Patel King RS, Rayburn H, Hynes RO. Defects in mesoderm, neural tube and vascular development in mouse embryos lacking fibronectin. Development 1993; 119: 1079–1091

39 Spring J, Beck K, Chiquet Ehrismann R. Two contrary functions of tenascin: dissection of the active sites by recombinant tenascin fragments. Cell 1989; 59: 325–334

40 Saga Y, Yagi T, Ikawa Y, Sakakura T, Aizawa S. Mice develop normally without tenascin. Genes Dev 1992; 6: 1821–1831

41 Lightner VA. Tenascin: does it play a role in epidermal morphogenesis and homeostasis? J Invest Dermatol 1994; 102: 273–277

42 Stamp GW. Tenascin distribution in basal cell carcinomas. J Pathol 1989; 159: 225–229

43 Koukoulis GK, Howeedy AA, Korhonen M, Virtanen I, Gould VE. Distribution of tenascin, cellular fibronectins and integrins in the normal, hyperplastic and neoplastic breast. J Submicrosc Cytol Pathol 1993; 25: 285–295

44 Fink TM, Jenne DE, Lichter P. The human vitronectin (complement S-protein) gene maps to the centromeric region of 17q. Hum Genet 1992; 88: 569–572

45 Cherny RC, Honan MA, Thiagarajan P. Site-directed mutagenesis of the arginine-glycine-aspartic acid in vitronectin abolishes cell adhesion. J Biol Chem 1993; 268: 9725–9729

46 Felding Habermann B, Cheresh DA. Vitronectin and its receptors. Curr Opin Cell Biol 1993; 5: 864–868

47 Albelda SM, Mette SA, Elder DE, et al Integrin distribution in malignant melanoma: association of the beta 3 subunit with tumor progression. Cancer Res 1990; 50: 6757–6764

48 Seftor RE, Seftor EA, Stetler Stevenson WG, Hendrix MJ. The 72 kDa type IV

collagenase is modulated via differential expression of alpha v beta 3 and alpha 5 beta 1 integrins during human melanoma cell invasion. Cancer Res 1993; 53: 3411–3415

49 Hardingham TE, Fosang AJ. Proteoglycans: many forms and many functions. FASEB J 1992; 6: 861–870

50 Murphy Ullrich JE, Schultz Cherry S, Hook M. Transforming growth factor-beta complexes with thrombospondin. Mol Biol Cell 1992; 3: 181–188

51 Taraboletti G, Belotti D, Giavazzi R. Thrombospondin modulates basic fibroblast growth factor activities on endothelial cells. Exs 1992; 61: 210–213

52 Simon AP, Kedinger M. Heterotypic cellular cooperation in gut morphogenesis and differentiation. Semin Cell Biol 1993; 4: 221–230

53 Liotta LA, Stetler-Stervenson WG. Tumor invasion and metastasis: an imbalance of positive and negative regulation. Cancer Res 1991; (Suppl) 51: 5054S

54 Stetler Stevenson WG, Liotta LA, Kleiner DE Jr. Extracellular matrix 6: role of matrix metalloproteinases in tumor invasion and metastasis. FASEB J 1993; 17: 1434–1441

55 Powell WC, Knox JD, Navre M, et al Expression of the metalloproteinase matrilysin in DU-145 cells increases their invasive potential in severe combined immunodeficient mice. Cancer Res 1993; 53: 417–422

56 Alvarez OA, Carmichael DF, DeClerck YA. Inhibition of collagenolytic activity and metastasis of tumor cells by a recombinant human tissue inhibitor of metalloproteinases. J Natl Cancer Inst 1990; 82: 589–595

57 Springman EB, Angleton EL, Birkedal Hansen H, Van Wart HE. Multiple modes of activation of latent human fibroblast collagenase: evidence for the role of a Cys73 active-site zinc complex in latency and a 'cysteine switch' mechanism for activation. Proc Natl Acad Sci USA 1990; 87: 364–368

58 Windsor LJ, Birkedal Hansen H, Birkedal Hansen B, Engler JA. An internal cysteine plays a role in the maintenance of the latency of human fibroblast collagenase. Biochemistry 1991; 30: 641–647

59 Chen LC, Noelken ME, Nagase H. Disruption of the cysteine-75 and zinc ion coordination is not sufficient to activate the precursor of human matrix metalloproteinase 3 (stromelysin 1). Biochemistry 1993; 32: 10289–10295

60 Girard MT, Matsubara M, Kublin C, Tessier MJ, Cintron C, Fini ME. Stromal fibroblasts synthesize collagenase and stromelysin during long-term tissue remodeling. J Cell Sci 1993; 104: 1001–1011

61 van den Brule FA, Engel J, Stetler Stevenson WG, Liu FT, Sobel ME, Castronovo V. Genes involved in tumor invasion and metastasis are differentially modulated by estradiol and progestin in human breast-cancer cells. Int J Cancer 1992; 52: 653–657

62 Murphy G, Cockett MI, Ward RV, Docherty AJ. Matrix metalloproteinase degradation of elastin, type IV collagen and proteoglycan. A quantitative comparison of the activities of 95 kDa and 72 kDa gelatinases, stromelysins-1 and -2 and punctuated metalloproteinase (PUMP). Biochem J 1991; 277: 277–279

63 Ogata Y, Pratta MA, Nagase H, Arner EC. Matrix metalloproteinase 9 (92-kDa gelatinase/type IV collagenase) is induced in rabbit articular chondrocytes by cotreatment with interleukin 1 beta and a protein kinase C activator. Exp Cell Res 1992; 201: 245–249

64 Nagase H, Ogata Y, Suzuki K, Enghild JJ, Salvesen G. Substrate specificities and activation mechanisms of matrix metalloproteinases. Biochem Soc Trans 1991; 19: 715–718

65 MacDonald NJ, Steeg PS. Molecular basis of tumour metastasis. Cancer Surv 1993; 16: 175–199

66 Engel J. Common structural motifs in proteins of the extracellular matrix. Curr Opin Cell Biol 1991; 3: 779–785

67 Wolf C, Rouyer N, Lutz Y, et al Stromelysin 3 belongs to a subgroup of proteinases expressed in breast carcinoma fibroblastic cells and possibly implicated in tumor progression. Proc Natl Acad Sci USA 1993; 90: 1843–1847

68 Ellis SM, Nabeshima K, Biswas C. Monoclonal antibody preparation and purification of a tumor cell collagenase-stimulatory factor. Cancer Res 1989; 49: 3385–3391

69 Ito A, Sato T, Iga T, Mori Y. Tumor necrosis factor bifunctionally regulates matrix metalloproteinases and tissue inhibitor of metalloproteinases (TIMP) production by human fibroblasts FEBS Lett 1990; 269: 93–95

70 Basset P, Wolf C, Chambon P. Expression of the stromelysin-3 gene in fibroblastic cells of invasive carcinomas of the breast and other human tissues: a review. Breast Cancer Res Treat 1993; 24: 185–193

71 Montgomery AM, De Clerck YA, Langley KE, Reisfeld RA, Mueller BM. Melanoma-mediated dissolution of extracellular matrix: contribution of urokinase-dependent and metalloproteinase-dependent proteolytic pathways. Cancer Res 1993; 53: 693–700

72 Okada Y, Morodomi T, Enghild JJ, et al Matrix metalloproteinase 2 from human rheumatoid synovial fibroblasts. Purification and activation of the precursor and enzymic properties. Eur J Biochem 1990; 194: 721–730

73 Murphy G, Nguyen Q, Cockett MI, et al Assessment of the role of the fibronectin-like domain of gelatinase A by analysis of a deletion mutant. J Biol Chem 1994; 269: 6632–6636

74 Garbisa S, Pozzatti R, Muschel RJ, et al Secretion of type IV collagenolytic protease and metastatic phenotype: induction by transfection with c-Ha-ras but not c-Ha-ras plus Ad2-E1a. Cancer Res 1987; 47: 1523–1528

75 Matrisian LM, McDonnell S, Miller DB, Navre M, Seftor EA, Hendrix MJ. The role of the matrix metalloproteinase stromelysin in the progression of squamous cell carcinomas. Am J Med Sci 1991; 302: 157–162

76 Hendrix MJ, Seftor EA, Grogan TM, et al Expression of type IV collagenase correlates with the invasion of human lymphoblastoid cell lines and pathogenesis in SCID mice. Mol Cell Probes 1992; 6: 59–65

77 Reponen P, Sahlberg C, Huhtala P, Hurskainen T, Thesleff I, Tryggvason K. Molecular cloning of murine 72-kDa type IV collagenase and its expression during mouse development. J Biol Chem 1992; 267: 7856–7862

78 Sato H, Kita M, Seiki M. v-Src activates the expression of 92-kDa type IV collagenase gene through the AP-1 site and the GT box homologous to retinoblastoma control elements. A mechanism regulating gene expression independent of that by inflammatory cytokines. J Biol Chem 1993; 268: 23460–23468

79 Azzam HS, Arand G, Lippman ME, Thompson EW. Association of MMP-2 activation potential with metastatic progression in human breast cancer cell lines independent of MMP-2 production. J Natl Cancer Inst 1993; 85: 1758–1764

80 Ciambrone GJ, McKeown Longo PJ. Vitronectin regulates the synthesis and localization of urokinase-type plasminogen activator in HT-1080 cells. J Biol Chem 1992; 267: 13617–13622

81 Shapiro SD, Griffin GL, Gilbert DJ, et al Molecular cloning, chromosomal localization, and bacterial expression of a murine macrophage metalloelastase. J Biol Chem 1992; 267: 4664–4671

82 Monteagudo C, Merino MJ, San Juan J, Liotta LA, Stetler-Stevenson WG. Immunohistochemical distribution of type IV collagenase in normal, benign, and malignant breast tissue. Am J Pathol 1990; 136: 585–592

83 Poulsom R, Pignatelli M, Steler-Stevenson W, et al Stromal expression of 72kDa type IV collagenase (MMP-2) and TIMP-2 mRNAs in colorectal neoplasia. J Pathol 1992; 167S: 150A

84 Campo E, Merino MJ, Liotta L, Neumann R, Stetler Stevenson W. Distribution of the 72-kd type IV collagenase in nonneoplastic and neoplastic thyroid tissue. Hum Pathol 1992; 23: 1395–401

85 Campo E, Merino MJ, Tavassoli FA, Charonis AS, Stetler Stevenson WG, Liotta LA. Evaluation of basement membrane components and the 72 kDa type IV collagenase in serious tumors of the ovary. Am J Surg Pathol 1992; 16: 500–507

86 Ura H, Bonfil RD, Reich R, et al Expression of type IV collagenase and procollagen

genes and its correlation with the tumorigenic, invasive, and metastatic abilities of oncogene-transformed human bronchial epithelial cells. Cancer Res 1989; 49: 4615–4621

87 Bonfil RD, Medina PA, Gomez DE, et al Expression of gelatinase/type IV collagenase in tumor necrosis correlates with cell detachment and tumor invasion. Clin Exp Metastasis 1992; 10: 211–220

88 Tryggvason K, Hoyhtya M, Pyke C. Type IV collagenases in invasive tumors. Breast Cancer Res Treat 1993; 24: 209–218

89 Brown PD, Levy AT, Margulies IM, Liotta LA, Stetler SW. Independent expression and cellular processing of Mr 72,000 type IV collagenase and interstitial collagenase in human tumorigenic cell lines. Cancer Res 1990; 50: 6184–6191

90 Poulsom R, Hanby AM, Pignatelli M, et al Expression of gelatinase A and TIMP-2 mRNAs in desmoplastic fibroblasts in both mammary carcinomas and basal cell carcinomas of the skin. J Clin Pathol 1993; 46: 429–436

91 Naylor MS, Stamp GW, D BD, Balkwill FR. Expression and activity of MMPs and their regulators in ovarian cancer. Int J Cancer 1994; 58: 50–56

92 Hewitt RE, Leach IH, Powe DG, Clark IM, Cawston TE, Turner DR. Distribution of collagenase and tissue inhibitor of metalloproteinases (TIMP) in colorectal tumours. Int J Cancer 1991; 49: 666–672

93 Noel AC, Polette M, Lewalle JM, et al Coordinate enhancement of gelatinase A mRNA and activity levels in human fibroblasts in response to breast-adenocarcinoma cells. Int J Cancer 1994; 56: 331–336

94 Monsky WL, Kelly T, Lin CY, et al Binding and localization of M(r) 72,000 matrix metalloproteinase at cell surface invadopodia. Cancer Res 1993; 53: 3159–3164

95 Afzal S, Lalani E-N, Baker T, et al Membrane localisation of activated gelatinases in adenocarcinomas. J Pathol 1994; 172: 101A

96 Afzal S, Lalani E-N, Foulkes W, et al Activated matrix metalloproteinase-2 (MMP-2) expression and synthetic MMP-2 inhibitor binding in ovarian carcinomas and tumour cell lines. Lab Invest 1996; 74: in press

97 Emonard HP, Remacle AG, Noel AC, Grimaud JA, WG S-S. Foidart JM. Tumor cell surface-associated binding site for the M(r) 72,000 type IV collagenase. Cancer Res 1992; 52: 5845–5848

98 Sato H, Takino T, Okada Y, et al A matrix metalloproteinase expressed on the surface of invasive tumour cells. Nature 1994; 370: 61–65

99 Nomura H, Sato H, Seiki M, Mai M, Okada Y. Expression of membrane-type matrix metalloproteinase in human gastric carcinomas. Cancer Res 1995; 55: 3263–3266

100 Duffy MJ. The role of proteolytic enzymes in cancer invasion and metastasis. Clin Exp Metastasis 1992; 10: 145–155

101 Keppler D, Abrahamson M, Sordat B. Secretion of cathepsin B and tumour invasion. Biochem Soc Trans 1994; 22: 43–94

102 Ravdin PM. Evaluation of cathepsin D as a prognostic factor in breast cancer. Breast Cancer Res Treat 1993; 24: 219–226

103 Haralson MA. Extracellular matrix and growth factors: an integrated interplay controlling tissue repair and progression to disease (editorial comment). Lab Invest 1993; 69: 369–372

104 Matrisian LM, Ganser GL, Kerr LD, Pelton RW, Wood LD, Negative regulation of gene expression by TGF-beta. Mol Reprod Dev 1992; 32: 111–120

105 Wang XF, Lin HY, Ng EE, Downward J, Lodish HF, Weinberg RA. Expression cloning and characterization of the TGF-beta type III receptor. Cell 1991; 67: 797–805

106 Lopez CF, Wrana JL, Massague J. Betaglycan presents ligand to the TGF beta signaling receptor. Cell 1993; 73: 1435–1444

107 Pelton RW, Johnson MD, Perkett EA, Gold LI, Moses HL. Expression of transforming growth factor-beta 1, -beta 2, and -beta 3 mRNA and protein in the murine lung. Am J Respir Cell Mol Biol 1991; 5: 522–530

108 Filmus J, Kerbel RS. Development of resistance mechanisms to the growth-inhibitory effects of transforming growth factor-beta during tumor progression. Curr Opin Oncol 1993; 5: 123–129

109 Newman MJ. Transforming growth factor beta and the cell surface in tumor progression. Cancer Metastasis Rev 1993; 12: 239–254

110 Flanders KC, Thompson NL, Cissel DS, et al Transforming growth factor-beta 1: histochemical localization with antibodies to different epitopes. J Cell Biol 1989; 108: 653–660

111 Mizoi et al 1993

112 Muir et al 1994

113 Heino et al 1989

114 Streuli CH. Extracellular matrix and gene expression in mammary epithelium. Semin Cell Biol 1993; 4: 203–212

115 Matrisian LM, Hogan BL. Growth factor-regulated proteases and extracellular matrix remodeling during mammalian development. Curr Top Dev Biol 1990; 24: 219–259

116 Salo T, Lyons JG, Rahemtulla F, Birkedal Hansen H, Larjava H. Transforming growth factor-beta 1 up-regulates type IV collagenase expression in cultured human keratinocytes. J Biol Chem 1991; 266: 11436–11441

117 Huhtala P, Tuuttila A, Chow LT, Lohi J, Keski OJ, Tryggvason K. Complete structure of the human gene for 92-kDa type IV collagenase. Divergent regulation of expression for the 92- and 72-kilodalton enzyme genes in HT-1080 cells. J Biol Chem 1991; 266: 16485–16490

118 Twining S. Regulation of proteolytic activity in tissues. Crit Rev Biochem Mol Biol 1993; 315–383

119 Gherardi E, Sharpe M, Lane K, Sirulnik A, Stoker M. Hepatocyte growth factor/scatter factor (HGF/SF), the c-met receptor and the behaviour of epithelial cells. Symp Soc Exp Biol 1993; 47: 163–181

120 Nabi IR, Watanabe H, Raz A. Autocrine motility factor and its receptor: role in cell locomotion and metastasis. Cancer Metastasis Rev 1992; 11: 5–20

121 Schor SL, Schor AM. Foetal-to-adult transitions in fibroblast phenotype: their possible relevance to the pathogenesis of cancer. J Cell Sci 1987; (Suppl) 8: 165–180

122 Williams R, Stamp GWH, Gilbert C, Pignatelli M, Lalani E-N. pS2 transfection of murine adenocarcinoma cell line (410.4) enhances dispersed growth. J Cell Sci 1996; 109: 63–71

123 Fiers W. Tumor necrosis factor. Characterization at the molecular, cellular and in vivo level. FEBS Lett 1991; 285: 199–212

124 Dvorak H. Tumors: Wounds that do not heal. N Engl J Med 1986; 1680–1659

125 Frater Schroder M, Risau W, Hallmann R, Gautschi P, Bohlen P. Tumor necrosis factor type alpha, a potent inhibitor of endothelial cell growth in vitro, is angiogenic in vivo. Proc Natl Acad Sci USA 1987; 84: 5277–5281

126 Gerlach H, Lieberman H, Bach R, Godman G, Brett J, Stern D. Enhanced responsiveness of endothelium in the growing/motile state to tumor necrosis factor/cachectin [published erratum appears in J Exp Med 1989 Nov 1; 170(5): 1793]. J Exp Med 1989; 170: 913–931

127 Malik ST, Griffin DB, Fiers W, Balkwill FR. Paradoxical effects of tumour necrosis factor in experimental ovarian cancer. Int J Cancer 1989; 44: 918–925

128 Sugarman BJ, Aggarwal BB, Hass PE, Figari IS, Palladino MA Jr, Shepard HM. Recombinant human tumor necrosis factor-alpha: effects on proliferation of normal and transformed cells in vitro. Science 1985; 230: 943–945

129 Naylor MS, Stamp GW, Balkwill FR. Investigation of cytokine gene expression in human colorectal cancer. Cancer Res 1990; 50: 4436–4440

130 Naylor MS, Stamp GW, Foulkes WD, Eccles D, Balkwill FR. Tumor necrosis factor and its receptors in human ovarian cancer. Potential role in disease progression. J Clin Invest 1993; 91: 2194–2206

131 Negus RP, Stamp GW, Relf MG, et al The detection and localization of monocyte

chemoattractant protein-1 (MCP-1) in human ovarian cancer. J Clin Invest 1995; 95: 2391–2396

132 G, Darling Fraker DL, Jensen JC, Gorschboth CM, Norton JA. Cachectic effects of recombinant human tumor necrosis factor in rats. Cancer Res 1990; 50: 4008–4013

133 Kahari VM, Chen YQ, Bashir MM, Rosenbloom J, Uitto J. Tumor necrosis factor-alpha down-regulates human elastin gene expression. Evidence for the role of AP-1 in the suppression of promoter activity. J Biol Chem 1992; 267: 26134–26141

134 Woessner JF Jr. Introduction to serial reviews: the extracellular matrix. FASEB J 1993; 7: 735–736

135 van Hinsbergh VW, van den Berg EA, Fiers W, Dooijewaard G. Tumor necrosis factor induces the production of urokinase-type plasminogen activator by human endothelial cells. Blood 1990; 75: 1991–1998

136 Hanemaaijer R, Koolwijk P, Le Clercq L, De Vree WJ, van Hinsbergh VW. Regulation of matrix metalloproteinase expression in human vein and microvascular endothelial cells. Effects of tumour necrosis factor alpha, interleukin 1 and phorbol ester. Biochem J 1993; 296: 803–809

137 Beranger, JY, Godeau G, Frances C, Robert L, Hornebeck W. Presence of gelatinase A and metalloelastase type protease at the plasma membrane of human skin fibroblasts. Influence of cytokines and growth factors on cell-associated metalloendopeptidase levels. Cell Biol Int 1994; 18: 715–722

138 Santala P, Heino J. Regulation of integrin-type cell adhesion receptors by cytokines. J Biol Chem 1991; 266: 23505–23509

139 Singh P, Rubin N. Insulinlike growth factors and binding proteins in colon cancer. Gastroenterology 1993; 105: 1218–1237

140 Keski OJ, Koli K, Lohi J, Laiho M. Growth factors in the regulation of plasminogen-plasmin system in tumor cells. Semin Thromb Hemost 1991; 17: 231–239

141 Ke Y, Fernig DG, Wilkinson MC, et al The expression of basic fibroblast growth factor and its receptor in cell lines derived from normal human mammary gland and a benign mammary lesion. J Cell Sci 1993;

142 Taub M, Wang Y, Szczesny TM, Kleinman HK. Epidermal growth factor or transforming growth factor alpha is required for kidney tubulogenesis in matrigel cultures in serum-free medium. Proc Natl Acad Sci USA 1990; 87: 4002–4006

143 Yayon A, Klagsbrun M, Esko JD, Leder P, Ornitz DM. Cell surface, heparin-like molecules are required for binding of basic fibroblast growth factor to its high affinity receptor. Cell 1991; 64: 841–848

144 Yamanaka Y, Friess H, Buchler M, et al Overexpression of acidic and basic fibroblast growth factors in human pancreatic cancer correlates with advanced tumor stage. Cancer Res 1993; 53: 5289–5296

145 Ponten F, Ren Z, Nister M, Westermark B, Ponten J. Epithelial-stromal interactions in basal cell cancer: the PDGF system. J Invest Dermatol 1994; 102: 304–309

8

Current concepts and misconceptions in hypertension

G. B. M. Lindop   A. G. Jardine

Hypertension research is at the forefront of several areas of biomedical science. Recent developments in genetics and in cell biology have identified novel pathogenetic mechanisms and it is now appropriate to re-evaluate classical observations on the pathology of hypertension. Many advances in research published in clinical and in basic science journals have not yet reached standard pathology texts; while other important observations in the older literature have been either ignored or misinterpreted. The purpose of this chapter is to update pathologists on current thought in the pathogenesis of hypertension and its complications, focusing on the main target tissues – the systemic arteries, the heart and the kidney.

Essential hypertension

Arteries

Growth and remodelling

The earliest effect of hypertension is medial hypertrophy in small arteries and arterioles – the 'resistance vessels'. The resulting increase in thickness of the vessel wall relative to the lamina diameter (wall-to-lumen ratio) restores the tension per unit area of media;[1] unfortunately an increase in wall-to-lumen ratio also confers increased contraction in response to a given pressor stimulus.[1,2] The simple structural change of increased wall-to-lumen ratio accounts for this phenomenon;[3,4] medial thickening in resistance arteries, traditionally given scant attention by pathologists, is therefore 'the vascular amplifier' that is crucial to the pathogenesis of hypertension.

Theoretically, increased wall-to-lumen ratio could have three causes:

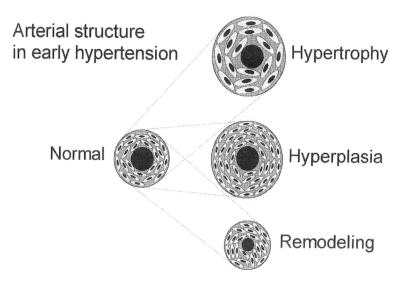

Fig. 8.1 Arterial structure in early hypertension

hypertrophy of existing smooth muscle cells, smooth muscle cell proliferation (hyperplasia) or even rearrangement of existing smooth muscle cells around a smaller lumen (remodelling) all of which would have a similar effect (Fig. 8.1).[5] By analogy with known biological responses of smooth muscle cells, both hypertrophy and hyperplasia probably occur, and to accommodate this, some degree of cellular rearrangement (remodelling) is required; however, the relative contribution of each remains unresolved and is still debated. In spontaneously hypertensive rats aortic smooth muscle cells become hypertrophied and polyploid, while proliferation contributes more to medial hypertrophy in resistance vessels; however, in human essential hypertension, resistance vessel remodelling may predominate over growth.[6]

Contraction and growth

It is now realized that circulating vasoactive agents and growth factors may have dual actions: first, most classical vasoconstrictors such as angiotensin II (Ang II) tend to promote vascular smooth muscle cell growth;[7] and second, circulating classical growth factors, such as platelet derived growth factor, are vasoconstrictors.[8] Both vasoconstrictors and growth factors can therefore increase blood pressure either directly, by vasoconstriction, or indirectly, by promoting growth of vascular smooth muscle, thereby adding a 'humoral amplifier' to the mechanical vascular amplifier (Fig. 8.2); as an example, the pathways by which Ang II may link contraction and growth

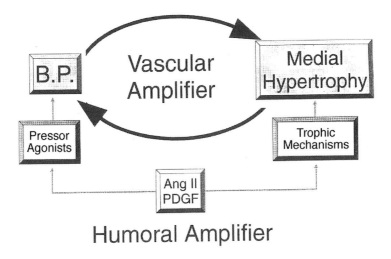

Fig. 8.2 Humoral Amplifier

have been reviewed.[7,9,10] Conversely, vasodilators such as nitric oxide tend to inhibit cell growth.[11] Vasodilators may therefore reduce pressure either directly by vasodilatation or, in the long term, via inhibition of vascular smooth muscle cell growth.

Vascular endothelium, smooth muscle cells and platelets all produce vasoactive agents and growth factors that affect vascular tone and potentially also structure.[12,13] Some of these agents were first investigated in the pathogenesis of atherosclerosis, where vascular smooth muscle cell growth and matrix production also occur. The hypothesis currently under active investigation is that vessel structure is modulated by products synthesized in the vessel wall as well as by circulating vasoactive agents.[13] The endothelium now emerges as a key player in controlling both vascular tone and structure. Therefore, in the short term, vascular tone is controlled by neuro-humoral influences, but in the long term, vessel structure is also modulated by responses to haemodynamic stimuli such as flow and pressure: the endothelium senses the former and the smooth muscle cells respond to the latter and to signals from the endothelial cells.[13-15] A list of candidate pathogenetic factors in the pathogenesis of hypertension now includes some agents that are generated in the vessel wall (Table 8.1). Their role in hypertension remains to be established; reviews of how they may interact and influence vessel structure are given.[10,13,16-18]

Arteriosclerosis

Medial hypertrophy is followed by hypertensive arteriosclerosis. Arteriosclerosis includes 'hyaline' arteriolosclerosis, which affects mainly arterioles,

Table 8.1 Vessel wall-generated candidate pathogenetic factors in hypertension

Cell type	Growth promoter	Growth inhibitor
Endothelial cell	PDGF FGF CSF IL-1 TGF-α TGF-β Endothelin Ang II TNF-α	PGI$_2$ No TGF-β IL-1 Heparinoids No
Smooth muscle cell	EGF FGF TGF-β IL-1 TNF-α PDGF IGF-1	No IL-1 TGF-β

Ang II, angiotensin II; CSF, cerebrospinal Fluid; EGF; FGF, fibronection growth factor; IGF-1; insulin-like growth factor-1; IL-1; interleukin-1; PDGF; platelet-derived growth factor; PGI$_2$, prostacyclin; TGF-α, transforming growth factor-α; TGF-β, transforming growth factor-β; TNF-α, tumour necrosis factor-α.

and arteriosclerosis, which affects the larger vessels in the rest of the arterial tree. Both biopsy[19] and autopsy[20] studies may fail to reveal any arterial lesions in hypertensive subjects, suggesting that arteriosclerosis develops slowly over many years. It appears to be identical to age-related arteriosclerosis.[21,22]

Hyaline is restricted to arterioles and the smallest arteries. There is considerable variation in tissue susceptibility; arterioles in the spleen, kidney, gut, retina and brain being worst affected while those in skeletal muscle, skin and the heart are usually spared.[23,24] In the kidney, the afferent arterioles and the terminal radial (interlobular) arteries are predominately affected.[25–27]

Hyaline is composed of accumulated proteins and lipid derived from the blood (plasmatic vasculosis) as well as proteins synthesized by vascular smooth muscle cells; its histochemical reactions[23] and ultrastructure[26] have been reviewed. More recent studies implicate arterial glycosaminoglycans in its pathogenesis. Hyaluronic acid molecules have a non-specific affinity for C3b component of complement, which then in turn binds immunoglobulin M (IgM) and other complement components.[28] This process may be only one of many mechanisms operating to cause slow retention of plasma proteins that pass through the vessel wall. Because animal models of diabetes and hypertension do not form hyaline (personal observations), other aspects of its pathogenesis remain uninvestigated.

In the brain, heart and kidneys, autoregulation ensures maintenance of constant flow over a wide range of pressure. In hypertension the autoregulatory curve is shifted to the right,[29] probably because of loss of compliance in the arterial tree caused by arteriosclerosis (Fig. 8.3). The susceptibility of the elderly to hypotension and shock is well known, and overtreatment of

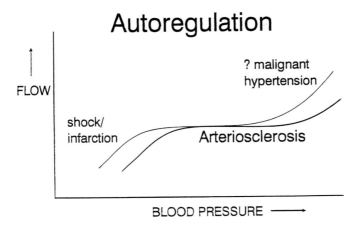

Fig. 8.3 Autoregulation

hypertension in the elderly may precipitate boundary (watershed) zone cerebral infarction owing to perfusion failure.[30] On the other hand, arteriosclerosis probably enables some elderly patients to tolerate high levels of blood pressure.

Heart – left ventricular hypertrophy

Once regarded as a beneficial compensatory response, left ventricular hypertrophy (LVH) is now viewed in a new light.[31,32] When severe, LVH has several drawbacks: larger cardiac myocytes have a greater diffusion distance for oxygen to reach their centre; increased myocardial stiffness caused both by myocyte hypertrophy and by accompanying interstitial fibrosis impairs diastolic relaxation and coronary artery filling; and, finally, hypertension predisposes to coronary atheroma. LVH is associated with a threefold increase in coronary artery disease and is an independent risk factor,[33] which further compromises coronary flow reserve and oxygen delivery. Clinical evidence of myocardial ischaemia is shown by the propensity of patients with LVF to develop angina with increased levels of lactate in coronary sinus blood at rest, even in the absence of coronary artery atheroma.[31] Ischaemia may account for their high incidence of ventricular arrhythmias and sudden death in patients with LVH.[31,32]

For a given rise in blood pressure, the degree of LVH varies; some patients with modest increments in pressure develop considerable ventricular hypertrophy. Genetic variation is likely to underlie this observation. Genes controlling the activity of the renin angiotensin system are currently under intense investigation because Ang. II is both a potent pressor hormone and promotor of cardiac as well as smooth muscle cell growth.[31]

Recently, 'functional' variants (polymorphisms) in the gene for angiotensin converting enzyme (ACE) have been identified. A deletion polymorphism in intron 16 of the ACE gene that leads to increased ACE activity is also associated with LVH in some studies,[34–36] although not with hypertension. Intriguingly, in some cases of LVH the hypertrophy may be asymmetrical.[37] Although reminiscent of hypertrophic cardiomyopathy, detailed pathological studies have not been reported and it is uncertain whether myocyte disarray, regarded as the diagnostic stigma of this condition,[38] is present. In hypertrophic cardiomyopathy there are diagnostic mutations in contractile protein genes;[38] molecular genetic studies will reveal whether hypertension may unmask a tendency to hypertrophic cardiomyopathy.

Kidney

It is a myth that essential hypertension gives rise to the 'finely granular kidney'. The best autopsy study included 420 cases of well-documented established hypertension and showed clearly that only half had granular kidneys.[20] There is no correlation with arteriosclerosis or with hyaline arteriolosclerosis.[20,39] The presence of contracted kidneys with small superficial scars correlates better with ulcerated aortic atheroma proximal to the renal arteries.[20,39] Ulcerated atheromatous plaques shed their contents and platelet emboli arise from their surface. Although most of this material is histologically invisible, careful autopsy examination reveals microscopically visible cholesterol emboli in up to 5% of elderly subjects and in 15–30% with aortic atheroma and aneurysms.[40] Severe athero-embolism can cause acute renal failure, malignant hypertension, and a vasculitis-like clinical syndrome.[40,41] Therefore, atheroembolism, rather than arteriosclerosis or hypertension per se, emerges as the prime candidate for causing superficial cortical scarring of the kidney – 'benign nephrosclerosis'.[39]

It is arguable whether mild to moderate hypertension causes renal impairment. Only severe essential hypertension causes histological changes in the kidney that lead to nephrosclerosis and progressive renal failure. Perhaps owing to effective treatment, end-stage renal failure caused by hypertensive nephrosclerosis is increasingly uncommon in developed countries; a possible exception being African-American patients.[42] In end-stage kidneys it is often difficult to establish whether renal damage is caused by severe essential hypertension or whether hypertension has supervened upon a primary glomerular disease.[42]

Glomerular hyperfiltration

The role of hypertension in progression of primary renal disease is now well established. When nephrons become fewer, renal vascular resistance rises, but glomerular filtration rate is preserved. This implies vasoconstriction of the glomerular efferent arterioles and increased glomerular filtration in the remaining nephrons. Theoretically, this pressure-dependent glomerular hyperfiltration with increased passage of macromolecules into the glomerular mesangium could lead to glomerulosclerosis.[43] In support of this idea, the pathological stigma of glomerular hypertension, focal and segmental glomerulosclerosis, complicates diseases associated with diminished nephron number; the immature kidney seems especially susceptible.[44,45] Rodent models involving surgical removal of five-sixths of the renal tissue lead to glomerulosclerosis and end-stage renal failure.[46,47] However, careful follow-up of kidney donors shows no increase in risk of renal failure in a solitary kidney suggesting that nephrectomy (or loss of half of the normal nephron number) does not reach the threshold for glomerular damage caused by hyperfiltration in adults.

As hypertension aggravates glomerulosclerosis, the role of growth factors and vasoactive agents in both conditions is under active investigation; progress has been recently reviewed.[48] The beneficial effect of ACE inhibitors on the progression of some forms of glomerulosclerosis implicates the renin-angiotensin system.[49] However, because these drugs also reduce glomerular capillary pressure it remains uncertain whether these agents act predominantly on glomerular haemodynamics or on cell growth. Glomerulosclerosis is caused by cell growth and migration followed by matrix production. Regardless of whether these processes act predominantly by locally generated or circulating humoral agents, or by haemodynamic factors such as hyperfiltration, or by a combination of both, hypertension remains the single most important risk factor in the progression of glomerular diseases in humans.[50]

Malignant hypertension

In developed countries malignant hypertension has become uncommon.[51] This is not universal; a notable exception is the susceptibility of the black races.[52] Once commoner in the young adults, in whom renal disease and untreated essential hypertension[53,54] are the most important predisposing factors, malignant hypertension is now relatively more common in the elderly population in whom atherosclerotic renovascular disease is an increasing problem.[55]

Arteries

The cerebral arteries on the surface of the brain have been examined during an acute rise in pressure following graded injections of Ang II.[56] The first response is transient vasoconstriction. This is followed by segments of forced dilatation as resistance arteries begin to fail. Finally, more generalized dilatation spreads distally along the vessel as autoregulation is overcome, and breakdown of the blood–brain barrier with tissue damage occurs as flow increases (Fig. 8.4). Tracer studies show that plasma penetrates into the dilated segments of the artery giving rise to the lesions of plasmatic vasculosis/fibrinoid necrosis familiar to pathologists.[57] These processes[58] have

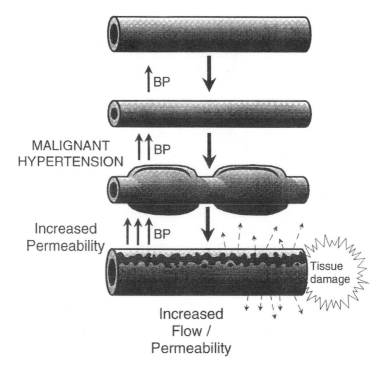

Fig. 8.4 Malignant hypertension

been studied mainly in the easily visualized cerebral and mesenteric arteries but there is some evidence that similar changes occur in renal resistance vessels.[59]

These arterial lesions simply indicate accumulation of plasma in the vessel wall, probably caused by endothelial damage. In hypertension it is pressure induced, with the rate of rise being more important than the absolute height. There is no dividing line between lesions best termed plasmatic vasculosis and those of fibrinoid necrosis; but confusion is avoided by reserving the term 'fibrinoid necrosis' for those lesions in which there is histological evidence of cellular necrosis. Although the cause of smooth muscle cell necrosis has never been established, it clearly indicates severe vascular damage as does penetration of red blood corpuscles into the vessel wall. Arterial fibrinoid necrosis is the hallmark of malignant phase hypertension, but may not be found in a renal biopsy in cases of clinical malignant hypertension when in the later stages intimal proliferation may predominate.[60]

Kidney

Malignant hypertension causes a previously normal kidney to become enlarged, oedematous and may have tiny 'flea bite' haemorrhages.[54] The minority of glomeruli are affected histologically.[55] Micro-injection studies indicate that acute vascular damage in the renal resistance vessels may be similar to experimentally induced lesions in the cerebral and mesenteric arteries.[59] This suggests that failure of autoregulation in individual afferent arterioles transmits pressure to its glomerulus. This accounts for the patchy nature of glomerular involvement. The commonest lesion is thickening of capillary walls owing to accumulation of fluid, probably the glomerular equivalent of plasmatic vasculosis of the afferent arterioles. A more severe lesion is focal fibrinoid necrosis of the glomerular tuft, which also corresponds to and may be continuous with the same lesion in the afferent arteriole, implying the same pathogenesis. Rarer lesions, once called 'blood cysts' are simply aneurysms of glomerular capillaries.[55] So-called focal 'infarction' of the glomerular tuft probably represents a combination of the above spectrum of lesions.

The transmission of raised pressure to the glomerular tuft accounts for all of the observed lesions and probably gives rise to the proteinuria and haematuria that are associated with malignant hypertension. Endothelial damage sometimes causes intravascular coagulation and microangiopathic haemolytic anaemia.[61] Therefore, individual nephrons may be subjected to hyperperfusion, while others become ischaemic owing to intravascular coagulation and, later, to intimal proliferation. Focal ischaemia contributes to the high levels of renin and to hypertrophy of the juxtaglomerular apparatus which are often, but not always, found in malignant hypertension.[62] The presence of arterial lesions led to the presumption that all downstream damage must be ischaemic in aetiology. While true in the endstage this has led generations of pathologists to come to the erroneous conclusion that the early renal lesions in malignant hypertension were also ischaemic in origin. Examination of the experimental evidence suggests the reverse.

Effects of treatment

This is strangely logical: lowering blood pressure reduces the complications that are most directly related to pressure, and has less effect on those caused by atheroma and thrombosis. The most important beneficial effects are prevention of heart failure, once the major cause of death in hypertensive patients, and reduced incidence of haemorrhagic stroke. Malignant hypertension is now readily treated; death is now uncommon in developed countries and the development of end-stage renal failure is largely dependent on the degree of renal insufficiency at presentation.[50] It is well established that treatment of severe hypertension is beneficial.[63] Disappointingly, but not surprisingly, treatment of mild to moderate hypertension does not lower the incidence of the complications of atheroma: namely, myocardial infarction, the commonest cause of death in hypertensive patients today.[63,64] The incidence of stroke is probably reduced but some analyses of the many clinical trials take a more sanguine view[65] than others.[66] Unfortunately, most trials do not distinguish between cerebral infarcts, which should not be closely linked to pressure, and haemorrhagic stroke which should.

Blood pressure can now be reduced effectively by a variety of drugs, alone, or in combination. Inhibitors of the renin-angiotensin system have rendered 'drug-resistant hypertension' uncommon. In the clinical trials treatment has probably been given too late to reverse or arrest atheroma in the target organs; although failure to target mechanisms common to the development of both atheroma and hypertension is an alternative hypothesis. The quest is now to discover which agents are most effective in preventing end-organ damage and in prolonging survival.

The future

Genes and growth in hypertension

In hypertension, cardiovascular hypertrophy is now seen as a potential cause or as well as a consequence of elevated pressure. The epidemiological observation that low birth weight infants who exhibit exaggerated 'catch-up' growth in early life also have higher blood pressures in childhood and in adulthood[67,68] has suggested that a generalized disorder of early growth may influence adult blood pressure. This fascinating observation fits with other findings that relate growth to hypertension.[10] Experimental studies suggest strongly that the developing renin-angiotensin system influences adult blood pressure, as blockade of its action in early life lowers adult blood pressure.[69,70] Although the mechanisms remain to be established, these important observations have exciting implications for potential therapeutic intervention.

Hypertension is probably inherited as a polygenic characteristic. Linkage analysis studies in essential hypertension are beginning to identify candidate genes. Angiotensinogen is a determinant of Ang II production and two large population studies have linked polymorphic markers in the gene for angiotensinogen with essential hypertension.[71,72] Polymorphisms in the ACE gene give rise to variation in the conversion of Ang I to Ang II and have been linked to a variety of disorders associated with cardiovascular growth[34-36] and to variation in the rate of progression of glomerulonephritis;[73] although this area remains controversial owing to insufficient sample size in some of the studies, other similar genetic associations will be revealed in the near future.

Finally, a remarkable success has been the elucidation of the genetic basis of a rare autosomal dominant form of hypertension – 'glucocorticoid remediable' or 'dexamethasone suppressible' hyperaldosteronism. This disorder presents with a previously enigmatic form of Conn's syndrome caused by hyperplasia of the zona glomerulosa rather than by an adenoma. The biochemical and clinical features are similar to but less severe than those of classical Conn's syndrome. A chromosomal translocation causes glucocorticoid response elements to become linked to the gene for aldosterone synthase.[74] Glucocorticoids then increase aldosterone production and cause hypertrophy of the zona glomerulosa. As the same genetic abnormality gives rise to differing clinical features, there must be differences in the expression of other genes which will, in turn, become candidate genes for the aetiology of essential hypertension.

Therapeutic approaches

The height and/or the rate of rise in blood pressure was once paramount in governing the outcome of hypertension. Modern treatment and good control of pressure ensures that end-organ changes such as LVH and renal impairment are now more important than blood pressure per se. Increasingly, genetic factors are implicated in the development of end-organ damage, and future drugs will specifically target cardiovascular and renal damage. Genetic testing will identify high-risk patients in whom earlier intervention to prevent end-organ damage may be indicated, perhaps even before 'clinically significant hypertension' occurs.

Conclusion

This is an exciting time in hypertension research. For almost a century, since the invention of the sphygmomanometer, research has been directed to the causes and consequences of elevated blood pressure. In the light of recent understanding of molecular genetics and the cell biology of the vessel wall, we must take a wider view of hypertension: pressure is not the only problem.

REFERENCES

1 Mulvaney MJ, Hansen PK, Aalkjaer C. Direct evidence that the greater contractility of resistance vessels in spontaneously hypertensive rats is associated with a narrowed lumen, a thickened media, and an increased number of smooth muscle cell layers. Circulat Res 1978; 43: 854–864

2 Owens GK, Schwartz SM, McCanna M. Evaluation of medial hypertrophy in resistance vessels of spontaneously hypertensive rats. Hypertension 1987; 11: 198–207

3 Folkow B. Physiological aspects of primary hypertension. Physiol Rev 1982; 62: 347–504

4 Lever AF. Slow pressor mechanisms in hypertension: A role for hypertrophy of resistance vessels? J Hyperten 1986; 4: 515–524

5 Owens GK. Differential effect of antihypertensive drug therapy on vascular smooth muscle cell hypertrophy, hyperploidy, and hyperplasia in the spontaneously hypertensive rat. Circulat Res 1985; 56: 525–536

6 Heagerty AM, Aalkjaer C, Bund SJ, Korsgaard N, Mulvany MJ. Small artery structure in hypertension. Dual processes of remodeling and growth. Hypertension 1993; 21: 391–397

7 Dzau VJ, Gibbons GH, Pratt R. Molecular mechanisms of vascular renin-angiotensin system in myointimal hyperplasia. Hypertension 1991; 18 (Supp.II): 100–105

8 Berk BC, Alexander RW, Brock TA, Gimbrone MA, Webb RC. Vasoconstriction: a new activity for platelet derived growth factor. Science 1986; 232: 87–90

9 Naftilan AJ. Role of angiotensin II in vascular smooth muscle cell growth. J Cardiovasc Pharmacol 1992; 20(Suppl.1): S37–S40

10 Lever AF, Harrap AB. Essential hypertension: a disorder of growth with origins in childhood? J Hyperten 1992; 10: 101–120

11 Moncada S, Higgs A. The L-anginine-nitric oxide pathway. N Eng J Med 1993; 329: 2002–2012

12 Ross R. The pathogenesis of atherosclerosis: a perspective for the 1990s. Nature 1993; 362: 801–809.

13 Gibbons GH, Dzau VJ. The emerging concept of vascular remodelling. N Engl J Med 1994; 330: 1431–1438

14 Langille BL. Remodeling of developing and mature arteries: endothelium, smooth muscle and matrix. J Cardiovasc Pharmacol 1993; 21(Suppl.1): S11–S17

15 Nerem RM, Harrison AD, Taylor WR, Alexander RW. Haemodynamics and vascular endothelial cell biology. J Cardiovasc Pharmacol 1993 21 (Suppl. 1): S6–S10

16 Bobik A, Campbell JH. Vascular derived growth factors: cell biology pathophysiology and pharmacology. Pharmacol Rev 1993; 45: 1–42

17 Newby AC, George SJ. Proposed roles for growth factors in mediating smooth muscle cell proliferation in vascular pathologies. Cardiovasc Res 1993; 27: 1173–1183

18 Lindop GBM, Boyle JJ, McEwen P, Kenyon CJ. Smooth muscle cell phenotype in hypertension. J Human Hyperten 1995; 9: 475–478

19 Salz M, Sommers SC, Smithwick RA. Clinicopathologic correlations of renal biopsies from essential hypertensive patients. Circulation 1957; 16: 207–212

20 Bell ET, Clawson BJ. Primary (essential) hypertension. A study of four hundred and twenty cases. Arch Pathol 1928; 5: 939–1002

21 Wright I. The microscopical appearances of human peripheral arteries during growth and ageing. J Clin Pathol 1963; 16: 499–522

22 Darmady EM, Offer J, Woodhouse MA. The parameters of the ageing kidney. J Pathol 1973; 109: 195–207

23 Dustin P. Arteriolar hyalinosis. In: Richter GW, Epstein MA, eds. Review of Experimental pathology. New York: Academic Press, 1962: 73–138

24 Smith JP. Hyaline arteriosclerosis in the kidney. Light and electron microscopic studies. J Pathol Bacterial 1959; 69: 147–168

25 Evans G. A contribution to the study of arteriosclerosis, with special reference to its relation to chronic renal disease. Quart J Med 1921; 214–282

26 Lindop GBM. The effects of hypertension on the structure of human resistance vessels. In: Swales J, ed. Textbook of Hypertension. London: Blackwells, 1994: 663–669

27 Moritz AR, Oldt MR. Arteriolar sclerosis in hypertensive and non-hypertensive individuals. Am J Pathol 1937; 13: 679–728

28 Gamble CN. The pathogenesis of hyaline arteriolosclerosis. Am J Pathol 1986; 122: 410–420

29 Strangaard S, Olesen J, Skinhoj E, Lassen NA. Autoregulation of brain circulation in severe arterial hypertension. Br Med J 1973; 1: 507–510

30 Graham DI. Ischaemic brain damage of cerebral perfusion failure type after treatment of severe hypertension. Br Med J 1975; 4: 791

31 McLenachen JM, Henderson E, Morris KL, Dargie HJ. Ventricular arrhythmias in patients with hypertensive LVH. N Engl J Med 1987; 317: 787–792

32 Koren MJ, Devereux RB, Casale PN, Savage DD, Laragh JH. Relation of left ventricular mass and geometry to morbidity and mortality in uncomplicated essential hypertension. Am Coll Physiol 1991; 114: 345–352

33 Chambers J. Left ventricular hypertrophy: an underappreciated coronary risk factor. Br Med J 1995; 311: 273–274

34 Marian AJ, Yu Q, Workman R, Grieve G, Roberts R. Angiotensin-converting enzyme polymorphism in hypertrophic cardiomyopathy and sudden death. Lancet 1994; 342: 1085–1086

35 Schunkert H, Hans-Werner H, Holmes SR, et al Association between a deletion

polymorphism of the angiotensin-converting enzyme gene and left ventricular hypertrophy. N Engl J Med 1994; 330: 1634–1638

36 Prasad N, O'Kane KPJ, Johnstone HA, et al The relationship between blood pressure and left ventricular mass in essential hypertension is observed only in the presence of the angiotensin-converting enzyme gene deletion. Quart J Med 1994; 87: 659–662

37 Strauer BE, Motz W, Schwartzkopff B, Vester E, Leschke M, Scheler S. The heart in hypertension. In: Swales JD, Ed. Hypertension. 1994: 712–731

38 Davies MJ, McKenna WJ. Hypertrophic cardiomyopathy – pathology and pathogenesis. Histopathology 1995; 26: 493–501

39 Moore S. The relation of superficial cortical scars of the kidney to aortic atherosclerosis: a hypothesis of renal ischaemia. J Pathol 1964; 88: 471–478

40 Racusen L, Solez K. Renal infarction, cortical necrosis, and atheroembolic disease. In: Tisher CC, Brenner BM, eds. Renal pathology: With clinical and functional correlations. Philadelphia: JB Lippincott Co., 1994: 810–831

41 McGowan JA, Greenberg A. Cholesterol athero-embolic renal disease. Am J Nephrol 1986; 6: 135–142

42 Freeman BI, Iskandar SS, Appel RG. The link between hypertension and nephrosclerosis. Am J Kidney Dis 1995; 25: 207–221

43 Brenner BM. Nephron adaptation to renal injury and ablation. Am J Physiol 1985; 248: F324–327

44 Bathena DB, Weiss JH, Holland NH, et al Focal and segmental glomerulosclerosis in reflux nephropathy. Am J Med 1980; 68: 886

45 Kiprov DD, Colvin RB, McCluskey RT. Focal and segmental glomerulosclerosis and proteinuria associated with unilateral renal agenesis. Lab Invest 1982; 46: 275–281

46 Anderson S, Rennke HG, Brenner BM. Therapeutic advantage of converting enzyme inhibitors in arresting progressive renal disease associated with systemic hypertension in the rat. J Clin Invest 1986; 77: 1993–2000

47 Anderson S, Meyer TW, Rennke HG, Brenner BM. Control of glomerular hypertension limits glomerular hypertension in rats with reduced renal mass. J Clin Invest 1985; 76: 612–619

48 Wolf G. Vasoactive substances as regulators of renal growth. Exp Nephrol 1993; 1: 141–151

49 Jardine AG. Angiotensin II in glomerulonephritis. J Hyperten 1995; 13: 487–492

50 Brown MA, Whitworth JA. Hypertension in human renal disease J Hyperten 1992; 10: 701–712

51 Kincaid-Smith P. What has happened to malignant hypertension? In: Bulpitt CJ, ed. Handbook of Hypertension. Vol 6. Amsterdam: Elsevier, 1985: 255–265

52 Seedat YK. Perspectives of hypertension in blacks: Black vs white differences. J Cardiovasc Pharmacol 1990; 16(Suppl.7): 67–70

53 Kincaid-Smith P, McMichael J, Murphy FA. The clinical course and pathology of hypertension with papilloedema (Malignant hypertension). Quart J Med 1958; 105: 117–163

54 Heptinstall RH. Malignant hypertension: a study of fifty one cases. J Pathol Bacteriol 65: 423

55 Helmchen U, Wenzel UO. Benign and malignant nephrosclerosis and renovascular disease. In: Tisher CC, Brenner BM, eds. Renal Pathology with Clinical and Functional Correlations. Philadelphia: JB Lippincott, 1994: 1201–1236

56 MacKenzie ET, Strandgaard S, Graham DI, Jones JV, Harper AM, Farrar JK. Effects of acutely induced hypertension in cats on pial arteriolar calibre, local cerebral blood flow, and the blood-brain barrier. Circulat Res 1976; 39: 33–41

57 Giese J. The pathogenesis of hypertensive vascular disease. Copenhagen: Munksgaard, 1966

58 Byrom FB The evolution of acute hypertensive vascular disease. Prog Cardiovasc Dis 1974; 17: 31–37

59 Wilson SK, Heptinstall RH. Effects of acute angiotensin induced hypertension on intra-renal arteries in the rat. Kidney Int 1984; 25: 492–501

60 Pitcock JA, Johnson JG, Share L et al Malignant hypertension due to musculomucoid intimal hyperplasia of intrarenal arteries. Circulat Res 1975; 36 & 37 (Suppl): 133–141

61 Yu SH, Whitworth JA, Kinkaid-Smith P. Malignant hypertension: Etiology and outcome. Clin Exp Hyperten 1986; [A]8: 1211–1230

62 Lindop GBM. The human renin secreting cell in health and disease. In: Robertson JIS, Nicholls MG, The Renin-angiotensin System. London: Gower Medical Publishing, 1992: 19.1–19.15

63 Hamilton M, Thompson EN, Wisniewski TKM. The role of blood pressure control in preventing complications of hypertension. Lancet 1964; I: 235–238

64 Collins R, Peto R, MacMahon S. Blood pressure, stroke and coronary heart disease II; short-term reduction of blood pressure: overview of randomised drug trials and their epidemiological context. Lancet 1990; 337: 827–838

65 Bronner LL, Kanter DS, Manson JE. Primary prevention of stroke. N Eng J Med 1995; 1392–1400

66 Robertson JIS, Ball SG. Benefits from treating hypertension. In: Hypertension for the Clinician. London: WD Saunders, 1995: 101–111

67 Barker DJP, Osmond C, Golding J, Kuh D, Wadsworth MEJ. Growth in utero, blood pressure in childhood and adult life, and mortality from cardiovascular disease. Br Med J 1989; 298: 564–567

68 Barker DJP, Bull AR, Osmond C, Simmonds SJ. Fetal and placental size and risk of hypertension in adult life. Br Med J 1990; 301: 259–262

69 Morton JJ, Beattie EC, MacPherson F. Angiotensin II receptor antagonist losartan has persistent effects on blood pressure in young spontaneously hypertensive rats: lack of relation to vascular structure. J Vasc Res 1992; 29: 264–269

70 Harrap SB, Van der Merwe WM, Griffin SA, MacPherson F, Lever AF. Brief angiotensin converting enzyme inhibitor treatment in young spontaneously hypertensive rats reduces blood pressure longterm. Hypertension 1990; 16: 603–614

71 Caufield M, Lavender P, Farrall M et al Linkage of angiotensinogen gene to essential hypertension. N Engl J Med 1994; 330: 1629–1633

72 Jeunmaitre X, Soubrier F, Kotelevtsev YV, et al Molecular basis of human hypertension: role of angiotensinogen. Cell 1992; 71: 169–180

73 Harden PN, Geddes C, Rowe PA, et al Polymorphisms in angiotensin-converting-enzyme gene and progression of IgA nephropathy. Lancet 1995; 345: 1540–1542

74 Connell JMC, Inglis GC, Fraser R, Jamieson A. Dexamethasone-suppressible hyperaldosteronism: clinical, biochemical and genetic relations. J Human Hyperten 1995; 9: 505–509

9

The pathologist in the 21st century: man or machine?

N. Mapstone   P. Quirke

Predicting the future is a pastime fraught with danger. Who would have guessed, in 1970, that the pathology laboratory 25 years ahead would be routinely using immunological methods to characterize antigen expression on many tumours or that it would be possible to detect small numbers of organisms or genetic lesions in archival paraffin material using a simple chemical reaction such as the polymerase chain reaction (PCR)? At a more prosaic level, who would have predicted that the simple clinical techniques of endoscopy and colposcopy would have yielded such a vast increase in the number of biopsies the laboratory would receive? Conversely, who would have foreseen that a tool of vast potential for the examination of the ultra-structure of cells, would be relegated to the specialized fields of renal biopsy work and neuropathology, with many pathologists (even academic pathologists) rarely darkening the door of their electron microscopy suite?

These examples are a warning to all who would predict the future of a scientific speciality. And yet, there are many intimations of what the future might hold. Once pathologists could only peer at by-products of a disease process, the artefacts of light microscopy. Now, with the advances of molecular biology, they have the potential to examine the root cause of those processes by detecting genetic aberrations, or the genes of specific infectious organisms.

The key areas that can be readily identified as radically affecting our future are the revolutions in information technology, molecular biology, robotics and clinical imaging. To this must be added the political, economic and social changes of the next 10–20 years. To predict the future is indeed a dangerous pursuit.

Currently, the histopathologist's quintessential function is the interpretation of microscopic images. If this could be equally performed by machines, or the information so acquired could be obtained from other sources, the histopathologist would be staring redundancy in the face. We consider at some length the likelihood of both of these possibilities.

Information technology

Computers: the pathological report

Information technology is critical to the business of pathology. Our product is information and if clinicians can obtain it in any other way that is more informative, quicker or cheaper then our service will wither and die. We need to grasp the information technology revolution and use it to benefit the patient, clinicians and ourselves.

At the moment the many faces of information technology may seem to have little application to the practising pathologist. He will still be dictating reports into a Dictaphone, or even hand writing them. His reports may well be filed on a computer, but he will still depend upon 'hard copy' printouts of them to convey the information to the clinicians.

It does not need an intimate knowledge of the potential of information technology to see that this state of affairs will have changed dramatically by the turn of the century. Voice recognition systems may have been rudimentary 5 years ago, but are becoming increasingly sophisticated and pressures of time and cost (especially secretarial costs) will ensure that all will be dictating their reports directly into computers in the foreseeable future. Current systems depend to a greater or lesser extent upon the use of 'rigid phrasing' and discrete speech, which the computer can recognize with ease. However, the use of free text in these systems is increasing[1] and continuous speech recognition, which is much closer to normal speech, is likely to be available in the next few years.

These reports will be immediately available to the clinicians once authorized on the hospital computer network. Much of this is already 'old technology', available in some forward-looking establishments. The voice will replace or co-exist with the written word; there will be direct voice control of computer systems and voice mail (or E-mail) will be as common as the normal postal service is today.

Computers: the pathological image

What format will the reports take? As will be discussed later, it seems likely that the amount of information that the pathologist will be able to provide about, for example, a colorectal carcinoma will increase. The clinician and pathologist will also be able to access pictures of the gross specimens, taken by digital camera during specimen receipt and dissection.[2] The only limitation on the use of digital pictures will be the memory space required to store them in. One of the few certainties of modern computing is that data storage becomes cheaper and more abundant every year. It will be possible to store images of macroscopic and microscopic appearances on the laboratory computer and to print key pictures on the report. This may obviate the need to store large numbers of glass slides, and may facilitate the review of previous material. High-resolution digital cameras will be able to record an entire haematoxylin and eosin slide for viewing on a high-resolution workstation that comes equipped with sophisticated morphometric analysis and expert systems.[3]

A variation would be an automated slide file from which the slides are accessed remotely by computer workstation either in the office or at home!

The ease of access of microscopic material to clinicians might raise an issue of 'demarcation' to pathologists uncertain of their positions. Radiologists have for many years had to cope with clinicians as amateur radiologists emboldened by their possession of the patient's X-rays. Will the pathologists have to run the same gauntlet of partly informed criticism?

Once digital imaging is more commonly used, digital cameras will be attached to many microscopes. This will be allied to improvements in display technology with flat screen monitors of large diameter. It will then be a relatively minor step to cut out the display 'middle man' – the eyepiece objective of the microscope. Pathologists will be making diagnoses from the video screen rather than directly down the lenses – but a video screen that far surpasses the monitors and televisions of today. This will obviously facilitate teaching and demonstration enormously.

The meeting of the computer and microscope on the pathologist's bench will eventually develop into a unified pathologist's workstation. These will be integrated systems at which the pathologist will be able to make his diagnoses, compose reports, refer cases directly to colleagues, access archival information, consult his electronic library and communicate with the rest of the world. As robotics becomes more commonplace, he may well be able to keep his workstation at home, put on his 'virtual reality' goggles and perform a cut-up many miles away. He may never learn what formalin smells like.

Computers: communication of ideas (the Internet)

Much has been written about the Internet. Is it likely to have any impact upon the practice of pathology? The internet is about putting information on-line and its exchange. If you believe that information is the business of pathology then it must have a major impact. Already a number of groups for the discussion of pathological material are available. Some departments have their own 'Web pages,' which are really no more than electronic prospectuses. However, the improvement in communications which the Internet heralds will have some influence on pathology. Once secure transmission of details is available on the Internet, the dissemination of reports and other material will be easier.

However, it is in the dissemination of research that the Internet is most likely to make major changes. When individual researchers or their groups have their own 'Web pages' or equivalents, it will be easier to get an idea of who is pursuing active research in any area. A personal 'Web page' will probably be similar to a curriculum vitae, detailing current and previous interests and achievements. The use of a World Wide Web search program will allow the rapid location of all researchers with, for example, the words 'tuberculosis' and 'PCR' in their Web page.

The universal use of electronic journals must be only a matter of a few years away. This will make research much more accessible, and at a more mundane level, drastically reduce the amount of time required to publish a paper as well as getting instantaneous feedback from other researchers. Sophisticated search programs will allow researchers to concentrate specifically upon papers that have a direct interest for them and to be automatically alerted when such papers are released. Indeed, the future of paper journals may be in doubt. General journals such as the British Medical Journal or the Lancet will always have a place in the paper publishing market. The more specialized scientific journals, which have recently proliferated, have a more restricted audience with greater access to computers. They may be more threatened by electronic journals. The critical difference between paper journals and electronic journals is peer review and the presence of publishers who derive profit from paper publications. If electronic journals of good repute appear then their instantaneous world-wide on-line publication with no limitation of space, no charges for colour and the possibility of multimedia, video, sound, help files, attached comments from readers, etc. would seem to sound the death knell of medical publishing as we know it. Electronic journals will either come from publishers, if they can find a way of charging, or from scientists themselves; after all, most of the work of producing the copy for the printers is done by members of the scientific community. Is this something the Wellcome trust or a consortium of university libraries ought to sponsor?

Computers: image communication (telepathology)

The technology for telepathology is already with us. The first examples of telepathology go back to 1992[4] but more recently, international telepathology and teleradiology enabled consultations between the United Arab Emirates and the USA.[5] The potential for long distance referral of difficult or unusual cases, the provision of frozen section services to outlying hospitals,[6] quality assurance and 'telecommuting' for histopathologists are obvious.

The current utopian ideal for telepathology is for a laboratory to produce slides that are placed on a microscope at that laboratory. The microscope is linked to a pathologist's computer, which might be next door or in another country, depending upon the mode of communication used. The diagnosing pathologist controls the microscope electronically. At present he requires a human assistant at the laboratory to change slides but the provision of robotic slide loaders must be within the scope of technological advance in 10 years time.

Should pathologists working in district general hospitals feel worried about this advance? Will the general pathologist be overtaken by specialist pathologists working at central laboratories serving a region? Not necessarily. Personal communication with clinicians is important in pathology as it is currently practised. An alternative scenario is that the generalist pathologist stays at his district general hospital and refers his difficult slides requiring a specialist opinion to a national expert. Where does that leave the specialist in his regional hospital? Even national boundaries should be no limit, and international experts might expect an increase in work at the expense of their national colleagues.

These scenarios all exclude the influence of personal relationships in diagnosis and referral practice. The opportunity to physically meet and talk to colleagues will continue to influence both clinical referral and pathologist-to-pathologist referral. It seems more likely that telepathology will allow greater use of case conferences and increased ease in referral practice, but will it ever completely replace the 'personal touch'?

Computers: image analysis (Morphometry)

'There's no point in becoming a pathologist nowadays. All the diagnoses will be made by computer in the foreseeable future.' Such comments were common many years ago, and the continuing presence of histopathology as a speciality refute the idea. Any examination of the current scope of morphometry should prove reassuring to the pathologist who feels that the skills of his eye and brain are under threat of redundancy.

Image analysis systems in cytology have been under development for the last 30 years. Despite this, a working system (Papnet),[7] which allows some screening of slides identifying the areas of greatest concern, has only just arrived. The presence of humans in histological diagnosis seems assured for many years to come. If pathologists need to look for a threat to classical, light microscopy-based pathology, they should be looking uneasily towards the molecular biologists rather than the morphometrists. Molecular biologists will be diagnosing the actual lesions that cause disease, whilst morphometry is often just a rather more sophisticated (and sometimes less dependable) way of detailing the cytological changes that those disease cause. Morphometry provides more information (and sometimes too much information) but is that information necessarily relevant or useful?

Whilst it seems unlikely that computers will overtake histopathological diagnosis, advances in the facility with which morphometrical measurements can be taken should be a boon to pathologists. Currently, the pathologist may put out a non-committal report suggesting that there may be, for example, an excess of intraepithelial lymphocytes in a specimen, but suggesting that there might not be enough lymphocytes to diagnose lymphocytic gastritis or colitis. His only alternative it to spend a significant period of time actually counting the cells or taking the slide to a semiautomated morphometric system. The advent of the pathologist's individual work station (q.v) connected to a powerful computer will allow him to quantify many such parameters quickly and without moving from his office. Measurement of parameters such as distance of tumour cells from resection margins should become more reliable.

Computers: teaching

Many of the potential advances that information technology heralds for teaching are already with us. CDroms, networks and the Internet have already increased the resources (and expenditure) of teachers. Improvements in microscopic display technology will facilitate postgraduate and, to a lesser extent, undergraduate teaching. Much greater use of multimedia will occur as well as the potential for virtual reality experiences for training e.g. the cut-up, the virtual reality autopsy, etc. It is possible that the lecture will become a thing of the past with students logging on to a multimedia experience or even be assigned an Internet tutorial or logging into the teaching or research pages of an international expert. The potential for small discussion groups of students and teachers conducted by E-mail is enormous, and easily organized, even with today's technology. However, it is rarely used. It seems that the 'personal touch' in referral practice will still be required in teaching for some time to come.

Pathology and the outside world

Political changes

We cannot predict the next three governments in the UK and their attitude to the National Health Service and histopathology. We can, however, extrapolate from the Strategic Review and the private finance initiative to show one possible face of the future. A system of privatized pathology laboratories competing for business locally and nationally where quality = value − cost. One large laboratory might emerge in each major city or conglomeration, with smaller centers surviving where communication links are poor or distances large. The opposite view is the slow development of the status quo or more radically the decentralization of pathologists as communications improve and home working becomes the norm.

The closer integration of Europe will lead to more European Union regulations and greater European collaboration. The decrease in British scientific output over the last 10 years will, however, lead to a loss of pre-eminence with a rise in the contribution to pathology from the Asian tiger economies.

Economic changes

All developed countries are attempting to decrease the percentage of gross national product spent on health. We can expect to see hard times ahead, which will lead to increased demands for efficiency that can only be met by automation, centralization and increased throughput. Universities will also become financially stretched and will only value pathology if it contributes to their research income. We need to look for new income-generating markets to finance our services (and our salaries). British pathology departments may need to look abroad for work.

Autopsies

How many autopsies will the pathologist perform in the future? Probably fewer than at present. The hospital autopsy is a threatened species in most areas, and in some hospitals in on the verge of extinction. Improvements in clinical imaging techniques have enveloped clinicians in an aura of false diagnostic security. This trend will increase as clinical imaging becomes more impressive and available. A cost-conscious government is, at some stage, likely to examine the expenditure on the coronial autopsy work. It is unlikely to support any increase in the numbers of autopsies performed.

These factors, together with negative social attitudes to the autopsy, will probably result in a major reduction of autopsies in most hospitals, unless there is a change of awareness amongst clinicians about the role of the autopsy in teaching, audit and routine practice.

Demographic changes

The population is aging and will carry a greater burden of pathology. Expectations of health will rise leading to more consultations and thus investigations. Increasing cure rates for cancer and earlier diagnosis and treatment of cardiovascular disease combined with a decrease in smoking will also change the patterns of disease. The greater concerns over the environment may lead to the necessity to recycle our waste products such as solvents.

Clinical changes

Probably the most unpredictable factor in the future of pathology is the effect of clinical changes. Clinicians with an increasingly scientific background are expecting more information from their pathology reports. The advent of endoscopy dramatically increased the numbers and changed the nature of pathology departments' workloads. Similar though less pronounced changes were seen following the introduction of the breast screening programme. New screening programmes for other organs may result in a similar disruption of the workload. Surgeons are becoming increasingly adept at the use of the endoscope, and 'remote control' surgery using robotic and miniaturization techniques would seem to be a logical development. This may result in biopsies from sites usually only seen in resection specimens, if at all. It has been commented that as time has progressed, pathologists are expected to say more and more about less and less material. It seems likely that this trend will continue.

Clinical imaging

To date clinical imaging has tended to increase our workload rather than decrease it. This may change in the future. Already sophisticated computing in combination with spiral computed tomography (CT) has enabled a CT colonoscopy where using a mouse and computer screen it has been possible to traverse a computer recreation of a patient's colon. The combination of such imaging technology with the biochemical analysis of nuclear magnetic resonance (NMR) might enable radiologists to diagnose lesions without recourse to biopsy. This, however, is likely to be outweighed by the increasing use of minimally invasive techniques such as guided fine needle aspirates with smaller and smaller samples for the morphologists. Improvements in endoscopic ultrasound will allow the earlier detection of lesions for biopsy, throwing up more histopathological challenges.

Technological matters

Specimen preparation

Current fixation techniques require a day or more for the preparation of specimens before they can be examined microscopically. Frozen sections, whilst allowing rapid diagnoses, are hampered by the often poor morphological preservation of tissue architecture and cytology. Attempts to routinely use, for example, microwaves for tissue fixation have their evangelists, particularly in neuropathology[8] but have failed the test of widespread acceptability.

Fixation is already assisted in some situations by increasing temperatures. The use of increased pressures may also allow more rapid fixation.

What would be the consequence of more rapid fixation and processing? We could expect there to be many more requests for urgent histopathological examination. On-call histopathologists would no longer be an underutilized resource.

Image acquisition

Much of the assumption so far has been that new technology will allow more sophisticated analysis of the morphometrical parameters that we already use in histological diagnosis. Perhaps other techniques will provide the same kind of information, or even more information, by using agents other than light waves. Ultrasound would seem to be too insensitive for such diagnosis, but positron emission technology and NMR can provide a wealth of information about the chemical composition of certain specimens. We may be able to differentiate lesions according to, for example, their sodium ion concentration.[9] The intracellular biochemical lesions associated with neoplasia follow the genetic lesions, and precede the morphological manifestations, so this, ideally, would provide a means of early tumour diagnosis. However, our experience of the changes in the use of electron microscopes have shown that merely having a great deal of information about the composition of a tissue at a very low level will not necessarily provide valuable diagnostic information. A more hopeful development is the atomic force microscope.[10] This instrument interacts with the sample, and can measure forces at the molecular level. It can even manipulate the molecules of the sample – nanomanipulation. The technique has been used for the study of the cytoskeleton, membranes and ion channels and in the future may allow direct visualization of and reading of DNA/RNA sequences.

Robotics

Advances in robotics are likely to have major effects upon the work of the routine laboratory. Automation for staining and coverslipping is already commonplace in many laboratories. Immunohistochemical staining and in situ hybridization[11] is being automated and one day sectioning will also be successfully automated.

If tissue sampling can be standardized (no more staples or sutures in the blocks), then the automation process may go from the receipt of the specimen (or even from the acquisition of the specimen from the patient)[12] to the pathologists' workstation – at least for the easier small endoscopic or skin biopsies, which comprise half of our workload.

Molecular biology

The genome projects

The genomes of the first free-living organisms, *Haemophilus influenzae*[13] and *Mycoplasma genitalium*[14] have been sequenced by the Institute for Genomic Research (TIGR) *Eschenchia coli Saccharomyces cerevisiae, Caenorhabidits elegans, Drosophilia* and *Homo sapiens* are well on their way to being completed. The first decade of the 21st century will see the completion of the human genome project. Between 100 000 and 300 000 genes will be identified and our knowledge of the genetic basis of many common diseases will be understood or greatly improved. The expressed sequence tag approach of Venter and colleagues from TIGR will speed up this process by identifying the expressed DNA sequences and thus the functioning genes. This approach with new techniques such as serial analysis of gene expression (SAGE)[15] will allow the relatively rapid assessment of mRNA expression pattern of a tissue. This may enable the disease phenotype to be characterized by looking at very large numbers of genes very rapidly. Molecular biology has been relatively limited in the past by its requirement to analyse each gene or part of a gene separately. Such new approaches will allow the rapid analysis of many genes simultaneously.

Disease detection

Current molecular methods are valuable when looking for a specific molecular lesion e.g. a known mutation/deletion, loss of heterozygosity or molecular phenotype such as microsatellite instability. It is poor in the routine detection of lesions or point mutations in large genes, multigenic diseases, large-scale screening, etc. This may change rapidly. New methods of DNA sequencing or point mutation detection are constantly being developed. The DNA repair protein method of identifying point mutations appears promising.[16] Multiplexing reactions are becoming more widespread and ligase methods of point mutation detection are being produced. A rapid 28-mutation test kit for cystic fibrosis is about to be marketed. It may well be possible to test for hundreds of mutations simultaneously. Such technologies will make the screening of single gene defects and multigenic diseases (such as myocardial infarction, hypertension and dementia) feasible.

Miniaturization and automation

New technologies are just around the corner. The United States Advanced Technologies Programme has funded research into DNA chips where thousands of oligonucleotides of different sequences will be attached to chips and on hybridization to a target DNA molecule a signal is emitted, which can be detected by computer. These chips could be manufactured cheaply and allow low-cost, rapid molecular biology.

The future holds out automation from the biological sample to the molecular pathologist. Automated DNA extraction is already available and this can be simply combined with robotic PCR machines and sensitive gel capillary analysis such as that provided by the Applied Biosystems 310 DNA analyser. The next step in the technology is to enable continuous capillary electrophoresis of the whole process avoiding carryover contamination. This will be available in the next 10 years.

Molecular analysis may just be a bolt on for an autoanalyser in 15 years. Sophisticated expert systems will be available to analyse the sequence/amplification data and make a provisional diagnosis.

Infectious diseases

Microbiologists are responsible for the laboratory diagnosis of the great majority of infectious diseases. There are, however, a significant proportion of infections that depend to a greater or lesser extent upon the diagnostic acumen of the histopathologist. This may be because culture is insufficiently sensitive (such as in *Helicobacter pylori* infection), difficult (such as in tuberculosis) or even currently impossible (such as in Whipple's disease).

Immunohistochemical stains may be easier to perform in some situations than a culture technique (such as in cytomegalovirus infection of the colon) or the disease may be so unexpected as to evade the list of cultures performed in the routine case (such as amoebic colitis in the UK). Technological advances, especially molecular techniques, make it likely that histopathologically diagnosed infections will increase in number.

Molecular techniques are becoming gradually ever more important in microbiology. PCR is a recognized means of detecting many viral infections, such as hepatitis C or human papillomavirus infection. Similar techniques are now used widely in the typing of bacterial infections. Whilst the microbiologists' culture techniques may eventually be superseded there is no reason why the histopathologist should not bring his skill to bear in any of these tests. The introduction of in situ PCR may, however, have a major impact upon the histopathologist's role in diagnosing infectious diseases. The histopathologist will usually receive the biopsy tissue sample, which immediately places a diagnostic responsibility upon him. If he has an in situ PCR test for a range of infectious organisms he may well be able to provide a diagnosis before the culture results are ready in situations such as infectious colitis. The microbiologist might have more to fear from molecular biology than the histopathologist!

Cancer

Advances in molecular biology may have minor effects upon the histopathologists' workload for infectious diseases. However, they will have a vastly greater effect upon the reporting of cancer cases. They may eventually be used in screening for neoplastic lesions, the definitive 'tissue' diagnosis, prognostic indices, assessment of tumour stage and grade, identification of chemotherapy sensitivity, sensitive determination of tumour recurrence, and even in the detection of resection margin involvement.[17] It seems very likely that within a few years any oncologist treating a patient who has had a resection will want a 'molecular profile' of his patient's cancer, for diagnostic, prognostic and treatment purposes. Whether or not screening, staging and determination of clearance will be performed by molecular methods will probably depend as much upon the cost of such techniques (in comparison with the cost of light microscopy) as upon their sensitivity and feasibility. Usually the histopathologist will have the sample, which will provide most of the material for these tests, and consequently it will probably fall to his lot to perform, supervise and interpret these tests.

To some extent haematopathology has led the field in the provision of molecular data for diagnostic purposes. Molecular techniques are routinely used in the detection of, for example, clonality in a range of lesions. The use of molecular techniques is radically changing the approach to, for example, acute myeloid leukaemia, from an arbitrary subdivision depending upon light microscopic diagnosis, to a classification based upon the genetic lesions, which are implicated in the disease. We may soon see the classification of carcinomas from other sites according to the genetic lesions they possess.

Summary

Changes in society are occurring more and more rapidly. The changes which have happened in the last 25 years will be easily outstripped by those in the next 25. The combination of advances in information technology, molecular biology and automation together with political changes in health care delivery make the future challenging to us all.

The one certainty about this chapter is that there will be many important omissions, and many of these changes will fail to come to pass. We can, however, be fairly certain that a committee of senior pathologists from many countries and subspecialties would omit as many crucial, unpredictable advances, and include as many technological 'advances' later to be demonstrated as cul-de-sacs. Our interpretation of the important factors likely to affect pathology over the next 20 years is inevitably personal. It will, we can confidently predict, raise a wry smile on the faces of our children when, in 25 years time, their Primary MRCPath looming, they dig out an old copy of *Progress in Pathology* for some last-minute revision (some things never change).

Acknowledgements

We would like to thank colleagues who shared ideas between Oxford and Leeds: Dr WA Reid, Dr AB Gledhill and Dr JI Wyatt in January 1995, and wish good luck to all of our colleagues over the next 25 years

References

1 Teplitz C, Cipriani M, Diconstanzo D, Sarlin J. Automated Speech recognition anatomic pathology (ASAP) reporting. Semin Diagn Pathol 1994; 11: 245–252

2 Schubert E, Gross W, Slderits R, Deckenbaugh L, He F, Bechich M. A pathologist designed imaging system for anatomic pathology signout teaching and research. Semin Diagn Pathol 1994; 11: 263–273

3 Brugal G, Dye R, Krief B, Chassery JM, Tanke H, Tucker JH. HOME: highly optimized microscope environment. Cytometry 1992; 13: 109–116

4 Cronenberger JH, Hsiao H, Falk RJ, Jennette JC. Nephropathology consultation via digitized images. Ann N Y Acad Sci 1992; 670: 281–292

5 Goldberg MA, Sharif HS, Rosenthal DI, et al Making global telemedicine practical and affordable: demonstrations from the Middle East. AJR. Am J Roentgenol 1994; 163: 1495–1500

6 Kayser K, Drlicek M, Rahn W. Aids of telepathology in intra-operative histomorphological tumor diagnosis and classification. In Vivo 1993; 7: 395–398

7 Ouwerkerk-Noordam E, Boon ME, Beck S. Computer-assisted primary screening of cervical smears using the PAPNET method: comparison with conventional screening and evaluation of the role of the cytologist. Cytopathology 1994; 5: 211–218

8 Ainley CD, Ironside JW. Microwave technology in diagnostic neuropathology. Neurosci Methods 1994; 55: 183–190

9 Coleman RE. Single photon emission computed tomography and positron emission tomography in cancer imaging. Cancer 1991; 67: 1261–1270

10 Lal R, John SA. Biological applications of atomic force microscopy. Am J Physiol 1994; 266: 1–21

11 Takahashi T, Ishiguro K. Development of an automatic machine for in situ hybridization and immunohistochemistry. Anal Biochem 1991; 196: 390–402

12 Markin RS. Clinical laboratory automation: concepts and designs. Semin Diagn Pathol 1994; 11: 274–281

13 Fleischmann R, Adams M, White O, et al Whole-genome random sequencing and assembly of Haemophilus influenzae. Science 1995; 269: 496–512

14 Fraser C, Gocayne J, White O, et al The minimal gene complement of Mycoplasma genitalium. Science 1995; 270: 397–403

15 Velculescu V, Zhang L, Vogelstein B, Kinzler K. Serial analysis of geneexpression. Science 1995; 270: 484–487

16 Ellis L, Taylor G, Banks R, Baumbergs N. MUT-S binding protects heteroduplex DNA from exonuclease digestion in-vitro – a simple method for detecting mutations. Nucl Acids Res 1994; 22: 2710–2711

17 Brennan JA, Mao L, Hruban RH, et al Molecular assessment of histopathological staging in squamous-cell carcinoma of the head and neck N Engl J Med 1995; 332: 429–435

10

Developments in microbiology: taxonomic change; new names, new methods and new microorganisms

J. Paul

The title of this chapter is to inform the reader, who is unlikely to be a microbiologist, of the presence of developments in microbiology that will be of importance to workers outside that discipline: the subtitle outlines the nature of these developments, which to some extent are inter-related.

Coping with new names and name changes

On a day-to-day basis, workers with an interest in infections are often confused by the appearance of unfamiliar scientific names for organisms. These include newly characterized organisms, known organisms with recently attributed medical importance, organisms of known medical importance, which are so rare or geographically restricted as to appear new to many workers and well-known organisms with well-understood medical significance whose names have been changed. Of these explanations, the final category, where there has been name changing of organisms with clearly defined medical importance of long standing, causes the most resentment from clinicians. It is important to have a strategy for dealing with unfamiliar names; the strategy amounts to learning a basic understanding of the rules that govern nomenclature, knowing where to find and how to use the key reference works on the subject and to understand the philosophy behind taxonomy, something of its origins and history and the scientific developments which have necessitated major taxonomic reconfigurations.

Taxonomy (systematics)

The discipline of taxonomy (taxis = arrangement, nomia = distribution), otherwise known as systematics, deals with the classification of organisms and aims to arrange them as orderly groupings, or taxa, according to degrees of similarity, into a hierarchical system based on relatedness. To allow a taxonomic system to operate, there must be an accompanying system of nomenclature. Such a system allows its users to identify organisms as belonging to particular taxa and refer to them by specific names. A universal taxonomy with precise definitions of its taxa allows workers to communicate with each other unambiguously using correct names of organisms. For many well-known groupings of plants and animals, the taxonomy and nomenclature are very stable. The situation with microorganisms is often unstable, there being a tendency for name change, which irritates clinicians, epidemiologists and others. Even medical microbiologists may be cynical about the nature of microbial nomenclature. However, it is important to comprehend that microbial taxonomy is working towards an ideal and that there are special problems associated with the discipline. An understanding may be reached by considering the historical background of systems of classification, the biological differences between microbes and larger animals and the results of recent molecular studies on these organisms. The scientific principles that guide microbial taxonomy are the same as those which allow the study of infectious disease and the diagnosis of microbial infection, and an understanding of these principles and of taxonomic criteria aids comprehension of more immediate and practical matters such as the diagnosis and treatment of patients.

Historical notes

John Ray (1627–1705) was a polymath, a Cambridge theologian, a lecturer in Greek and mathematics and an outstanding naturalist with personal field experience of the botany, entomology and ornithology of large areas of Britain. He produced a trilingual dictionary of English, Latin and Greek[1] and emphasized the importance of correct usage of classical words for organisms. His encyclopaedic knowledge allowed him to write comprehensive accounts of many aspects of natural history. With such a background, Ray was ideally placed to devise a system of taxonomy and nomenclature. His system was a landmark in the application of universal principles and nomenclature but it was cumbersome and lacked the constancy, simplicity, practicality and insight of that of Linnaeus, who using Ray's work among his source material, developed the foundation for modern systematics and nomenclature. Linnaeus, who was professor of medicine and botany at Uppsala developed a taxonomic system that he applied to all living things which were known to him, published as two separate works for plants and animals. The tenth edition of his *Systema Naturae* (1758)[2] is used as the basis for modern zoological nomenclature. Using numbers of characters seen or unseen in different organisms his system divides and subdivides down to the generic level within which species are listed. Many Linnaean binomial names of medical importance are unchanged, such as the tapeworm *Taenia solium*.

Classification

The orderly grouping of organisms according to degrees of similarity into a hierar-
chy (including: kingdoms, orders, families, tribes, genera, species).

The Linnaean approach relies on an intuitive ability to see similarity or difference, which is aided by our living in the same world as the organisms to
be classified. Hence, we know as a matter of common sense that a sheep is
not a cow but we have no insight into the relationship between
Pseudomonas aeruginosa and *Burkholderia cepacia* through natural experience.
Because of our intuitive ability to group animals naturally, Linnaeus and his
followers tended to group them in the manner of a family tree and
although Linnaeus believed animals had been created in that way, his
arrangement closely matches our present phylogenetic grouping of animals
based on genetic analysis and the fossil record. In fact his presentation may
have been subversive: its clarity and arrangement would have facilitated
evolutionists' thinking in phylogenetic terms. The animal classification,
especially larger animals like mammals, is now very stable: over a period of
200 years, hundreds of zoologists have performed revisionary studies, each
time aided by new scientific evidence and by their intuition to give us our
present system.

Bacterial classification is by comparison unstable: bacteriology is a new
discipline, about 100 years old; the organisms are so different from ourselves
that we have poor insight into understanding their relatedness; new data are
being acquired at a great rate – probably only a fraction of all species have
been described; there is no fossil record or embryological development to
guide one. Bacterial classification has required the use of arbitrary characters, such as cell wall structure, which may be of phylogenetic importance,
or may not be. As a result, unrelated organisms may appear superficially to
be related. One way to break from the grouping of bacteria based on intuition and unfounded personal bias is to use numerical taxonomic methods
in which hundreds of different characters, including biochemical differences, morphology, growth rates, presence of spores and so on, from each of
many different bacteria may be compared by computer.[3] From the phenetic
hyperspace a scheme of classification may be obtained that avoids human
bias but it is doubtful that such an approach necessarily leads to a natural
grouping of organisms as it is reliant on those characters that can be measured and there must be a degree of randomness as to the final outcome.
Furthermore, there is no fossil record to check that the scheme relates to
the evolutionary relatedness of the taxa. In the absence of fossils, genetic
material within bacteria has been used as a measure of relatedness.
DNA–DNA hybridization has been used to determine how much genetic
material is shared by different bacteria and has led to the arbitrary definition
of conspecifity of two bacteria being determined by their sharing 70–100%
of their genome as shown by DNA–DNA hybridization.[4] The main
problems with this are, of course, that it is an arbitrary definition and that

bacteria are notorious for exchanging large segments of DNA, even between quite different taxa and that on the other hand genetically similar bacteria may be of different and distinctive medical importance. Examples of bacteria that would be regarded as single species by DNA–DNA similarity are *Neisseria gonorrhoeae* and *Neisseria meningitidis, Yersinia pestis* and *Yersinia pseudotuberculosis* and *Shigella* spp. and *Escherichia coli*. It would be dangerous for medical practitioners to have to regard these pairs as single species and furthermore, although they are highly related, with rare exceptions the species within these pairs maintain their distinctiveness. It is almost as though the niche occupied by a bacterium defines and controls its specific characteristics, which may remain constant despite the exchange of large amounts of genetic material, suggesting that large regions of a bacterium's genome contribute little to its sense of identity.

Ribosomal RNA

Without fossils there is a need for a molecular clock. Ribosomal RNA (rRNA) has been found to be of exceptional value. All organisms have rRNA and it plays more or less the same role in all of them. Therefore it is a molecule that may be compared in all species. It is a large molecule with many domains. There are highly conserved regions and relatively variable regions. Conveniently, it may be sequenced directly with reverse transcriptase. As a result of the sequencing and comparison of rRNA it has been possible to develop a tool to detect and classify uncultivable organisms; to find uncultivable agents in tissue and associate them with disease syndromes; and to construct a universal phylogenetic tree (Fig. 10.1). The latest and most comprehensive version of the *Tree of Life* exists within the World Wide Web (http://phylogeny.arizona.edu/tree/phylogeny.html).[5] Ribosomal RNA structure is believed to be such a good predictor of bacterial phylogeny that it has been necessary to reclassify certain groups of bacteria, which appeared to be similar, by traditional laboratory test protocols.[6] An extreme example is the genus *Pseudomonas*, which has been split into five different rRNA homology groups,[7] four of which have been assigned new generic names (Table 10.1). One species, clearly not a true *Pseudomonas*, has shifted genus twice in recent years; *Pseudomonas Pseudomonas maltophilia* was moved to *Xanthomonas*, a genus of plant pathogens, with which it shares some features but following further study it has been moved to a new genus, *Stenotrophomonas*. This is just the sort of thing that irritates clinicians.

Nomenclature

'The primary purpose of nomenclature is to permit us to know as exactly as possible what another clinician, microbiologist, epidemiologist, or investigator is referring to . . .'

Clinical Infectious Diseases 1995; 21: 263

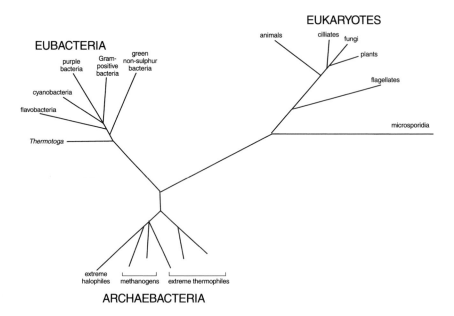

Fig. 10.1. The phylogeny of living organisms as inferred from rRNA sequences'

Table 10.1 rRNA homology groups of former *Pseudomonas* spp. and their new names

Group I Includes	*Pseudomonas* *P. aeruginosa, P. fluorescens, P. stutzeri, P. putida*
Group II Includes	*Burkholderia* *B. cepacia, B. mallei, B. pseudomallei, B. pickettii*
Group III Includes	*Comamonas* *C. acidovorans, C. testosteroni*
Group IV Includes	*Brevundimonas* *B. diminuta, B. vesicularis*
Group V Includes	*Stenotrophomonas* *S. maltophilia*

It is important to remember that correct names, with the exception of viral names, are written as Linnaean binomials, the generic names with first letter in upper case, specific name in lower case; both names underlined or printed in italics e.g. <u>Escherichia coli</u>, *Escherichia coli*.

Different governing bodies exist, which establish rules for the naming of animals, plants, fungi, bacteria and viruses. All of them use superficially similar systems with Linnaean binomials with the exception of the virologists who have rejected Linnaean binomials in favour of a descriptive naming system that is written in plain text. The rules for bacteria are stated in the *International Code of Nomenclature of Bacteria* (the Bacteriological Code, 1976 revision). To find correct bacterial names one must refer to the *Approved Lists of Bacterial Names* (1980); this is the starting point for nomenclature. An amended edition was published in 1989.[8] All taxonomic changes since 1989, whether they be name changes of known bacteria or descriptions of new taxa must be published in the *International Journal of Systematic Bacteriology* (ISJB). Even if described in another journal, a proposed name is not valid until listed in the IJSB. This makes it very easy to use correct names but requires access to the Approved Lists and to the IJSB, which are unlikely to be available in the standard histopathology library. In an effort to disseminate names to clinicians, various unofficial lists have been published. Of course, they cannot be completely up to date but are nearly so and are widely available. The chapter dealing with newer and unusual bacteria in the latest *Oxford Textbook of Medicine*[9] lists many of the more obscure medically important bacteria against concise clinical information and with references but is already a little out of date. The journal *Clinical Infectious Diseases* has started a programme of listing correct names.[10–14] It is extremely comprehensive but gives no additional information or references. For microbiologists, there is a concise list of new names in the *Public Health Laboratory Service Microbiology Digest*.[15]

Identification

Identification has traditionally been based on phenotypic characteristics, for example Gram's stain, acid-fast stain, presence of spores, growth conditions, growth rate, metabolism, fermentation reactions, colonial morphology, etc. Genetic identification, such as polymerase chain reaction (PCR) methods to amplify conserved genomic regions with sequencing, is already being used in routine clinical medicine. There are obvious benefits in the diagnosis and subsequent public health follow-up of cases of culture-negative bacterial meningitis, and rapid PCR methods will be useful for organisms that grow slowly, such as mycobacteria, or not at all, such as the Whipple's disease agent. Various bacteria have areas of the genome that are susceptible to genetic identification methods. Analysis of 16S rRNA genes, however, is probably the most versatile. All medically important bacteria have small subunit ribosomes (16S) whose ribonucleic acid (rRNA) is encoded by 16S rRNA genes. The deoxyribonucleic acid (DNA), which composes these genes, is a patchwork of highly variable and highly conserved sequences. The highly conserved regions may be used as targets for primers to amplify regions of the 16S rRNA gene, by PCR, from any bacterium. The sequences of the variable portions may be analysed and compared with reference sequence data from known bacteria.

'New' agents

Bacillary angiomatosis and cat-scratch disease

Bacillary angiomatosis in acquired immune deficiency syndrome (AIDS) patients is a recently characterized disease in which vascular proliferative lesions occur at various sites and in which bacilli may be seen in silver-stained histological sections. It was noted that the lesions bore some resemblance to the skin lesions of verruga peruana caused by *Bartonella bacilliformis*. In the elegant studies of Relman and co-workers,[16] using PCR-based amplification of 16S rRNA from affected tissue, genetic material was identified whose sequence resembled that of *Rochalimaea quintana* (as it was then known), the cause of trench fever, a louse-borne infection. An organism related to *R. quintana* was cultured using lysis–centrifugation methodology from the blood of febrile human immunodeficiency virus (HIV). seropositive patients by Slater and co-workers,[17] and Koehler and co-workers[18] isolated *Rochalimaea* spp. from the lesions of bacillary angiomatosis. One of these was *R. quintana* and the other a new species *Rochalimaea henselae*.[19] Subsequently, another species, *Rochalimaea elizebethae*, was described by Daly and co-workers[20] from an endocarditis patient. Although initial 16S rRNA sequence comparison methods showed isolates to be conspecific with the known taxon *R. quintana*, and the novel related organisms *R. henselae* and *R. elizebethae* were placed in the same genus, later comparison with *B. bacilliformis* showed such a degree of relatedness that all *Rochalimaea* spp. have been moved into the genus *Bartonella*.[21] Cat-scratch disease was long suspected as being an infectious disease. Patients suffer from fever and lymphadenopathy and bacilli may be seen in silver-stained histological tissues. Both *Bartonella henselae* and another 'new' bacterium, *Afipia felis*, have been isolated using careful culture methods, suitable for the isolation of fastidious organisms, from cat-scratch tissue. The confusing mosaic of organisms – *Bartonella* spp. (*Rochalimaea* spp.) and *Afipia felis* – and diseases – verruga peruana, Oroya fever, trench fever, bacillary angiomatosis, cat-scratch fever and endocarditis – are shown in Table 10.2.

Table 10.2 *Bartonella* spp., *Afipia* and associated diseases

Organism	Disease
Bartonella bacilliformis	Oroya fever Verruga peruana
Bartonella quintana	Trench fever Bacillary angiomatosis
Bartonella henselae	Bacillary angiomatosis Cat-scratch disease
Bartonella elizebethae	Endocarditis
Afipia felis	Cat-scratch disease

Whipple's disease

Whipple's disease is a systemic illness, typically of middle-aged white males, giving signs and symptoms of arthralgia, diarrhoea, abdominal pain, weight loss, lymphadenopathy, fever and skin pigmentation. Histologically, lesions show infiltrations of macrophages containing bacilli, which may be seen by silver staining and electron microscopy. The organism is not amenable to culture. Relman and co-workers[22] examined lymph nodes or duodenal tissue from five affected patients and used broad-range 16S cRNA primers to obtain a 904 base pair product, which was cloned and sequenced. Its sequence implied that the uncultivable Whipple's bacillus was related to the actinomycetes showing similarity to the genera *Actinomyces, Rothia* and *Dermatophilus.* The new agent has been named as *Tropheryma whippelii.*

Diseases in search of an infectious causative agent

A number of important, relatively common diseases are of uncertain aetiology but have clinical, histological and epidemiological features suggestive of an infectious cause. In the absence of a known cause, such illnesses may be defined by clinical, histological, radiological or immunological characteristics or combinations of these. As a consequence, diagnosis of cases must rely on the same methods. Histology may play an important role in confirming diagnosis. The identification of causative infectious agents of any of these illnesses would be of great importance as it would redefine diagnostic criteria of these diseases or perhaps certain subsets of these disease groupings and might shift the emphasis in diagnosis to microbiological cultural or molecular methods. The identification of infectious agents might also have important preventive or therapeutic consequences. The circumstantial evidence that suggests infectious aetiologies for sarcoid, Crohn's disease and Hodgkin's disease is open to various forms of interpretation and work in these areas is ongoing.

Sarcoid

> *'Sarcoidosis is a disease characterized by the formation in all of several affected organs or tissues of epithelioid cell tubercles, without caseation though fibrinoid necrosis may present at centres of a few, proceeding either to resolution or to conversion into hyaline fibrous tissue.'*

Scadding and Mitchell.[23]

The frequent presentation of sarcoid as a disease of the lungs and thoracic lymph nodes, where granulomatous lesions occur, suggests that it might be caused by an infectious agent which enters the body by the respiratory route. Circumstantial evidence that it has a mycobacterial aetiology includes: the reported visualization of acid-fast bacilli in tissues, that mycobacteria have been isolated from animals inoculated with sarcoid tissue, that mycobacterial phages have been isolated from sarcoid tissue and that sarcoid and tuberculosis may co-exist. Recently, molecular techniques have been used in attempts to associate the presence of mycobacterial genetic material with the disease. Bocart and co-workers[24] searched for mycobacterial DNA in granulomatous tissue from patients with sarcoidosis using PCR with specific primers to amplify a gene coding for a 65 kDa mycobacterial antigen. Sixteen sarcoid patients and 13 control patients were studied. Sarcoid tissues tested were all non-caseating granulomas from lymph nodes (eight), lung (three), skin (three), spleen and liver (one) and pituitary (one). Only two patients yielded positive results. The DNA sequences appeared compatible with *Mycobacterium tuberculosis*, suggesting possibilities which include laboratory contamination or that some cases might have been caused by *M. tuberculosis*. By PCR, Fidler and co-workers[25] found *M. tuberculosis* DNA in tissues affected by sarcoidosis in seven of 16 sarcoid patients compared with one of 16 matched controls and suggested that sarcoid might be caused by cell wall-deficient *M. tuberculosis*, thus explaining its apparent presence by PCR and absence by microscopy of stained tissue. Cell wall-deficient bacteria, which reverted to slow-growing mycobacteria, were isolated from samples of sarcoid tissue by Al-Zaatari and co-workers[26] Using specific PCR assay these isolates were identified as belonging to the *Mycobacterium avium* complex. Hence, there is a growing body of evidence associating various mycobacterial species with cases of sarcoid.

Crohn's disease

Crohn's disease is an inflammatory condition, which may affect any part of the alimentary canal but especially the terminal ileum. It has the histological appearance of non-caseating tuberculosis-like granulomatous disease. The present general consensus on Crohn's is that the condition is multifactorial, that its causation is related both to host factors (immune response) and to exposure to one or more agents, which may be infective, and that a number of aetiologies may lead to what is seen as a single clinical entity. There is circumstantial evidence that Crohn's may be the human equivalent of Johne's disease, a chronic intestinal infection of cattle caused by *Mycobacterium paratuberculosis*. The very slow growth rate of this organism has hampered structured studies to investigate this possible association but a slow-growing paratuberculosis-like mycobacterium was cultured from Crohn's disease tissue by Chiodini and co-workers.[27] The characterization of a *M. paratuberculosis*-specific insertion sequence, IS*900*, has facilitated study.[28] Johne's disease causes clinical disease in 1–2% and asymptomatic infection in about 3% of British cattle.[29] There is evidence that the organism occurs in pasteurised milk and IS*900* has been detected in two-thirds of a sample of Crohn's disease bowel specimens and one-third of a sample of long-term Crohn's specimen cultures, compared with 10% of normal gut tissue specimens, leading to the hypothesis that in Crohn's disease, the organism occurs as a cell wall-deficient variant, which cannot be readily visualized in sections or cultured.[30] However, even if *M. paratuberculosis* does commonly occur in viable form in retail milk supplies, it should in theory be detectable, at least occasionally, from gut tissues from the bulk of the human population and there may be other environmental sources of exposure besides milk. Carefully matched comparative studies would be needed to demonstrate, convincingly, an association. There is mounting epidemiological evidence of an association between measles infection during pregnancy and subsequent Crohn's disease in children thus exposed to the virus.[31] The measles and mycobacterial hypostheses are not mutually exclusive and much remains to be understood about the aetiology of Crohn's disease.

Hodgkin's disease

Although Hodgkin's lymphoma is a neoplastic disease that affects the reticuloendothelial system the disease shows some clinical and epidemiological features suggestive of its having an infectious aetiology: these include chronic lymphadenopathy, often with affected nodes draining the respiratory tract, which might suggest the route of acquisition of an infectious agent; the occurrence of fevers and night sweats, as occurs with some chronic infectious diseases; and the observation of cases affecting multiple family members. Vianna and co-workers[32] conducted a study to provide denominator-based epidemiological evidence for transmission of Hodgkin's disease. They compared the incidence of new cases of the disease in schools where there had been a primary case with schools where there had been no cases. In five of eight schools with a primary case, there was a secondary case during the study period, compared with no cases in the matched control schools. Such findings suggested that the disease might be caused by common exposure, in the affected schools, to some causative agent. The search for an infectious agent in Hodgkin's has been hampered by the presence of different histological types of disease, and confusion over the relationship of these types to one another and with the non-Hodgkin lymphomas. Clearly if different types are the manifestations of fundamentally different diseases and if any one of them is caused by a particular infectious agent, it is important to conduct the search for the agent on a type-specific basis. The present understanding is that lymphocyte-depleted Hodgkin's is a discrete form of the disease and that the relationships between the other types and with non-Hodgkin lymphomas may be blurred.[33] Weiss and co-workers[34] demonstrated the presence of Epstein-Barr viral DNA in tissues from four of 21 cases of Hodgkin's disease compared with none of 30 cases of non-Hodgkin's lymphoma. That Epstein-Barr virus is the cause of Hodgkin's is an appealing hypothesis: infectious mononucleosis increases the risk of Hodgkin's and the virus is closely associated with other neoplastic disorders – Burkitt's lymphoma, lymphomas in the immunocompromised, nasopharyngeal carcinoma – and it can be shown to immortalize B lymphocytes in vitro. Furthermore, several recent studies have revealed viral DNA in Hodgkin's tissue and the location of the DNA has been localized to the

Hodgkin's and Reed-Sternberg cells.[35] However, Epstein-Barr virus is ubiquitous in human populations, so if there is a role for it in the aetiology of Hodgkin's disease there must be variation in host factors, such as immune response for example, the mode of infection or the virus is one of a number of cofactors. Sauter[36] proposed crown gall disease — a disease of plants caused by a bacterium, *Agrobacterium tumefaciens* — as a model for Hodgkin's. In crown gall disease, bacterial DNA becomes incorporated into plant DNA. *A. tumefaciens* can be shown by ribosomal RNA analysis to be related to the group of bacteria that includes *Bartonella* and *Brucella*, which are known to parasitize mammalian cells. Hence, Hodgkin's may be a late result of chronic bacterial lymph node infection when there is incorporation of bacterial DNA, leading to malignant change. Johnson and co-workers[37] proposed mycoplasma-like-organisms, which are non-cultivable cell wall-deficient intracellular bacteria, as the cause of Hodgkin's. Such bacteria infect plants and also intraocular leukocytes in the condition chronic idiopathic intraocular inflammation. It has been shown that such organisms invade cells, destroy the nucleus and cause proliferation. They produce lipid compounds called hopanoids, which resemble mammalian cholesterol and it was suggested that hoponoids might cause a granulomatous reaction.

Notes on cell wall-deficient bacteria

When a hypothesis states that bacteria might be present in a tissue and there is evidence that such tissues contain bacterial DNA but no bacterium may be visualized, an explanation must be provided. In the three examples described — sarcoid, Hodgkin's and Crohn's — those in support of bacterial aetiologies have explained the invisibility of bacteria by their lack of cell walls, which renders them impossible to stain by conventional methods. The presence of cell wall-deficient bacteria must be demonstrated by other techniques. A number of medically important bacteria naturally lack cell walls, notably *Mycoplasma*, *Ureaplasma* and to a variable degree *Streptobacillus moniliformis*. In addition to these, a large number of other bacterial species have been found in vivo or have been created in vitro as cell wall-deficient variants.[38] Such forms are described variously as pyroplasts, spheroplasts or L-forms (after the Lister Institute). L-forms are not cultivable on routine media as, lacking walls, the cells lyse without the use of special osmotic support media. They have received plenty of attention, although they are currently unfashionable, because it is recognized that L-forms may be recovered from patients who have received antibiotics that act on cell walls. By lacking walls such organisms are able to resist certain antibiotics and may act as microbial persisters or reservoirs of infection. As cell wall-deficient bacteria are hard to visualize and culture it is not unreasonable to suppose that the role of such organisms in some diseases may have been overlooked. Molecular detection, possibly followed by confirmation by electron microscopy, special culture or immunofluorescent methods may offer the best chance of clarifying such situations.

REFERENCES

1 Ray J. Dictionariolum trilingue. London: The Ray Society (facsimile, 1981), 1675

2 Linnaeus C. Systema naturae. 10th edn. London: British Museum (Natural History facsimile, 1956), 1758

3 Sneath PHA. Numerical taxonomy. In: Krieg NR, Holt JG, eds. Bergey's manual of systematic bacteriology. Vol. 1. Baltimore: Williams and Wilkins, 1984

4 Johnson JL. Nucleic acids in bacterial classification. In: Krieg NR, Holt JG, eds. Bergey's manual of systematic bacteriology. Vol. 1. Baltimore: Williams & Wilkins, 1984

5 Morell V. Web-crawling up the Tree of Life. Science 1996; 273: 568–570

6 Woese CR. Bacterial evolution. Microbial Rev 1987; 51: 221–271

7 Palleroni NJ. Family 1. Pseudomonadaceae. In: Krieg NR, Holt JG, eds. Bergey's manual of systematic bacteriology. Vol. 1. Baltimore: Williams & Willkins, 1984

8 Skerman VBD, McGowan V, Sneath PHA. Approved lists of bacterial names (amended edition). Washington: American Society for Microbiology. 1989

9 Paul J. 'Newer' and unusual bacteria. In: Weatherall D, Ledingham J, Warrell D, eds. Oxford textbook of medicine. 3rd edn. Vol. 1. 778–796. Oxford: Oxford University Press, 1995

10 Bruckner DA, Colonna P. Nomenclature for aerobic and facultative bacteria. Clin Infect Dis 1995; 21: 263–272

11 Summanen P. Mircrobiology terminology update: clinically significant anaerobic Gram-positive and Gram-negative bacteria (excluding spirochetes). Clin Infect Dis 1995; 21: 273–276

12 McGinnis MR, Rinaldi MG. Selected medically important fungi and some common synonyms and obsolete names. Clin Infect Dis 1995; 21: 277–278

13 Miller MJ. Viral taxonomy. Clin Infect Dis 1995; 21: 279–280

14 Garcia LS. Classification of human parasites, vectors, and similar organisms. Clin Infect Dis 1995; 21: 281–282

15 Holmes B. Why do bacterial names change? PHLS Microbiol Dig 1996; 12: 195–197

16 Relman DA, Loutit JS, Schmidt TM, Falkow S, Tompkins LS. The agent of bacillary angiomatosis: an approach to the identification of uncultured pathogens. N Engl J Med 1990; 323: 1573–1580

17 Slater LN, Welch DF, Hensel D, Coody DW. A newly recognised fastidious Gram-negative pathogen as a cause of fever and bacteremia. N Engl J Med 1990; 323: 1587–1593

18 Koeler JE, Quinn FD, Berger T, LeBoit PE, Tappero JW. Isolation of *Rochalimaea* species from cutaneous and osseous lesions of bacillary angiomatosis. N Engl J Med 1992; 327: 1625–1631

19 Regnery RL, Olson JG, Perkins BA, Bibb W. Serological response to 'Rochalimaea henselae' antigen in suspected cat-scratch disease. Lancet 1992; 339: 1443–1445

20 Daly JS, Worthington MG, Brenner DJ, et al. *Rochalimaea elizabethae* sp. nov. isolated from a patient with endocarditis. J Clin Microbiol 1993; 31: 872–881

21 Brenner DJ, O'Connor SP, Winkler HH, Steigerwalt AG. Proposals to unify the genera *Bartonella* and *Rochalimaea* with descriptions of *Bartonella quintana* comb. nov., *Bartonella vinsonii*, comb. nov., *Bartonella henselae*, comb. nov. and *Bartonella elizebethae*, comb. nov., and to remove the *Bartonellaceae* from the order Rickettsiales. Int J Syst Bacteriol 1993; 43: 777–786

22 Relman DA, Schmidt TM, MacDermott RP, Falkow. Identification of the uncultured Whipple's bacillus. N Engl J Med 1992; 327: 293–300

23 Scadding JG, Mitchell DN. Sarcoidosis. 2nd edn. London: Chapman & Hall, 1985

24 Bocart D, Lecossier D, De Lassence A, et al. Search for mycobacterial DNA in granulomatous tissues from patients with sarcoidosis using the polymerase chain reaction. Am Rev Resp Dis 1992; 145: 1142–1148

25 Fidler H, Rook GA, McJohnson N, McFadden J. *Mycobacterium tuberculosis* DNA in tissue affected by sarcoidosis. Br Med J 1993; 306: 546–549

26 El-Zaatari AK, Naser SA, Markesich DC, et al. Identification of *Mycobacterium avium* complex in sarcoidosis. J Clin Microbiol 1996; 34: 2240–2245

27 Chiodini RJ, Van Kruiningen HJ, Merkal RS, Thayer WR, Coutu JA. Characteristics of an unclassified *Mycobacterium* species isolated from patients with Crohn's disease. J Clin Microbiol 1984; 24: 966–971

28 Green EP, Tizard MLV, Moss MT, et al. Sequence and characteristics of IS*900*, an insertion element identified in a human Crohn's disease isolate of *Mycobacterium paratuberculosis*. Nucl Acids Res 1989; 17: 9063–9072

29 Çetinkaya B, Egan K, Harbour DA, Morgan KL. An abattoir-based study of the prevalence of subclinical Johne's disease in adult cattle in south west England. Epidemiol Infect 1996; 116: 373–379

30 Hermon-Taylor J. Crohn's disease is *Mycobacterium paratuberculosis* enteritis in humans; implications for prevention and treatment. First European congress of chemotherapy. Glasgow. Expert lecture 6, 1996

31 Vianna NJ, Polan AK. Epidemiological evidence for transmission of Hodgkin's disease. N Engl J Med 1973; 289: 499–502

32 Ekbom A, Daszak P, Kraaz W, Wakefield AJ. Crohn's disease after in-utero measles virus exposure. Lancet 1996; 348: 515–517

33 Krajewski AS, Jarrett RF. Progress in Hodgkin's disease. In: Kirkham N, Hall P, eds. Progress in pathology. Vol. 1. Edinburgh: Churchill Livingstone, 1995

34 Weiss LM, Strickler JG, Warnke RA, Purtillo DT, Sklar J. Epstein-Barr viral DNA in tissues of Hodgkin's disease. Am J Pathol 1987; 129: 86–91

35 Niedobitek G, Young LS. Epstein Barr virus and lymphomas: an overview. In: Kirkham N, Lemoine NR, eds. Progress in pathology. Vol. 2. Edinburgh: Churchill Livingstone, 1995

36 Sauter C. Is Hodgkin's disease a human counterpart of bacterially induced crown-gall tumours. Lancet 1995; 346: 1433

37 Johnson L, Wirostko E, Wirostko W, Wirostko B. Mycoplasma-like organisms in Hodgkin's disease. Lancet 1996; 347: 901–902

38 Guse LB. Microbial protoplasts, spheroplasts and L-forms. Baltimore: Williams & Wilkins, 1968

11

Synovial fluid in health and disease

S. Rogers

Synovial joints are located mainly in the limbs and consist of the hyaline cartilage-covered ends of bones joined together by a fibrous capsule. The inner aspect of the joint capsule is lined by synovium, and the space created by this anatomical arrangement contains the synovial fluid. Normal synovium is made up of a discontinuous surface layer of synoviocytes, type A cells, which are of the monocyte-macrophage lineage, and type B cells, which are fibroblastic, overlying fibrovascular connective tissue.

Synovial fluid itself consists of a dialysate of plasma with the addition of macromolecules (hyaluronic acid–proteoglycan) derived mainly from synovium and cartilage. It is the hyaluronans, derived from type B cells, that are responsible for the high viscosity of normal synovial fluid. The articular cartilage is bathed directly in synovial fluid and this is important for the nutrition of chondrocytes.

Normal joints contain only a small volume of straw-coloured, transparent synovial fluid, which contains few cells (approximately 100 cells. mm^{-3}). Normal cellular constituents include synoviocytes, chondrocytes, fibroblasts, mononuclear cells of the immune system and neutrophil polymorphs.[1]

In joint disease, changes occur in both the fluid and cellular phases of synovial fluid and in its overall volume. The relative accessibility of synovial fluid by joint aspiration makes it ideal for exploiting in diagnosis of joint diseases, yet it remains an under-used investigation.[2] Synovial biopsy has its place in diagnosis and is invaluable in the recognition of conditions such as crystal arthropathies, amyloid, pigmented villonodular synovitis and detritic arthritis.[3] However, in the differential diagnosis of inflammatory arthropathies, synovial biopsy is often of limited value. For example, the changes

Table 11.1 Differential diagnosis of an acute monoarthropathy

Inflammatory arthritis
   Rheumatoid disease
   Seronegative arthritis
Osteoarthritis
Crystal-induced arthritis
Infection
Trauma

observed in rheumatoid disease, ankylosing spondylitis, psoriatic arthritis and Reiter's syndrome are usually indistinguishable. A typical non-specific inflammatory pattern shows synovial hyperplasia with infiltration by lymphocytes and plasma cells, and formation of lymphoid follicles. This is one area in which synovial fluid cytology has a role to play. From the clinician's point of view, synovial fluid analysis is a relatively non-invasive means of investigating the cause of monoarthropathies (see Table 11.1) and to distinguish between inflammation and non-inflammatory joint disease. In experienced hands, the refined techniques of synovial fluid analysis can provide clinically relevant information quickly.

In recent years, much work has been undertaken in both research and diagnosis using synovial fluid – these advances will be reviewed and some practical aspects of synovial fluid analysis will be discussed.

Practical aspects of synovial fluid analysis

Most laboratories will have the necessary equipment for undertaking synovial fluid analysis. This includes a haemocytometer for calculating total nucleated cell counts and a microscope equipped with good quality polarizers and a first-order red compensator.

Specimen collection

Only small volumes of fluid are required for analysis (minimum 1 ml). Normal synovial fluid has no fibrinogen or clotting factors. However, in disease states, the fluid may contain fibrinogen and is liable to clot. Therefore fluid should be collected into a tube containing a suitable non-crystalline anticoagulant, such as lithium or sodium heparin.[4] The container should not contain any glass beads as these can interfere with subsequent crystal analysis. Ideally, the fluid should be analysed as soon as possible after aspiration. However, if necessary, the specimen may be transported and stored under refrigerated conditions at 4°C for 24–48 h before analysis without significantly altering diagnostic accuracy.[5]

Gross analysis

Viscosity

Viscosity can be estimated 'at the bedside' by expressing the fluid from the end of the syringe, having removed the needle after aspiration, or in the laboratory by 'dropping' the fluid from a glass pipette. Normal synovial fluid produces a stringing effect with a long tail, owing to high viscosity; with poor viscosity the fluid will produce a raindrop pattern with a short tail. In general, normal and non-inflammatory fluids have a high viscosity, whereas low viscosity is associated with inflammatory arthropathies. The low viscosity is caused by the depolymerization of the long chains of hyaluronate, which occurs in association with inflammation.

Colour

Colour should be assessed by placing the fluid in a clear glass tube and observing against a white background. Normal synovial fluid is usually colourless or faintly straw-coloured. In inflammatory and non-inflammatory disease states the fluid becomes yellowish or straw-coloured; inflammation is accompanied by increased diapedesis of red blood cells and this is responsible for the xanthochromic effect. In septic arthropathies the fluid may be yellow or green and frank pus may be aspirated; confusion may occur with fluids containing large numbers of crystals or rice bodies because these may be mistaken for pus on gross examination. Fresh bleeding results in a homogeneous red synovial fluid.

Clarity

Clarity is best assessed by placing a white background with black print behind the tube of fluid. With decreasing clarity, the print will become less readable through the tube. Normal synovial fluid is transparent; this changes from translucent to opaque with increasing numbers of particles in the synovial fluid, e.g. white blood cells, crystals, tissue aggregates and detritic debris.

Mucin clot test

If synovial fluid is mixed with a few drops of 2% acetic acid a white precipitate ('mucin clot') forms. In general, normal and non-inflammatory fluids form a good mucin clot, which can be wrapped around the end of the pipette as a long strand. In inflammatory arthropathies, and in the presence of haemorrhage, a poor, friable mucin clot forms owing to the fragmentation of the hyaluronate–protein complexes.

Total cell count

Total nucleated cell count can be measured using a standard haematological counting chamber. It is unwise to attempt to use an automated cell counter for this purpose because the machine may become clogged by the viscous fluid. Normal synovial fluid has a cell count of around 100 cells. mm^{-3}. In non-inflammatory arthropathies it is usually < 1000 cells mm^{-3}. Very high cell counts (in excess of 60 000 cells. mm^{-3}) generally indicates one of the following conditions: gout, sepsis, reactive arthropathy or rheumatoid disease (see Table 11.2).

Wet preparation

For the wet preparation a few drops of synovial fluid are placed on a clean microscope slide and a coverslip is applied and pressed down to flatten the cells. The gap between the slide and the coverslip can be sealed with clear nail varnish to retard dehydration of the fluid and reduce streaming of cells.[4] The wet preparation is required for detection of crystals and tissue fragments and for the identification of ragocytes.

Ragocytes are cells that contain cytoplasmic granules.[6] They can be recognized and distinguished from ordinary granulocytes on high power by closing down the condenser iris of the microscope to enhance the refractility of the cytoplasmic inclusions. The ragocyte granules are larger than neutrophil granules and change colour from black to apple green on focusing up and down. The percentage of white cells that are ragocytes is estimated and provides useful diagnostic information. Although these cells were originally thought to be specific for rheumatoid disease, it is now known that they are associated with a number of conditions. High counts (greater than 60%) can be found in patients with rheumatoid disease, gout, pseudogout and septic arthritis. It is therefore important to take account of the other features of the synovial fluid analysis before suggesting a diagnosis.

For crystal analysis, a microscope equipped with cross polarizers and a first-order red compensator is required. The compensator should be mounted above the bottom polarizer, and for microscopes with a conventional fixed stage, the compensator should be able to rotate through 90° overlying the polarizer. This arrangement allows for differentiation between positively and negatively birefringent crystals (see Fig. 11.1).

Monosodium urate crystals are needle-shaped, 2–10 μm long and when viewed under compensated polarized light they exhibit strong negative birefringence. They appear bright yellow against a red background when the long axis of the crystal is parallel to the compensator (Fig. 11.1a). The compensator will have an arrow marked on the handle which indicates the slow vibration direction of the compensator (see arrow on Figs 11.1a and 11.1b). Calcium pyrophosphate dihydrate crystals are rhomboidal in shape, variable in size from < 1 μm up to 10 μm and exhibit weak positive birefringence. They show a weak blue colour against the red background when the long axis of the crystal is parallel to the compensator (Fig. 11.1b).[7]

Table 11.2 Synovial fluid characteristics

	Normal	Non-inflammatory	Inflammatory	Purulent	Haemorrhagic
Colour	Clear	Straw-coloured	Straw-coloured	Variable: white, yellow, green	Red or xanthochromic
Clarity	Transparent	Transparent	Transparent/opaque	Opaque	Transparent/opaque
Viscosity	High	High	Low	Variable: usually low	Intermediate
Mucin clot	Good	Good	Friable	Friable	Friable
WBC. mm⁻³	100	100–1000	1500–60 000	> 50 000	1000–8000
Culture	Negative	Negative	Negative	*Positive	Negative
Examples		Osteoarthritis Traumatic arthritis Detritic arthritis Avascular bone necrosis Amyloidosis	Rheumatoid disease Crystal-induced arthritis Seronegative spondylarthropathies Connective tissue diseases Juvenile chronic arthritis Low-virulence infections e.g. viruses, fungi, mycoplasma, Lyme disease	*Septic arthritis Acute gout Acute pseudogout *Tuberculous arthritis Reactive arthritis	Trauma Bleeding diathesis Aseptic bone necrosis Pigmented villo-nodular synovitis

* only examples which would have positive cultures

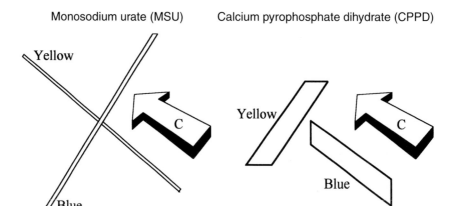

Monosodium urate (MSU)   Calcium pyrophosphate dihydrate (CPPD)

Fig. 11.1a MSU crystals viewed under compensated polarized light will exhibit a bright yellow colour when the long axis of the crystal is parallel to the compensator (C) and blue when it is perpendicular.

Fig. 11.1b CPPD crystals viewed under compensated polarized light will exhibit a weak blue colour when the long axis of the crystal is parallel to the compensator (C) and yellow when it is perpendicular.

The microscope set-up for crystal analysis should be checked by using reference slides, for example, a urate tophus, as a standard.

For detection of calcium hydroxyapatite crystals, which are not naturally birefringent and may be mistaken for dust, Alizarin red is instilled beneath the coverslip. These crystals form a birefringent red complex with the dye and are recognized by their morphology as fine granules.[8]

Diagnostic pitfalls in crystal analysis of joint fluids relate to the misinterpretation of artefactual crystals. In particular, crystals produced by plastics in sample tubes and steroid crystals from intra-articular injections may cause confusion. The latter may be mistaken for calcium pyrophosphate crystals; they can be distinguished from these by their absence of birefringence and failure to react with Alizarin red.

Other particles may be seen in the wet preparation; indeed, if recognizable macroscopically the particles should be selected out from the fluid for scrutiny. These include fragments of cartilage, which have been shed from the articular surface, synovial villi, meniscal fragments and wear debris from prosthetic joints.

Cytocentrifuge preparations

To obtain a cell monolayer in a cytocentrifuge preparation it may be necessary to dilute the synovial fluid with normal saline. The optimum concentration is 400 cells. mm^{-3} and the suspension should be centrifuged at 800 r.p.m. for 15–30 min and then air-dried for giemsa staining.[9] If there is a suspicion of infection, further slides may be required for Gram, para-aminosalicylic acid (PAS) or Zn staining.

There is a great diversity of cells which, with practice, can be identified in synovial fluid using giemsa-stained cytocentrifuge preparations; these include polymorphs, LE cells, mast cells, eosinophils, macrophages, cytophagocytic macrophages and synoviocytes. The presence or absence of the various cell types is noted and their numbers expressed as a percentage of the total nucleated cells by counting a random sample of 100 cells to produce a differential cell count.[10]

Inflammatory arthropathies

Rheumatoid disease

Rheumatoid disease usually manifests as a chronic inflammatory joint disease of unknown aetiology, which typically causes a peripheral, symmetrical polyarthritis. It is likely that the disease is triggered in genetically predisposed individuals by exposure to an unknown microbial agent. Once the acute arthritis has been initiated, there is a continuing autoimmune reaction involving T cells and local release of inflammatory mediators and cytokines, which leads to joint damage.[11] The presence of rheumatoid factor (IgM anti-IgG) activity in the serum is associated with disease severity. Rheumatoid disease characteristically has a prolonged course punctuated by exacerbations and remissions. Synovial fluid analysis is most likely to be of use in cases with atypical clinical presentations and during acute exacerbations to exclude a superimposed infective arthropathy and to distinguish active rheumatoid disease from secondary osteoarthritic changes.

Synovial fluid findings are variable, but in typical rheumatoid disease, the synovial fluid is translucent and forms a poor mucin clot; the cell count varies from $5-30 \times 10^3$ mm^{-3} with a ragocyte count of around 70%. The neutrophil polymorph is the predominant cell, often with marked apoptosis. Cytophagocytic macrophages are characteristically not seen.[9]

Serial synovial fluid analysis in patients with rheumatoid disease can provide prognostically useful information.[12] Synovial fluids in which lymphocytes and not neutrophils are the predominant cell type are associated with a more favourable prognosis, whereas high nucleated cell counts and high ragocyte counts point to a poorer outcome. Ragocyte granules represent immune complexes that have been ingested from the synovial fluid. It is thought that the subsequent release of lysosomal enzymes, which follows phagocytosis, plays a major part in the joint destruction of rheumatoid disease and this may explain why the outcome is worse where ragocyte counts are high.

Microscopic rice bodies consist of fibrinous particles formed by the entrapment of inflammatory cells in the dense fibrin network within inflamed joints. They occur in chronically inflamed joints in a number of conditions but are most frequently associated with rheumatoid disease.[13] Rice bodies can be detected by histological examination of synovial fluid sediments.

Seronegative spondylarthropathies

The seronegative arthropathies are a group of diseases including ankylosing spondylitis, Reiter's syndrome, psoriatic arthritis and enteropathic arthritis, which are characterized by the absence of serum rheumatoid factors and a clinical and genetic (association with HLA-B27) relationship to ankylosing spondylitis. These conditions also share similar findings on synovial fluid analysis. In most cases, this manifests as a typical, non-specific inflammatory picture with > 1000 cells. mm^{-3} and neutrophil polymorphs predominating. However, in some cases the synovial fluid findings are more specific for a seronegative inflammatory arthropathy, with lymphocytes and macrophages predominating and the presence of mast cells and/or cytophagocytic macrophages.[14]

Cytophagocytic macrophages are large macrophage-like cells with intracytoplasmic inclusions of effete cells or nuclear debris. These cells were first described in Reiter's syndrome and became known as Reiter or Pekin cells.[15] They are now known to occur in a variety of conditions, including septic arthritis and crystal arthropathies. Nevertheless, their presence in high numbers (> 5% of large mononuclear cells), or in association with mast cells, is indicative of a seronegative arthropathy. It has been proposed that cytophagocytic macrophages may play a regulatory role in synovial fluid by ingesting apoptotic neutrophil polymorphs, thereby preventing autolysis and limiting subsequent tissue damage.

Infective arthritis

Infective arthritis is important to recognize because untreated it can lead to rapid joint destruction. Normal joints seldom become infected unless the joint space is penetrated by a foreign body. More often, the patient has pre-existing joint disease or some other predisposing factor such as immuno-suppression or co-existing infection elsewhere. The normal route of infection is via the bloodstream.

In acute septic arthritis cells counts are very high (> 50 000 cells. mm^{-3}) with neutrophils predominating and there is a high proportion of ragocytes (> 90%). Bacteria are usually seen. However, synovial fluid leukocyte counts in the 'inflammatory range' have been described in immunocompromised patients with culture-proven infective arthritis. A high degree of suspicion for infectious arthritis should be maintained in at-risk patient groups such as intravenous drug abusers, patients with malignant disease and those on steroid therapy.[16]

Less common forms of infective arthritis include tuberculosis, viral and fungal infections and Lyme disease.

Lyme disease is transmitted by the bite of deer flies or ticks, for example *Ixodes dammini*, and the causative organism is the spirochaete, *Borrelia burgdorferi*. In about 50% of cases, Lyme disease is associated with the development of an oligoarthritis affecting large joints. The synovial fluid findings have been described as being similar to those of rheumatoid disease and, in a few cases, synovial fluid eosinophilia (> 2% eosinophils) has been reported.[17] Synovial fluid eosinophilia has also been reported in a variety of parasitic arthritidies, such as infection with *Strongyloides stercoralis, Ascaris lumbricoides* and *Enterobius vermicularis*, and in patients with rheumatoid and psoriatic arthritis and in association with hypereosinophilic syndromes.

Crystal-induced synovitis

The most commonly encountered crystals, which are relevant to joint disease, are monosodium urate, calcium pyrophosphate dihydrate and hydroxyapatite. The methods used for their identification have been described above. These crystals can cause acute inflammatory arthritis and/or chronic destructive joint disease (see Table 11.3).

Gout

Gout has been known about since Egyptian times. In 1797, William Hyde Woolaston, himself a gout sufferer, identified uric acid in gouty tophi.[7] Release of monosodium urate crystals into the joint space causes an acute inflammatory arthropathy. Affected patients usually have hyperuricaemia. Hyperuricaemia may be caused by increased intake of purines in the diet, overproduction of uric acid or renal/gut undersecretion of uric acid. Uric acid overproduction may be primary as in the X-linked deficiency of the enzyme hypoxanthine guanine ribosyl transferase, idiopathic, or secondary to myeloproliferative disorders, haemolysis or carcinomatosis. Renal undersecretion may be idiopathic or secondary to a variety of conditions such as chronic renal failure, hyperparathyroidism, diuretic therapy, lactic acidosis, lead poisoning and myxoedema.[7]

Table 11.3 Crystal-induced synovitis

	Gout	Acute pseudogout	Destructive pyrophosphate arthropathy
Colour	Yellow/white	Yellow/white	Straw-coloured
Clarity	Opaque	Opaque	Clear
Viscosity	Low	Low	High
Mucin clot	Friable	Friable	Good
WBC. mm^{-3}	> 20 000	> 20 000	< 1 000
Predominant cell type	Polymorphs	Polymorphs	Lymphocytes, macrophages, synoviocytes
% Ragocytes	> 40%	> 40%	< 5%
Crystal type	Monosodium urate	Calcium pyrophosphate dihydrate	Calcium pyrophosphate dihydrate (CPPD) and hydroxyapatite
Crystal shape	Needle-shaped	Rhomboidal	CPPD: rhombodial
Birefringence	Strong negative	Weak positive	CPPD: weak positive. Hydroxyapatite forms a birefringent complex with Alizarin red

Gout principally affects men over 40 years of age and postmenopausal women. The disease is typically characterized by recurring attacks of acute inflammation usually affecting a single joint in the lower leg. In its classical form gout presents no problem in diagnosis to the clinician. It is, however, not always an easy diagnosis to make and it is in such atypical cases that synovial fluid analysis is of particular diagnostic benefit.

During an acute attack, crystals of monosodium urate monohydrate are precipitated within the synovial fluid. The crystals become coated with immunoglobulins and are ingested by polymorphonuclear leukocytes, with subsequent disruption of their phagolysosomes and cell membranes leading to release of chemotactic factors and destructive lysosomal and cytoplasmic enzymes. With repeated attacks, urate crystals become deposited within and around the joint leading to permanent joint deformity and the formation of gouty tophi. Diagnosis from synovial fluid analysis rests on the finding of the characteristic crystals within the fluid, which may be intra- or extracellular. The cell count is in the inflammatory range (see Table 11.1) and is predominantly neutrophilic. The ragocyte count is often raised.

Calcium pyrophosphate deposition disease

Crystals of calcium pyrophosphate dihydrate (CPPD) may be detected in the synovial fluid in three different clinical settings: acute pseudogout, destructive arthropathy and occasionally in joints affected by chondrocalcinosis. The latter is a common condition in the elderly in which cartilage becomes calcified and occasionally CPPD crystals will be shed into the synovial fluid. This is of no clinical consequence and is not associated with inflammation. It may lead to diagnostic confusion if over-interpreted, especially when there is a coincident, unrelated joint disease affecting the same joint.

Acute pseudogout, on the other hand, is an important condition, which clinically resembles gout. It has a much shorter history, being first recognized in the early 1960s by analysis of synovial fluid of joints from patients with a gout-like syndrome, but in whom there was a tendency for more proximal joints to be affected. The knees are the commonest site for acute pseudogout. Pyrophosphate arthropathy has been associated with hypothyroidism, haemochromatosis, hyperparathyroidism and steroid therapy.[7] Acute pseudogout is probably initiated by shedding of crystals from a pre-formed deposit into the joint space, thereby initiating an inflammatory reaction, with a similar response to that described for urate crystals. The synovial fluid findings are similar to those of gout except that the crystals differ. That is, the cell count is high with neutrophils predominating and with a high proportion of ragocytes (see Table 11.3).

Chronic destructive pyrophosphate arthropathy may be clinically indistinguishable from osteoarthritis. Again, the knees are the commonest site, followed by wrists, hands, shoulders and ankles. It has been postulated that local joint damage, in the form of minor osteoarthritic changes may predispose to CPPD deposition, which causes inflammation and leads to a vicious cycle of joint damage, which is often severe and destructive.

The synovial fluid in such cases shows a non-inflammatory picture with < 1000 cells. mm^{-3}, predominantly mononuclear cells, and a low ragocyte count. Owing to the destructive nature of this arthropathy the CPPD crystals may be accompanied by large numbers of hydroxyapatite crystals.

Hydroxyapatite

Hydroxyapatite − $Ca_5(PO_4)_3(OH)$ − is the most stable crystalline form of calcium phosphate in vivo. It forms the main mineral constituent of bone and occurs at sites of pathological calcification throughout the body, including joints. It is deposited in soft tissues around the shoulder and is commonly found in joints affected by osteoarthritis and rheumatoid disease. The crystals themselves are not visible by light microscopy. However, they tend to form aggregates in joint fluid and are visible by 'pseudophase' microscopy. They are best demonstrated by instillation of Alizarin red under the coverslip of a wet preparation.

Non-inflammatory arthropathies

Osteoarthritis

Osteoarthritis is a common, progressive joint disease that most commonly affects the hands, knees and hips. The initial pathological changes occur in the articular cartilage of affected joints. The chondrocytes proliferate to form clones and there is an increase in water content and a reduction in proteoglycans in the cartilage matrix. This is followed by surface fibrillation and vertical fissuring, fragments of damaged cartilage slough off exposing the underlying bone, which becomes eburnated as bone articulates with bone in the damaged joint. Thin-walled cysts form in the subchondral bone and osteophytes form at the joint margins in an attempt to restore joint stability. The synovium, by comparison, shows minor changes with fibrosis, hyperplasia of synoviocytes and scattered chronic inflammatory cells, predominantly lymphocytes.[18]

Osteoarthritis does not usually present a diagnostic problem to the clinician. However, there are occasions when diagnostic joint aspiration may be indicated as a consequence of an acute flare-up in a joint which presents clinically with pain and swelling. In these circumstances, synovial fluid analysis can help by distinguishing between inflammatory and non-inflammatory conditions.

The synovial fluid in osteoarthritis typically shows a non-inflammatory picture being clear and viscous with a good mucin clot. The total nucleated cell count is low. Exposure of subchondral bone may lead to release of hydroxyapatite crystals and fragments of cartilage may be present. In severely damaged joints, haemorrhage may occur as a result of intra-articular fractures of the thin-walled subchondral bone cysts.

Trauma

The commonest manifestation of trauma to joints is the production of a traumatic haemarthrosis. The synovial fluid findings in such cases depend on whether or not the haemorrhage is accompanied by fluid exudation across the damaged synovium. In cases where there is haemorrhage, but little or no exudate, the synovial fluid findings will show a cell count of approximately 8000 cells mm^{-3}, with blood-derived polymorphs predominating. In the presence of fluid exudation the cell count will be low.

The finding of intracellular lipid in synovial fluid has been reported in association with intra-articular fracture. In these cases, the lipid droplets contained needle-shaped crystals on polarized microscopy. The lipid is assumed to be bone marrow-derived and to be a useful pointer to the presence of fracture in joints with a low cell count and haemorrhage.[19,20]

In cases of unexplained haemarthrosis with no history of trauma, or in patients with recurrent intra-articular bleeding, other causes of haemorrhage should be considered. Non-traumatic haemarthrosis may occur as a result of a bleeding diathesis and in patients with pigmented villo-nodular synovitis.

Artificial joints

Joint replacement surgery is now commonplace and fluid may be aspirated from such joints. Joint infection is a risk with all artificial joints, particularly in the first 6 months post- implantation. It can usually be traced to intra-operative bacterial contamination, and the usual causative organisms are *Staphylococcus aureus, Staphylococcus epidermidis* and *Streptococcus*. Late infection, occurring after 6 months, is usually a consequence of haematogenous spread of bacteria from a site elsewhere in the body. In chronic infection, the usual causative organism is *Staphylococcus epidermidis*.

Wear particles may be released into the joint space during function of joint prostheses. The particles depend on the type of prosthesis used and include bone cement debris (polymethacrylate and X-ray contrast medium), polyethylene particles, alumina ceramic particles and, in small joint prostheses, silicone wear particles. The fate of such wear particles is dependent upon their size. Small ones (< 30 µm) are phagocytosed by macrophages, larger particles may be incorporated into the soft tissues where they excite a foreign body giant cell reaction. Synovial fluid from joints with worn prostheses may contain identifiable particles. Polyethylene particles are thread-like, varying in diameter from 0.5–1 mm and exhibit birefringence in polarized light. Methylmethacrylate particles are refractile but not birefringent. Special techniques such as electron probe microanalysis may be employed as a research tool for the identification of metal particles.[21]

The cytological characteristics of synovial fluid from prosthetic joints are very variable, depending on the functional state of the joint. With impending joint failure, the features may be those of a traumatic haemarthrosis or those of a non-specific inflammatory arthropathy.

Malignancy

Malignant cells in joint effusions are rare and virtually all reports occur in the setting of metastatic disease. Activated lymphocytes of rheumatoid disease should not be confused with malignant cells. Squamous cell carcinoma is one of the most frequently described metastatic malignancies – the cytological features being typical with the presence of 'tadpole' and 'fibre' cells.[22] In difficult cases, immunocytochemistry may be needed to establish the diagnosis. Interpretation of the immunostaining should rely on detecting positivity in the obviously malignant cells because both synoviocytes and mesothelial cells may exhibit positive keratin staining.

More commonly, cancer patients may develop joint symptoms as a secondary phenomenon, e.g. gout in haematological malignancies and as a consequence of hyperuricaemia following chemotherapy, or CPPD deposition as a result of hypercalcaemia.

Key points for clinical practice

- Synovial fluid analysis is useful in investigating the cause of mono- and oligoarthropathies.
- Synovial fluids can be classified as inflammatory, non-inflammatory, purulent or haemorrhagic on the basis of gross appearances, total cell counts and culture.
- In some instances, synovial fluid findings may point to a specific cause within the groups of inflammatory or non-inflammatory joint disease.
- Very high cell counts, > 60 000 cells. mm^{-3} indicate one of the following conditions: gout, sepsis, reactive arthritis or rheumatoid disease.
- High ragocyte counts > 60% are associated with rheumatoid arthritis, gout, pseudogout or sepsis.
- In immunocompromised patients, maintain a high degree of suspicion for infectious arthritis.
- Monosodium urate crystals are needle-shaped and exhibit strong negative birefringence under compensated polarized light.
- Calcium pyrophosphate dihydrate crystals are rhomboidal in shape and exhibit weak positive birefringence under compensated polarized light.

REFERENCES

1 Serre G, Vincent C, Mauduyt MA, Soleilhavoup J-P, Planel H. Morphologic, quantitative and cytoenzymologic studies of synoviocytic and monocytic cells in synovial fluid. Anal Quantit Cytol 1984; 6: 227–237

2 Freemont AJ. Synovial fluid analysis. The forgotten investigation. Eur J Med 1993; 2: 323–326

3 Revell PA. The synovial biopsy. In: Anthony PP, MacSween RMN, eds. Recent Advances in Histopathology. Edinburgh: Churchill Livingstone, 1987: 79–94

4 Gatter RA. A practical handbook of joint fluid analysis. Philadelphia: Lea and Febiger, 1984

5 Jones STM, Denton J, Holt PJL, Freemont AJ. Refrigeration preserves synovial fluid cytology. Ann Rheum Dis 1993; 52: 384

6 Hollander JL, McCarty DJ, Astorga G, Castro-Murillo E. Studies of the pathogenesis of rheumatoid joint inflammation. The 'RA cell' and a working hypothesis. Ann Intern Med 1965; 62: 271–280

7 Dieppe PA, Calvert P. Crystals and joint disease. London: Chapman and Hall, 1983

8 Cunningham T, Uebelhart D, Very JM, Fallet GH, Vischer TL. Synovial fluid hydroxyapatite crystals: detection threshold of two methods. Ann Rheum Dis 1989; 48: 829–831

9 Freemont AJ, Denton J. Atlas of synovial fluid cytopathology. Dordrecht: Kluwer Academic Publishers, 1991

10 Freemont AJ, Denton J, Chuck A, Holt PJL, Davies M. Diagnostic value of synovial fluid microscopy: a reassessment and retionalisation. Ann Rheum Dis 1991; 50: 101–107

11 Sewell KL, Trentham DE. Pathogenesis of rheumatoid arthritis. Lancet 1993; 341: 283–286

12 Davis MJ, Denton J, Freemont AJ, Holt PJL. Comparison of serial synovial fluid cytology in rheumatoid arthritis: delineation of subgroups with prognostic implications. Ann Rheum Dis 1988; 47: 559–562

13 Galvez J, Sola J, Ortuno G, et al. Microscopic rice bodies in rheumatoid synovial fluid sediments. J Rheum 1992; 19: 1851–1858

14 Freemont AJ, Denton J. The disease distribution of synovial fluid mast cells and cytophagocytic mononuclear cells in inflammatory arthritis. Ann Rheum Dis 1985; 44: 312–315

15 Pekin TJ, Malinin TI, Zvaifler WJ. Unusual synovial fluid findings in Reiter's syndrome. Ann Intern Med 1967; 66: 677–684

16 McCutchan HJ, Fisher RC. Synovial leukocytosis in infectious arthritis. Clin Ortho Rel Res 1990; 257: 226–230

17 Kay J, Eichenfeld AH, Athreya BH, Doughty RA, Schumacher HR. Synovial fluid eosinophilia in Lyme disease. Arthritis Rheumatol 1988; 31: 1384–1389

18 Hamerman D. The biology of osteoarthritis. N Engl J Med 1989; 320: 1322–

19 Baer AN, Wright EP. Lipid laden macrophages in synovial fluid: a late finding in traumatic arthritis. J Rheumatol 1987; 14: 848–851

20 Freemont AJ, Denton J. Synovial fluid findings early in traumatic arthritis. J Rheumatol 1987; 15: 881–882

21 Lohrs U, Bos I. The pathology of artificial joints. In: Berry CL, ed. Current topics in Pathology. Berlin: Springer-Verlag, 1994: 1–51

22 Flint A, Remick DG. Metastatic squamous cell carcinoma: diagnosis by synovial fluid aspiration. Acta Cytol 1984; 6: 776–777

12

The current status of the autopsy

R. D. Start   D. W. K. Cotton

The Greek word autopsy means 'to see for one's self' and therefore has no specific reference to a post mortem examination; consequently the preferred synonym is necropsy, which means 'to see after death'. Whichever terminology is employed, the autopsy retains an important and yet often unrecognized role in modern medical practice. The aim of this review is to promote the role of autopsy and to identify those other areas in which autopsies can make a useful contribution to a variety of medical disciplines.

Autopsy rate definitions

Standardization of the methods used to calculate autopsy rates is essential in order to facilitate useful comparative studies and all discussions of specific autopsy rates should begin by establishing which definitions of autopsy rates are appropriate.[1] There are two main types of autopsy in the UK: medico–legal autopsies are performed at the request of the local coroner or equivalent authority; whilst clinical (hospital or consent) autopsies are performed after permission has been obtained from relatives of the deceased. It should be remembered that coroner's autopsies take precedence in the sense that hospital autopsies can only be requested when it has been decided that the coroner has no interest in the case. For instance, a hospital autopsy cannot be requested in order to determine the cause of death because if the cause of death is unknown, the case must automatically be referred to the coroner.

The overall or total autopsy rate for a hospital, clinical department or individual clinician is simply defined as the total number of autopsies divided by the total number of deaths. The separate autopsy rates for medico-legal and clinical or hospital autopsies are occasionally referred to as differential autopsy rates,[2] but there appears to be some confusion in relation to their precise definition. In all cases when a death certificate cannot be completed, the death must be referred to the coroner or equivalent authority; the medico-legal autopsy rate being defined as the number of medico-legal autopsies divided by the total number of deaths. The assertion that 'non-sudden death' medico-legal cases should be included in the clinical autopsy rate, because clinical autopsies might have been requested if the cases had not fallen within medico-legal jurisdiction, makes too many assumptions regarding clinician's autopsy request behaviour to have any validity. The clinical autopsy rate is more complicated and at least two definitions are currently in use. The clinical autopsy rate may be defined as the number of clinical autopsies divided by the total number of deaths or, alternatively, as the number of clinical autopsies divided by the number of deaths remaining after medico-legal autopsies have been subtracted. The discrepancies between clinical autopsy rates calculated by the two methods are variable and there is potential for misleading comparisons if clinical autopsy rates are not defined clearly. The information provided by the two methods is different and the inclusion of both rates would not only augment autopsy audit but would also remove a potential source of confusion.

Trends in autopsy rates

Approximately one in four of all registered deaths is followed by a medico-legal autopsy and this medico-legal autopsy rate has remained relatively constant during the last few decades. Clinical autopsy rates have declined during each decade since the 1950s.[2,3] Less than 10 000 clinical autopsies are now performed each year in England and Wales and these numbers represent less than 2% of all deaths.[4] Similar trends have been seen in other countries whilst relatively few, mainly those where consent is not required, have managed to maintain high autopsy rates.[5] There are also no satisfactory definitions of what constitutes an adequate autopsy rate. An overall figure of 35% has been suggested,[6] but the acceptable proportions of clinical and medico-legal autopsies within such an overall total have yet to be defined and even then the lack of standardization in the use of autopsy rate definitions might prevent valid comparisons between different centres.

Many factors have contributed to the steady decline in clinical autopsy rates, the most important of which has been a failure to change the attitudes of clinicians towards the autopsy. The level of a clinician's interest in autopsies appears to be the most important factor in the decision to request an autopsy.[7] The new 'high-tech' diagnostic modalities available in modern medicine have increased the clinician's confidence in clinical diagnoses with the result that autopsies are often considered to be obsolete and unnecessary. Many clinicians, particularly physicians, are sceptical of persisting high levels of discrepancy between clinical and autopsy diagnoses.[8-11] They do not see a major role for autopsy in clinical audit and are reluctant to acknowledge the importance of autopsy to the accuracy of mortality statistics, medical education and the monitoring of the effects of new treatment regimens and diagnostic procedures.

Pathologists are themselves not blameless, and some, overburdened by other duties, would vigorously oppose attempts to increase clinical autopsy rates.[12] Apathy, low standards of autopsy practice and poor communication have understandably failed to stimulate interest from clinicians who need to be convinced of the continuing relevance of the autopsy.[13] This lack of interest results in a reluctance to request autopsies, which is reinforced by unpleasant demonstration facilities, a lack of proper request procedures and hostile relatives who have themselves been influenced by the medical community's failure to appreciate the role of the autopsy.

Whilst the factors contributing to the decline in clinical autopsy rates can be identified, the reasons for the increases in medico-legal autopsy rates can rarely be identified easily. An increased public awareness of opportunities for litigation and the influences of individual coroners may be important factors. Another suggestion is that some clinicians are using medico-legal autopsies as substitute for clinical autopsies.[3] These clinicians may be unaware of the legal constraints that prevent the retention of tissues from medico-legal autopsies and therefore limit the scientific and educational value of this type of autopsy. The reciprocal changes in the clinical and medico-legal autopsy rates mean that the medico-legal autopsy is now the major component of autopsy practice in some teaching centres. If the current trend continues and the maintenance of satisfactory overall autopsy rates becomes consistently dependent on a high proportion of medico-legal autopsies, then the availability of reports and material from these cases could become critically important for medical education, audit and research.

The autopsy and medical education

The involvement of medical students in the autopsy suite as a routine part of their curriculum has declined steadily in the last few decades. It is generally agreed that the many and difficult issues surrounding death, dying and bereavement should receive more attention in modern integrated undergraduate medical education.[14] Regardless of specialist interests, all doctors require a basic understanding of the variety of cultural attitudes that exist towards death. The role of autopsy should form an integral part of this knowledge base, and the utility of the information provided by autopsies should be presented at all appropriate opportunities with practical instruction in specific related communication skills, such as how to break bad news and how to approach relatives for autopsy consent.[14] Beginning as medical students and junior trainees, doctors must consider and appreciate the need for autopsies, with suitable encouragement provided through observations of senior clinicians making autopsy requests to grieving relatives. The responsibility for autopsy requests remain with the consultant in charge of the case and the delegation of this duty should be a positive process and not merely left to the most inexperienced junior clinicians.[15] Little of the factual content of consultations at the time of death may remain with the relatives, but they will remember much of the delivery style.[16]

Some units, particularly those involved in transplantation or in paediatrics, operate clearly defined autopsy-request policies. Others request autopsies on a single-case basis and autopsy requests are more likely when patients are young and confidence in clinical diagnoses is low.[7] Surgeons seem to have a special interest in autopsies when patients die before surgery or as a result of postoperative complications. This interest appears to incorporate a personal audit of the individual surgeon's complications of surgery and the suitability of surgical intervention in particular clinical situations. The suggestion that accreditation for training could be linked to the demonstration of an adequate autopsy rate requires consideration, but would be difficult to enforce in practice.[15] First, there is the lack of standardized autopsy rate definitions with no agreement on what constitutes an adequate autopsy rate and second, clinical autopsy rates are dependent on consent from relatives. Age, religious and cultural influences can produce low autopsy rates despite the most sensitive request procedures. It may be more useful to monitor autopsy request rates but this type of information is rarely available in most centres.

Hospitals also have a duty towards public education and, in cases where consent is given for autopsy, relatives may want to be informed of the results of this investigation. It is important that autopsy findings are communicated without delay. This can be achieved through a post-autopsy conference with the relatives, as is often carried out in the case of sudden infant death syndrome (SIDS), or through the family doctor. Pathology departments can and should routinely send copies of clinical autopsy reports to family doctors. The Royal College of Pathologists has issued guidelines for the speed (or 'timeliness') with which clinical autopsy reports should be issued and clinicians must insist on the observance of these targets, which include a summary to be issued within 2 days and a final report, including histology, to be issued within 3 weeks of the autopsy date.[17] The provision of medico-legal autopsy reports to clinical teams is dependent on agreement of the local coroner or equivalent authority and some will not even release such reports for the purposes of the National Confidential Enquiry into Perioperative Deaths (NCEPOD).[18] This practice is obstructive, particularly when relatives are legally entitled to obtain copies of these autopsy reports directly from the same authority.

Medical education must therefore also address the medico-legal aspects of death. The opportunities to teach important practical skills, such as death certification and the indications for the referral of deaths to coroners, are decreasing under pressure from other subjects within the undergraduate curriculum. Postgraduate education is uncommon because of a lack of appreciation of the importance of these issues. These attitudes are reinforced by the virtual absence of medico-legal topics in many current professional examinations and the common practice of delegating these duties to junior clinicians. Such behaviour may explain why some senior clinicians appear to have less knowledge of the medico-legal aspects of medicine than the juniors under their supervision.[19] Some pathologists monitor the circumstances of all hospital deaths, whilst also ensuring the accuracy of death certification.[20] This system would not be practicable or acceptable in many centres and an accessible advice service combined with better postgraduate education and the regular circulation of written guidelines should be adequate solutions.

It is important to bear in mind the fact that national statistics regarding disease incidence and prevalence are based to some extent on death certificates, including those completed without benefit of autopsy.

In an educational sense, the autopsy provides a useful opportunity to develop problem-solving skills. Autopsies provide ready-made clinical problems through which the basic science of pathology can be linked to applied clinical situations. Autopsy demonstrations should be informal sessions in which there is an opportunity to enhance interest and knowledge through discussions and interaction.[21] Some autopsy rooms will never be able to overcome negative aesthetic considerations and there is scope for alternative and improved presentation of autopsy material. Still-video or closed-circuit television recordings of autopsy findings can be combined with radiological and biochemical information to create fully integrated teaching material for all levels of medical education.[22,23] The same records of autopsy findings can be shown during regular clinico-pathological meetings to those clinicians unable to attend autopsy demonstrations because of other inescapable duties. Clinical autopsies can be a valuable educational tool for trainee surgeons who can further their clinical anatomy knowledge through assisting with autopsies. Practical skills, such as fibreoptic examination of the upper gastrointestinal and respiratory tracts, can be developed and refined during clinical autopsies. New surgical procedures can be devised, tested and improved using cadavers at autopsy. Major orthopaedic, cardiothoracic and ear, nose and throat (ENT) surgical procedures are particularly suited to clinical autopsy-based development.

The decline in autopsy rates has provoked a critical evaluation of the current role of autopsy in clinical practice. This appraisal has in turn stimulated the development and application of a wide range of technical innovations, which together have enabled the autopsy to maintain its importance within modern medicine.[24] Some observers believe that the autopsy remains largely a gross anatomical technique, which has changed little since its development in the era of descriptive anatomy. This view ignores all of the new dissection methods described for sites previously rarely examined in detail,[25,26] and also ignores the growing practice of sectioning tissues in planes similar to those studied by modern imaging techniques, such as echocardiography and computed tomography, in order to facilitate direct correlation of autopsy findings with earlier investigations during life.[27] The introduction of these and other procedures such as cytology, toxicology, angiography and other imaging techniques reflects the continuing evolution of the autopsy, which is essential if the ever-changing requirements of modern clinical practices are to be met.[28,29] Pathologists should be familiar with new autopsy techniques, and an ability to adapt the standard autopsy examination for specific conditions not only prevents the loss of important information but is also appreciated by the clinicians responsible for making the autopsy request. In cases where relatives wish to restrict the extent of an autopsy, the option of a needle-core biopsy autopsy might be acceptable and laparoscopic autopsy has been developed in some centres.[30,31]

The autopsy and research

Effective audit programmes based on the information from autopsies provides an ideal mechanism for identifying those areas of clinical practice that could benefit from further research. The NCEPOD has facilitated recognition of the persisting problems of thromboembolism in surgical practice,[18,32] whilst other autopsy studies have demonstrated difficulties in the accurate diagnosis of intra-abdominal sepsis, visceral performations and the complications of previous surgical intervention.[8–11]

The effects of the established decline in clinical autopsy rates on autopsy-based output and the possible implications for the provisions of material for future research applications are difficult to assess.[33] Few formal measurements of the utility of autopsy-derived material in research programmes are available to support or refute suggestions that research activities may be compromised by declining clinical autopsy rates. Many of the modern concepts of disease and health evolved from detailed observations collected from large numbers of autopsies. Although the rate at which new diseases and conditions have appeared has slowed in recent decades, the contribution of autopsies to the clarification, discovery and treatment of these conditions has been significant. Contemporary examples would include human immunodeficiency virus (HIV)-related diseases and organ transplantation. The largest subject categories within autopsy-related research are represented by the neurosciences, including ophthalmology and cardiovascular disease.[33] The study of bone and joint disease is also highly dependent on autopsy material. Such observations are clearly an indication of the difficulties of obtaining human tissues for many research applications from sources other than clinical autopsies.

In spite of involvement in clinical research, many investigators, both medically and scientifically qualified, seem to be unaware of the potential for research material derived from autopsies. Some of the molecular biological techniques are limited when applied to autopsy material, others can be applied to fresh or archival autopsy-derived tissues.[34] This material can be collected in a cost-effective manner and could be linked to appropriate information stored in an autopsy databank.[35] The challenge for pathologists is to convince others engaged in medical research that autopsies can still provide valuable material and information. Many expensive clinical trials of therapeutic regimens used in the treatment of a variety of cancer types have been designed without reference to autopsy findings. Large prospective studies of other conditions, with the possible exception of transplantation, often do not include autopsy as an integral part of outcome evaluation.[36] The low autopsy rates in such research must surely limit the accuracy of subsequent findings with consequential problems for interpreting and assessment. No health care interventions can be based, with any confidence, on clinical research data gathered without appropriate reference to autopsies. Coroners must be persuaded to supply medico-legal autopsy reports and material to surgical teams for inclusion in the NCEPOD and other systems of audit and research.

The autopsy and audit

In all medical disciplines audit is now an established part of clinical activity and forms a useful mechanism for the identification of specific educational requirements. The process of audit must be linked to postgraduate education and professional development. The Royal College of Surgeons of England and Wales has frequently endorsed a central role for autopsy within medical audit, particularly through contributions to the NCEPOD and the Joint Working Party, which produced 'The Autopsy and Audit' report in conjunction with the Royal College of Physicians and Royal College of Pathologists.[15,18] Unfortunately, these formal recognitions of the importance of autopsies within surgical audit have not been followed by any significant changes in autopsy practice and clinical autopsy rates continue to decline. The reasons for this disparity are complex but must result in part from the outdated and poor quality autopsy services provided by many pathology departments. Physicians tend to be more resistant than surgeons to the role of autopsy in audit and this may be because physicians deal with functional derangements that often have no gross anatomical sequelae visible at autopsy.

The attitudes of local clinicians can be influenced by regular and active feedback of autopsy results.[37] This should begin with attendance by the clinical team at the autopsy and the inclusion of autopsy material in routine clinico-pathological meetings. Regular clinical speciality audit meetings based on hospital deaths are a valuable educational resource and the use of video technology by pathology departments can enhance these forums by the presentation of macroscopic autopsy findings. Pathologists must provide prompt autopsy reports that contain clinically relevant information correlating clinical findings with the pathological processes leading to death. A carefully designed autopsy consent form, which allows the clinician to specify the main areas of interest, facilitates this process.[15]

The small proportion of hospital deaths currently investigated by autopsy represents a non-random sample and therefore cannot be considered to be representative of the hospital population as a whole. Using random sampling of hospital deaths for clinical audit when there is no other indication for performing an autopsy has yet to become acceptable or practicable.[15] The ability of an autopsy service to contribute to clinical audit is affected by staffing levels, funding and the attitudes of local clinicians, coroners, pathologists and relatives. Clinicians have not been impressed by repeated presentations of high discrepancy rates between clinical diagnoses and autopsy findings. There may be more benefit in presenting this type of audit information in a positive rather than negative fashion. The emphasis has generally been placed on missed or wrong diagnoses, whilst low rates of discrepancies for many conditions have been ignored.[8-11] Few studies have attempted to show how improvements in diagnostic accuracy could be achieved in the identified problem areas. Demonstrations of the practical utility of the information provided by autopsies are essential if clinicians are to be encouraged to adopt formal systems for monitoring the accuracy of clinical diagnoses through autopsies. The classification of diagnostic discrepancies is a contentious issue.[8] Clinical diagnoses result from a complex decision-making process, which is often reliant on information from more than one source, and pathologists may not always be capable of assessing the clinical significance of a discrepant diagnosis. Some centres use a multi-disciplinary panel of consultants to classify discrepancies.[38] This allows the clinical aspects of cases to be considered in more detail and assists in the identification of those areas of clinical practice that require further investigation.

Autopsy-based clinical audit systems can also generate information that can be used for patient-care-related risk management purposes.[39] Risk management is the process of minimizing or preventing those activities that have the potential to create liability for complaints or compensation claims. Monitoring of treatment outcomes and diagnostic accuracy could help to identify possible sources of future claims. Autopsies can help to eliminate suspicion by the avoidance of suggestions of concealment and the provision of objective findings that separate the effects of treatment from the effects of disease. Many malpractice claims arise in an atmosphere of supposition and speculation created by a lack of communication combined with a fear of litigation. An autopsy facilitates the substitution of facts for conjecture and can often provide an explanation for the unfavorable outcome of a procedure. Trivial and malicious claims can be pre-empted by the use of autopsies and independent pathologists already perform autopsies arising from cases of alleged negligence in some centres. Some clinicians are opposed to increasing autopsy rates because of the false assumption that ignorance is preferable to knowledge and that more autopsies will produce more lawsuits. The very basis of risk management is to make use of all relevant information and the availability of autopsy findings has been shown to reduce both the number of claims and the costs of settlements where liability existed.

Key points for clinical practice

- Medico-legal autopsies now represent the major component of autopsy practice and the availability of reports and material from these autopsies could become critically important for education, audit and research purposes. There are currently few indications to suggest that change is imminent or that is strongly desired by the majority of doctors.
- The complete loss of clinical autopsies is unlikely in the foreseeable future and a low level of activity will persist in larger teaching centres where many clinicians and researchers still remain unconvinced of the potential contribution of the modern autopsy to all areas of medical practice, including surgery.
- How much further clinical autopsy rates can decline without compromising the ability of the autopsy to maintain its contribution to modern clinical practice remains to be seen.
- More autopsies will only result from more autopsy requests, which themselves will only arise from increased clinical interest in autopsies.
- Autopsies remain the most specific method of monitoring clinical management, judgement and technique in medical practice today.

REFERENCES

1 Start RD, Underwood JCE. Defining necropsy rates. Bull R Coll Pathologists 1992; 78: 14–15
2 Peacock SJ, Machin D, Duboulay CE, Kirkham N. The autopsy: a useful tool or an old relic? J Pathol 1988; 156: 9–14
3 Start RD, McCulloch TA, Benbow EW, Lauder I, Underwood JCE. Clinical necropsy rates during the 1980s: the continued decline. J Pathol 1993; 171: 63–66
4 Office of Population Censuses and Surveys. Mortality statistics – General, England and Wales. 1992, DH1: 27
5 World Health Organisation. 1992 World Statistics Annual. Geneva: WHO, 1993
6 Yesner R, Robinson MJ, Goldman L, Reichert CM, Engel L. A symposium on the autopsy. Pathol Ann 1985; 20: 441–477
7 Start RD, Hector-Taylor MJ, Cotton DW, Startup M, Parsons MA, Kennedy A. Factors which influence necropsy requests: a psychological approach. J Clin Pathol 1992; 45: 254–257
8 Shanks JH, McCluggage G, Anderson NH, Toner PG. Value of the necropsy in perioperative deaths. J Clin Pathol 1990; 43: 193–195
9 Mosquera DA, Goldman MD. Surgical audit without autopsy: tales of the unexpected. Ann R Coll Surg London 1993; 75: 115–117
10 Stothert JC Jr., Gbaanador G. Autopsy in general surgery practice. Am J Surg 1991; 162: 585–588
11 Barendregt WB, de Boer HH, Kubat K. Autopsy analysis in surgical patients: a basis for clinical audit. Br J Surg 1992; 79: 1297–1299
12 Besanceney CF. Perspectives on the autopsy. Hum Pathol 1990; 21: 1083–1084
13 Whitty P, Parker C, Prieto-Ramos F, Al-Kharusi S. Communication of results of necropsies in North-east Thames region. Br Med J 1991; 303: 1244–1246
14 Sherwood SJ, Start RD. Asking relatives for permission for a post mortem. Postgrad Med J 1995; 71: 269–272

15 Joint Working Party of the Royal College of Pathologists, the Royal College of Physicians of London and the Royal College of Surgeons of England. The Autopsy and Audit. London: RCPath, RCP, RCS, 1991

16 Charlton R. Autopsy and medical education: a review. J Royal Soc Med 1994; 87: 232–236

17 The Royal College of Pathologists. Guidelines for post mortem reports. London: RCPath, 1993

18 Campling EA, Devlin HB, Hoile RW, Lunn JN. The Report of The National Confidential Enquiry into Perioperative Deaths. London: The National Confidential Enquiry into Perioperative Deaths, 1993.

19 Start RD, Delargy-Aziz Y, Dorries CP, Silcocks PB, Cotton DWK. Clinicians and the coronial system: ability of clinicians to recognise reportable deaths. Br Med J 1993; 306: 1038–1041

20 Leadbeatter S, Knight B. Reporting deaths to coroners. Br Med J 1994;

21 Du Boulay C. In defence of the post-mortem demonstration. J Pathol 1994; 174: 309–311

22 Cross SS, Laidler P. Computer-assisted learning in morbid anatomy. A simulation of autopsy procedures and death certification. Med Sci Law 1990; 30: 115–118

23 Sloka K, Schilt G. Utilization of the postmortem examination with emphasis on audiovisual aids. Arch Pathol Lab Med 1987; 111: 883–884

24 Cotton DWK, Cross SS. The hospital autopsy. Oxford: Butterworth-Heinemann, 1993

25 Geddes JF, Gonzalez AG. Examination of spinal cord in diseases of the craniocervical junction and high cervical spine. J Clin Pathol 1991; 44: 170–172

26 Bromilow A, Burns J. Technical method: technique for the removal of the vertebral arteries. J Clin Pathol 1985; 38: 1400–1402

27 Donchin Y, Rivkind AI, Bar-Ziv J, Hiss J, Almog J, Drescher M. Utility of postmortem computed tomography in trauma victims. J Trauma 1994; 37: 552–55

28 Forrest AR. ACP Broadsheet no 137: April 1993. Obtaining samples at post mortem examination for toxicological and biochemical analyses. J Clin Pathol 1993; 46: 292–296

29 Suvarna KS, Start RD. Cytodiagnosis and the necropsy. J Clin Pathol 1995; 48: 443–446

30 Underwood JC, Slater DN, Parsons MA. The needle necropsy. Br Med J 1983; 286: 1632–1634

31 Avrahami R, Watemburg S, Hiss Y, Deutsch AA. Laparoscopic vs conventional autopsy. A promising perspective. Arch Surg 1995; 130: 407–409

32 Lindblad B, Eriksson A, Bergqvist D. Autopsy-verified pulmonary embolism in a surgical department: analysis of the period from 1951 to 1988. Br J Surg 1991; 78: 849–852

33 Start RD, Firth JA, Macgillivray F, Cross SS. Have declining necropsy rates reduced the contribution of necropsy to medical research? J Clin Pathol 1995; 48: 402–404

34 Phang TW, Shi CY, Chia JN, Ong CN. Amplification of cDNA via RT-PCR using RNA extracted from postmortem tissues. J Forensic Sci 1994; 39: 1275–1279

35 Reid WA, Harkin PJ, Jack AS. Continual audit of clinical diagnostic accuracy by computer: a study of 592 autopsy cases. J Pathol 1987; 153: 99–107

36 Hill RB, Anderson RE. Contributions of the autopsy to modern medical science. In: Hill RB, Anderson RE, eds. The autopsy – medical practice and public policy. Stoneham, Massachusetts: Butterworths, 1988: 43–66

37 Champ C, Tyler X, Andrews PS, Coghill SB. Improve your hospital autopsy rate to 40–50 per cent, a tale of two towns. J Pathol 1992; 166: 405–407

38 Start RD, McCulloch TA, Silcocks PB, Cotton DWK. Post mortem macroscopic examination, the clinician's missing practice. J Pathol 1994; 173: 381–382

39 Start RD. Risk management, loss control and the autopsy. Br J Hosp Med 1993; 50: 576–578

13

Genomic imprinting in human pathology

B. Tycko

Most genes are expressed equally from the two parental alleles, but a small subset of human genes are differentially expressed depending on whether they have been inherited from the mother or the father. The process that differentially marks the two alleles in the parental germlines is termed genomic imprinting. Substantial evidence implicates both normal and aberrant genomic imprinting in the pathogenesis of human genetic diseases and embryonal tumours. Here I review our current understanding of the molecular biology of genomic imprinting and highlight the involvement of imprinting in human pathology.

What is genomic imprinting?

According to Mendel's laws the activity of a gene should not depend on its parental origin. In violation of these laws, there is a growing list of observations that point to differences in the activity of certain genes depending on whether they have been inherited from the mother or the father. The process by which alleles are marked in the two parental germlines for differential expression in the offspring is referred to as genomic imprinting or, alternatively, as parental or gametic imprinting. Genes whose expression is inhibited after passage through the mother's germline are conventionally said to be 'maternally imprinted' and conversely genes whose expression is inhibited when transmitted by fathers are referred to as 'paternally imprinted'. The inhibition of gene expression at imprinted loci is often virtually complete, so that imprinted genes are monoallelically expressed in somatic tissues of the offspring: this endpoint of monoallelic gene expression is termed the functional imprint. Genomic imprinting is reversible – a gene that has been imprinted by passage through one type of parent will be reactivated on passage through the opposite type of parent. Comprehensive reviews of genomic imprinting have appeared recently, with either basic [1] or clinical [2] emphasis. This chapter is an updated version of a previous review.[3]

Historical aspects

An early observation pointing to the existence of genomic imprinting in mammals was the finding of aberrant development of isoparental embryos in mice.[4-6] True parthenotes, induced by ethanol exposure of oocytes, or gynogenones made by replacement of male pronuclei with female pronuclei, grew to early somite stages before involuting. Up to this stage, the conceptuses were relatively normal in size and appearance, but they showed inadequate placental tissues. An inverse situation was seen in androgenones that were induced by transplantation of male pronuclei into ova from which the female pronucleus had been removed; these developed to the late preimplantation stage but often failed to implant; the small percentage that were able to implant gave rise to predominantly extraembryonic placental tissues, with severely stunted development of the embryo proper. It was concluded that maternal and paternal genomes are both essential for the development of mice past early embryonic stages and that their contributions to growth of the early conceptus are non-equivalent. In particular, it was proposed that certain genes that are essential for growth of trophoblastic tissue are expressed preferentially or exclusively from the paternally transmitted genome, i.e. are maternally imprinted, and that conversely there might exist paternally imprinted genes whose activity is essential for the development of the embryo proper.

Additional evidence for non-equivalence of maternal and paternal genomes came from experiments using mice that carried various chromosomal translocations. In genetic crosses meiotic non-disjunctions produced uniparental disomies for particular chromosomes or chromosomal regions.[7-9] For example, one type of cross generated fetuses containing two copies of a large portion of the maternal chromosome 7 but no copies of the corresponding portion of the paternal chromosome 7. These fetuses were developmentally retarded, showed small placentas and died in utero at midgestation. The reciprocal cross, resulting in two paternal and no maternal chromosome 7 homologues, produced conceptuses that died at a much earlier stage.[9] By this approach several different chromosomes and subchromosomal regions were scored for their ability to produce an abnormal phenotype when they were inherited as uniparental disomies. As only a subset of chromosomal regions showed evidence of harbouring imprinted genes by this assay, these studies allowed the construction of a low-resolution 'imprinting map' of the mouse genome.[10] Chromosomal mapping of imprinted disease loci in humans has suggested that for at least some syntenic chromosomal regions there might be good agreement between the mouse and human 'imprinting maps' Table 13.1.[11]

Table 13.1 Imprinted genes[a] in mice and humans[1]

Gene/locus	Chromosome	Silent allele	Gene product
Igf2 (mu)[b]	mu 7 (distal)	Maternal	Growth factor
IGF2 (hu)[c]	hu 11p15.5	Maternal	
H19 (mu)[b]	mu 7 (distal)	Paternal	RNA
H19 (hu)[c]	hu 11p15.5	Paternal	
Mash2 (mu)[b]	mu 7 (distal)	Paternal	Transcription factor
Kip2 (mu)[b]	mu 7 (distal)	Paternal	Cyclin-cdk inhibitor
Ins2 (mu)[b]	mu 7 (distal)	Maternal; not imprinted in pancreas	Growth factor/metabolic regulation
Igf2R (mu)[b]	mu 17 (proximal)	Paternal	*Igf2* clearance receptor/mannose 6-phosphate receptor
Mas (mu)[b]	mu 17 (proximal)	Maternal	Tyrosine kinase protoon-cogene
Snrpn (mu)[b]	mu 7 (central)	Maternal	Splicing factor
SNRPN (hu)[c]	hu 15q11–13	Maternal	
IPW (hu)[c]	hu 15q11–13	Maternal	RNA
PAR1, PAR5 (hu)[c]	hu 15q11–13	Maternal	RNAs
Xist	mu X	Maternal; functional imprint in placenta only	RNA
WT1 (hu)[c]	hu 11p13	Paternal; not functionally, imprinted in kidney	Transcription factor
U2af-rs/-bpL (mu)[b]	mu 11 (homologue on hu 5q23–q31)	Maternal	Splicing factor? (intronless gene)
Ins1 (mu)[b]	mu 6	Maternal	*Ins2* homologue
Peg1/Mest (mu)[b]	mu 6	Maternal	Hydrolase enzyme?

[a] Gene clusters corresponding to possible imprinted domains are grouped together in the table. Only genes with proven monoallelic expression are included.
[b] Genes of mouse origin.
[c] Genes of human origin.

A series of reports in the late 1980s showing that in certain lines of transgenic mice the transgene is subject to allele-specific DNA methylation and in some cases allele-restricted mRNA expression provided the first evidence for defined, albeit artificial, DNA sequences that were subject to parent-of-origin specific modifications.[12–15] These experiments also raised the possibility that DNA methylation might be involved in imprinting. As the imprinting observed at transgene loci is not a perfect model for natural genomic imprinting, the field was briefly stalled by the lack of defined examples of endogenous imprinted genes. It was the finding of such genes in the early 1990s that brought about the current phase of research.

Imprinted genes in mice and humans

The expectation that some endogenous genes would be found to be imprinted was fulfilled when experiments with either gene 'knock-out' or naturally occurring strains of mice in which the two parental alleles could be distinguished showed that the insulin-like growth factor 2 (*Igf2*) gene was expressed only from the paternal allele and that the genes encoding the *Igf2*/mannose 6-phosphate receptor (*Igf2R*) and a differentiation-related fetal RNA (*H19*) were expressed only from the maternal alleles.[16–18] Two of these genes, *IGF2* and *H19*, were then shown to be monoallelically expressed in humans, with evolutionary conservation of the parental 'direction' of the imprinting in both cases.[19–23] Several additional imprinted genes have since been characterized (Table 13.1). At least one of these, *SNRPN*, encoding a protein involved in mRNA splicing, also shows conservation of imprinting between mice and humans[24,25] and another, *ZNF127*, encoding a zinc-finger family transcription factor, is predicted to show such conservation based on its functional imprinting in mice[26] and its allele-specific DNA methylation in humans.[27] Evolutionary conservation of functional imprinting seems not to be entirely predictable because the human *IGF2R* gene is biallelically expressed, i.e. not subject to functional imprinting, in several tissues of most[28] but not all[29] individuals.

The evolutionary conservation of imprinting suggests that the phenomenon might provide some selective advantage. Several possible advantages of imprinting for the success of the species have been proposed, all of which are speculative.[3] Among the 'theories of imprinting' one stands out, not necessarily as having a greater likelihood of being correct, but rather as being testable. This is the proposal that imprinting arose in mammals as an evolutionary concomitant of the placental mode of reproduction.[30] It is argued that a particular paternal genome will be more successful in propagating itself if it can promote the growth of a large placenta and fetus, while the maternal genome is under an opposite pressure – to restrain excessive placental and fetal growth so that multiple pregnancies can be sustained over the lifetime of the mother. The theory proposes that the maternal germline will have imprinted certain genes, which act to promote growth of the placenta and fetus, while the paternal germline will have imprinted certain genes which can restrain the growth of the placenta and fetus. In fact, three genes with growth-promoting activity: those encoding insulin-like growth factor II, insulin itself and the mas oncoprotein, are maternally imprinted in at least some developing tissues of the mouse. Conversely, two genes with growth-restraining activity, *Igf2R* and *H19*, are paternally imprinted in both mice and humans and a third gene with predicted growth-inhibitory activity, *Kip2*, is paternally imprinted in mice.[31] How the other known imprinted genes and additional imprinted genes yet to be isolated will fit into this picture remains to be seen.

Progress in defining the size of the set of imprinted genes, and the shared characteristics, if any, of the genes in this set, will depend on the development of efficient screening methods for identifying imprinted genes. Recently, two such methods have been developed. Using a two-dimensional gel system the mouse genome was scanned for DNA restriction sites that were differentially methylated depending on their parental origin.[32] A search for transcripts arising near one such site identified a gene, *U2af1-rs/U2afbpL*, which may encode a protein involved in mRNA splicing and is expressed exclusively from the paternal allele. Another laboratory carried out cDNA subtraction and differential cDNA screening starting from mRNAs of gynogenetic versus androgenetic mouse conceptuses. At least one novel imprinted gene, *Peg1/Mest*, transcribed exclusively from the paternal allele and encoding a protein homologous to certain hydrolase enzymes, was isolated in this screen.[33]

DNA methylation and imprinting

Any biochemical modification of the DNA or chromatin, which can account for imprinting, must satisfy four requirements. The modification must be made prior to fertilization, it must be able to confer transcriptional silencing, it must be stably transmitted through mitosis in somatic cells and it must be reversible on passage through the opposite parental germline. Some fairly exotic possibilities are consistent with these requirements. For example, imprinted genes could conceivably contain DNA sequences that undergo a reversible physical rearrangement, such as a precise inversion, during oogenesis and spermatogenesis, but physical mapping of imprinted loci has shown no evidence for such rearrangements. A second possibility is that imprinted genes could interact with hypothetical oocyte or spermato-cyte-specific DNA or chromatin-binding proteins, which could establish transcriptional silencing complexes capable of persistence and replication in somatic cell divisions but also be susceptible to displacement during the next cycle of gametogenesis. Chromatin proteins that show this type of behaviour have been described,[34] but such proteins have not yet been implicated in genomic imprinting.

By contrast, a third model, which invokes site-specific DNA methylation as the imprinting mechanism, is supported both by *a priori* considerations and by experimental evidence. Methylation of DNA in mammalian cells occurs at cytosine residues in CpG dinucleotides. CpG-methylation of genes, particularly in their promoter regions, can render them transcriptionally silent and the methylation pattern is transmitted through cell divisions by the action of the maintenance DNA methyltransferase. While the modification is stably propagated in the presence of an active methyltransferase, it can, in principle, be reversed when DNA replicates under conditions in which the methyltransferase is inhibited or sequestered, as may be the case in early development.[35] The loss of methylation of many DNA sequences in the immediate post-zygotic period and during the formation of the germ cells is well documented[36–39] and some investigators feel that the extent of this loss cannot be accounted for by passive mechanisms and instead reflects an active process involving a putative demethylase enzyme, but an enzyme of this type has yet to be isolated from mammalian cells. In the mature gametes, for several different types of sequences, the DNA in sperm is known to be CpG-methylated in a different pattern from the DNA in ova.[36,38–41] While much of this difference is lost from somatic cells in early development, allelic methylation differences might well persist at certain demethylation-resistant sites. Direct evidence for persistence of gametic methylation differences at specific CpG dinucleotides during early development has been produced for the murine *H19*[42] and *Igf2r*[43] genes. The simplest methylation model for imprinting posits that, because of a critical positioning and/or density of CpGs found at imprinted genes, gametic methylation differences are preserved at demethylation-resistant sites in or near these genes in early somatic development and that these critical sites somehow nucleate the formation of more widespread hypermethylation and inactive chromatin, leading to gene silencing.

Allele-specific DNA methylation has been found for every imprinted transgene and for all of the endogenous imprinted genes which have been examined. For *H19*, allele-specific DNA methylation has been shown in fetal and adult tissues, with hypermethylation of the imprinted allele within the promoter sequences and through the entire extent of the gene.[21,44–46] In humans, the *H19* gene in sperm is extensively methylated while in gynogenetic ovarian teratomas the gene is largely unmethylated.[21] Moreover, partial methylation of the *H19* promoter inhibits its ability to activate transcription of a reporter gene in transfection experiments[21] and demethylation of imprinted *H19* alleles by exposure of cells to the DNA methyltransferase inhibitor 5-azacytidine (AzaC) can reactivate transcription from these alleles (T. Moulton and B. Tycko, unpublished observations). Allele-specific methylation is also present at several CpGs in the *Igf2*[45] and *Igf2R*[43] genes of mice but, in contrast to *H19*, the active *Igf2* and *Igf2R* alleles were found to be hypermethylated at some of the sites examined. However, the inactive *Igf2* allele may be hypermethylated at other regulatory sites because, as with *H19*, imprinting of *Igf2* could be erased by AzaC.[47] Also consistent with an important role for methylation in the imprinting of these genes, mouse embryos with a targeted deletion of the DNA methyltransferase gene showed abnormal functional imprinting of all three genes.[48]

Because of the potential for indirect effects of experimental manipulations that cause demethylation and because of difficulties in separating cause from effect in relating CpG methylation to transcriptional activity, it will be difficult to prove that allele-specific DNA methylation is sufficient to account for genomic imprinting. Nonetheless, as discussed below, changes in the methylation of imprinted genes are useful markers for aberrations of functional imprinting in human genetic diseases and neoplasms. Also, because DNA methylation can be manipulated with drugs like AzaC it is conceivable that the design of less mutagenic analogues of these drugs could eventually provide a pharmacological approach to the treatment of diseases involving aberrant functional imprinting.

Regional imprinting

One feature of genomic imprinting, which is not explained by the simple methylation model, and which is likely to be crucial for understanding both the mechanism of imprinting and the basis of diseases involving imprinting is the physical clustering of imprinted genes. In mice and humans at least three chromosomal regions contain more than one imprinted gene (Table 13.1). In an area of mouse chromosome 7, which is syntenic with human chromosome 11p15.5 and which may encompass less than a megabase (mb) of DNA, there are five known imprinted genes: *Mash2*,[49] *Ins2, Igf2, H19*, and *Kip2*. The opposite imprinting of *Igf2* and *H19* seems to reflect competition of the promoters of these two genes for the same enhancer element(s), so that only one of the two genes can be active on a given chromosome.[46,50,51] On mouse chromosome 17 the *Igf2r* and *Mas* genes are located within 300 kb of each other and are both imprinted, although again in opposite parental directions.[52] On human chromosome 15q11–q13, a region that is frequently deleted in the Angelman and Prader-Willi syndromes, there appears to be an 'imprinted domain' of about 1–2 mb in size, which contains at least four maternally imprinted genes or transcripts: *SNRPN, IPW, PAR1* and *PAR5*[25,53,54] and is very likely to contain at least two more imprinted genes, *ZNF127*,[26] and at least one as yet uncloned oppositely imprinted gene (see below).

If confirmed by additional mapping, the regional clustering of imprinted genes will suggest a parallel between imprinting and the clearly regional phenomenon of X-chromosome inactivation, in which many genes are coordinately silenced in a process that initiates at an 'inactivation centre' and spreads in cis to the remainder of the chromosome.[55] As is true for imprinting, X-inactivation is correlated with CpG-hypermethylation of gene sequences and maintenance of transcriptional silencing on the inactive X chromosome depends on this hypermethylation, although there is evidence suggesting that the process of X-inactivation is initiated in early development by a methylation-independent mechanism involving chromatin condensation.

On the human inactive X chromosome an increasing number of genes are being identified, which either partially or completely escape inactivation, and regional imprinting also may be able to skip over intervening genes. The mouse *Th* gene, situated between *Ins2* and *Mash2*, is biallelically expressed, at least in some tissues.[56] In addition, several other genes near, although not necessarily within, the apparent clusters of imprinted genes are not affected by functional imprinting: the human *L23MRP* gene lies only 40 kb downstream of *H19* but is biallelically expressed in a variety of fetal and adult tissues,[57] the ribonucleotide reductase M1 subunit gene (*RRM1*), also located in the same chromosomal band as human *IGF2* and *H19*, has been shown not to be functionally imprinted in kidney[58] and several genes near *Igf2r* on mouse chromosome 17 are biallelically expressed.[17]

Genes in imprinted chromosome domains and genes on the inactive X chromosome share another characteristic – altered timing of their replication during the cell cycle. Genes on the inactive X chromosome replicate later than those on the active X chromosome, and for each of the three known imprinted domains it has been shown that alleles on the maternal chromosome replicate at a different time in S-phase than those on the paternal chromosome.[56] Whether this DNA replication asynchrony is a cause or an effect of the functional imprint remains to be seen.

Imprinting and RNA

There are hints of an association of non-coding RNAs with genomic imprinting. While most spliced and polyadenylated RNAs contain open reading frames (ORFs), which are translated to give rise to proteins, several genes have been identified that give rise to spliced and polyadenylated RNAs, which lack long or conserved ORFs and are probably not translated. Three of these, from the *H19*,[59] *IPW*[53] and *XIST*[60] genes, have not been assigned any precise biochemical functions. As these genes are subject to functional imprinting and map to imprinted domains one can speculate that non-coding RNA might have some general function in the imprinting mechanism. What this function might be is unclear and the fact that *XIST* RNA is retained in the nucleus[60] while *H19* RNA is predominantly cytoplasmic[59] further obscures the picture.

Variation in functional imprinting

Potentially significant for understanding the effects of imprinting in disease are observations that the functional imprint can vary among different tissues and even between different individuals. The maternal allele of the murine *Igf2* gene is silent in all tissues except choroid plexus and meninges, where the functional imprint is not present and this allele is expressed[16] and in humans the maternal *IGF2* allele is repressed in most fetal tissues, including fetal liver, but is expressed in the adult liver, in which there is transcription from an alternative upstream promoter.[61,63] There is also evidence for relaxation of imprinting of human *IGF2* in embryonal tumours[20,63] but in this setting the mechanism of biallelic expression appears to involve disruption of enhancer competition with *H19*, rather than alternative promoter usage (see below). The murine *Ins2* gene is functionally imprinted in the yolk sac but not in the pancreas[64] and the *Mas* gene is functionally imprinted in adult muscle, but not in a variety of other tissues.[51] In humans the *WT1* gene is not subject to functional imprinting in its primary site of expression, the developing kidney,[19] but this gene appears to be monoallelically expressed in certain poorly expressing tissues such as brain.[65] Similarly, paternal imprinting of human *H19* is relaxed in trophoblast of hydatidiform moles[66] and in normal placenta as well.[19,67]

The efficiency of imprinting also depends on genetic background: in transgenic mice the presence or absence of methylation imprinting of the transgene can be strain dependent, suggesting the existence of imprinting modifier genes.[68,69] Also, imprinting of the Tme trait, linked to the *Igf2r* gene in mice, is under the control of a strain-specific modifier locus,[70] and the human *Igf2R* gene appears to be subject to variable functional imprinting in different individuals.[29] Whether imprinting modifier genes correspond to variants of the DNA methyltransferase or the putative DNA demethylase enzyme or are genes that indirectly regulate DNA methylation via effects on chromatin structure are interesting unanswered questions.

Imprinting in human genetic disease

Clinical observations can suggest a role for genomic imprinting before molecular data are available. An example is a disease observed at equal frequencies in males and females but transmitted exclusively or preferentially from one type of parent. A variation on this pattern are conditions in which both types of parents can transmit the phenotype, but a particularly severe form of the disease results from transmission by one type of parent. A second type of evidence for imprinting is a disease phenotype recurrently associated with uniparental disomies for a particular chromosome or chromosomal region.

In a review published in 1990, at least 10 distinct human genetic diseases and syndromes were listed as candidates for involvement of genomic imprinting.[71] Some of these have withstood the test of time better than others (Table 13.2). The clearest examples of imprinted genetic diseases in

Table 13.2 Human disorders with evidence for genomic imprinting[a]

Disease	Chromosome	Evidence for imprinting
Prader-Willi syndrome	15q11–q13	Paternal deletions; maternal UPD
Angelman syndrome	15q11–q13	Maternal deletions; paternal UPD
Russel-Silver syndrome (short stature)	7(q?)	Maternal UPD
Wilms' tumour	11p15.5	Loss of maternal alleles
Hepatoblastoma	11p15.5	Loss of maternal alleles
Embryonal Rhabdomyosarcoma	11p15.5	Loss of maternal alleles
Beckwith-Weidemann syndrome	11p15.5	Maternal transmission; paternal UPD
Insulin-dependent diabetes mellitus	11p15.5 (INS locus)	Paternal transmission
Neuroblastoma	1p36	Loss of maternal alleles
	2p24.3 (*MYCN* locus)	Amplification of paternal alleles
Osteosarcoma	13q14.3 (*RB1* locus)	Loss of maternal alleles
Retinoblastoma	13q14.3 (*RB1* locus)	Hypermethylation of paternal alleles in some tumours
Paraganglioma syndrome	11q23–qter	Paternal transmission

[a] A partial list containing some of the best studied conditions. Diseases such as those caused by triplet repeat expansions in which the imprinting effects do not fit the most restrictive definition are not included.

humans are the Prader-Willi (PWS) and Angelman (AS) syndromes. Both syndromes include mental retardation (mild to moderate in PWS and severe in AS) but the associated stigmata are entirely distinct: individuals with PWS are slow moving and become overweight owing to severe hyperphagia; individuals with AS are thin and hyperactive, and have a characteristic 'happy puppet' appearance, with inappropriate laughter. Both syndromes often result from chromosomal deletions in bands 15q11–q13 and the deletions in the two syndromes can be cytogenetically indistinguishable. A role for genomic imprinting in producing the distinct phenotypes was raised when it was found that the deleted DNA in the two syndromes was of opposite parental origin: in each case of PWS the deletion had occurred on the paternal chromosome 15, while for each case of AS it had occurred on the maternal homologue.[72] Additional evidence for opposite imprinting in the two syndromes was the finding that cases of PWS with maternal disomy for the entire chromosome 15 are fairly frequent[73] and that rare cases of AS can be caused by paternal disomy of this same chromosome.[74] One hypothesis was that a single PWS/AS gene, imprinted paternally in some cell types and maternally in others, might account for both syndromes, but more recent high-resolution mapping of the minimal deleted regions has shown that PWS and AS are caused by losses of two very closely linked but distinct genes (or probably a gene cluster for PWS), which are oppositely imprinted.[75,76]

Three maternally imprinted genes in the PWS minimal deleted region, SNRPN,[24,77] encoding a protein component of a ribonucleoprotein thought to be involved in brain-specific mRNA splicing, ZNF127,[78] encoding a putative nucleic-acid binding protein, IPW, encoding an abundant noncoding RNA[52] and two less well characterized maternally imprinted transcripts, PAR1 and PAR5[53] have been identified to date. Which, if any, of these genes is essential for the PWS clinical phenotype is not yet resolved, but patients with PWS show a bimaternal pattern of DNA methylation, on Southern blot analysis with probes, throughout this chromosome 15q11–q13 region and a finding of this pattern in the appropriate clinical context is considered as molecular support for a diagnosis of PWS. The AS gene, predicted to be paternally imprinted, has yet to be identified. Rare PWS families have recently been identified in which the disease is caused by small (40–60 kb) DNA deletions at the upstream border of SNRPN. In these cases there is altered functional and methylation imprinting not only of SNRPN but also of other genes and DNA markers over more than a mb of DNA, suggesting that the deletions have disrupted an 'imprinting centre'.[79] The smallest region of overlap of the deletions is being characterized and this may prove to be very informative in terms of the imprinting mechanism.

Imprinting effects are not restricted to simple genetic diseases; the important complex genetic disease insulin-dependent diabetes mellitus (IDDM) has been found to show a higher incidence of paternal as opposed to maternal transmission[80] and genetic associations strongly suggest that a locus responsible for this bias is the insulin gene itself, in particular a poly-morphic tandem DNA repeat in the INS promoter region.[81–83] A hypothe-sis is that increased expression of insulin early in fetal or postnatal life predisposes to later immune system-mediated islet cell destruction and that the paternal allele is expressed preferentially. As mentioned above, the *Ins2* gene is in fact maternally imprinted in mice, although the functional imprint is restricted to the yolk sac and is not present in the pancreas.

An important group of human diseases, which have been suspected to show imprinting effects, are the so-called triplet-repeat diseases. These inherited disorders, including Fragile-X mental retardation (FRAX), myotonic dystrophy (DM) and Huntington's disease (HD) among others, result from the presence of unstable repetitive trinucleotide DNA sequences in or near the disease genes. While parent-of-origin effects on severity or rapidity of onset in these diseases initially raised the possibility of a role for genomic imprinting, there is as yet no direct evidence for classical imprinting of the genes involved in these diseases.[84]

Imprinting in neoplasia

The early studies of androgenetic and gynogenetic embryos in mice were mirrored by studies of human hydatidiform moles and benign ovarian ter-atomas or dermoid cysts, which showed uniparental origins of these tumours. Moles, which are composed mostly of trophoblastic tissue, were found to lack maternal chromosomes and to contain a reduplicated paternal complement of chromosomes,[85,86] while cytogenetic analysis showed that dermoids, which differentiate into a broad spectrum of somatic tissues but which never show placental elements, invariably contained a reduplicated complement of maternal chromosomes derived from an unfertilized oocyte.[87] Consistent with this, teratomas and teratocarcinomas can be produced in mouse ovaries by inducing ova to undergo parthenogenesis in situ.[88]

Classical genetic evidence for imprinting in tumorigenesis can precede the identification of candidate genes. In at least one familial tumour syn-drome, the inherited paraganglioma or glomus tumour syndrome, the phe-notype, usually bilateral carotid body tumours, is only manifested after transmission of the disease gene from fathers.[89] As the high frequency of affected individuals in the pedigrees is otherwise consistent with autosomal dominant transmission, it has been predicted that the chromosome 11q23–qter gene accounting for this syndrome will turn out to be a mater-nally imprinted/paternally expressed dominant oncogene.[90]

The retinoblastoma (*RB*) gene is the protoype tumour-suppressor gene predicted in the classical 'two-hit' model for recessive oncogenesis. Surprisingly, in view of the necessity for biallelic inactivation of *RB* in the development of retinoblastomas, there are also hints that the *RB* locus might be subject to genomic imprinting. Evidence for imprinting of *RB* has come from observations in the *RB*-related tumour, sporadic osteosarcoma. In these tumours there is a strong bias in the parental origin of *RB* allele losses. In one study 90% of cases showed loss of the maternal *RB* allele, presumably with mutation of the retained paternal allele.[91] As the tumours were of relatively late onset and were not preceded by retinoblastomas they probably contained somatic rather than germline *RB* mutations. From this it was concluded that, rather than resulting from a parental bias in the germline mutation rate, the observed bias in *RB* allele losses probably reflects bona fide genomic imprinting. While evidence for differences in DNA methylation at maternal versus paternal *RB* alleles in leukocytes and fibroblasts has been reported,[92] whether there are allelic differences in the level of *RB* mRNA expression in osteosarcoma precursor cells or other cell types is not yet known. If an allelic bias exists it may be restricted to those rare individuals who subsequently develop osteosarcoma, and indeed may predispose them to this tumour by allowing the first genetic 'hit' of the *RB* gene, when it occurs on the more highly expressed allele, to partially release the cell from normal growth regulation. Observations that about 10% of unilateral retinoblastomas show hypermethylation of the *RB* promoter and first exon and that the hypermethylation is restricted to the paternal allele, give some support to this.[92-95]

There is also evidence suggesting parental imprinting of both a dominant oncogene and a putative tumour-suppressor gene involved in human neuroblastoma. Amplification of a large segment of DNA containing the *MYCN* proto-oncogene is a frequent finding in neuroblastomas, where the presence of amplification confers a poor prognosis. When the parental origin of the amplified DNA was examined, 12 of 13 cases showed amplification of the paternal *MYCN* allele.[96] Whether this parental bias reflects an allelic bias in N-*myc* mRNA expression in neuroblasts remains to be determined. Neuroblastomas also frequently show loss of DNA in chromosomal band 1p36, implicating one or more tumour-suppressor genes in this region. In one study[97] the lost 1p36 DNA was found to be selectively of maternal origin (13 of 15 cases), but this bias was not found in a second study.[96] This discrepancy may have been resolved by an analysis of a larger set of cases, in which the maternal bias in 1p36 losses was confirmed, but only among tumours that lacked concurrent *MYCN* amplification.[98]

Finally, a role for genomic imprinting in tumorigenesis is firmly established by findings in the Beckwith-Wiedemann syndrome (BWS) and in a group of embryonal tumours associated with this syndrome. BWS is diagnosed by the presence of variable somatic manifestations, including exomphalos, macroglossia, visceromegaly (including organomegaly affecting tongue, kidney, liver and adrenal), hemihyperthrophy and gigantism, all of which reflect overgrowth of developing tissues, and about 7% of affected individuals will develop Wilms' tumor (WT), adrenocortical carcinoma (ADCC), hepatoblastoma (HB) or embryonal rhabdomyosarcoma (ER). The evidence for imprinting in BWS takes several forms. In some families, the trait is associated with constitutional chromosomal inversions or translocations at 11p15.3–p15.4 or 11p15.5, but the phenotype is only expressed after passage of the structurally abnormal chromosome through the maternal germline.[99,100] More frequently the syndrome can be transmitted within families with no cytogenetic abnormalities but with genetic linkage to chromosome 11p15.5, and here too the phenotype is usually seen after passage of the disease gene through the maternal germline.[101–103] In a third substantial group of cases the syndrome occurs de novo in association with paternal disomy for 11p15.5.[104–106] In fact, mice that are constructed as genetic mosaics for paternal disomy of the homologous chromosomal region are a potential animal model for BWS and show increased body size.[107] Lastly, numerous studies indicate that each of the four types of embryonal tumours, which are associated with BWS, show frequent loss of heterozygosity (LOH) for DNA markers at 11p15.5 and, importantly, in series of WTs, ERs and HBs (consisting primarily of sporadic rather than BWS-associated cases) there is a very strong (95–100%) bias towards loss of maternal 11p15.5 alleles.[20,21,108–114]

Several observations are consistent with the hypothesis that BWS is caused by the abnormal expression of one particular imprinted gene, *IGF2*. This gene maps to 11p15.5 and is normally expressed only from the paternal allele. According to the 'IGF2 hypothesis', paternal disomies or duplications of chromosome 11p15.5 lead to a twofold increase in *IGF2* protein production and a corresponding increased growth of *IGF2*-responsive tissues, accounting for the characteristic organomegaly. The chromosomal rearrangements, deletions or putative point mutations in the 11p15.3–15.5 region, which account for the remaining cases of BWS, most of which show selective maternal transmission, are postulated either to somehow cause a failure of imprinting of the maternal *IGF2* allele, thereby leading to the same endpoint of increased *IGF2* protein production, or to somehow superactivate the paternal allele. In fact, two early reports described BWS patients with significantly increased circulating somatomedin (bioactive *IGF2*) levels.[115,116] The finding of biallelic *IGF2* mRNA expression, i.e. erasure of functional imprinting, in fibroblasts and tongue tissue of some,[117] although not all[22] BWS patients who lacked paternal 11p15 disomies, supports the *IGF2* hypothesis. As structural lesions of DNA within the *IGF2* gene were not found, the disruption of imprinting may be a long-range chromosomal effect. A chromosomal domain effect is also supported by the fact that patients with BWS frequently show neonatal hypoglycaemia, which might reflect increased insulin production caused by co-ordinate activation of the closely linked INS and *IGF2* genes. In contrast to the *IGF2* hypothesis, some investigators favour the alternative that the 11p15.3–p15.4 and perhaps also the 11p15.5 chromosomal rearrangements physically disrupt two or more as yet unidentified growth suppressor genes whose role in the syndrome might be more fundamental than *IGF2*.[118,119]

The finding of recurrent LOH in a particular chromosomal region in tumours is usually taken as evidence for the existence of a tumour-suppressor gene in that location and it is likely that at least one embryonal tumour-suppressor gene (designated 'WT2' to distinguish it from the previously identified *WT1* gene) resides at chromosome 11p15.5. Based on the selective loss of maternal 11p15.5 alleles in embryonal tumours, one criterion for candidate genes is that they be expressed only from the maternal allele in fetal kidney, but it is also possible that '*WT2*' might not be imprinted and that the observed selective loss of maternal alleles might be caused solely by pressure to retain the active paternal copy of *IGF2*.[120] In fact, most WTs and ERs (and probably HBs), which have lost maternal alleles at 11p15.5, are also found to contain duplicated paternal alleles. This results in two transcriptionally active copies of *IGF2* per cell, and in two early studies nearly all WTs were found to express high levels of *IGF2* mRNA.[121,122] Recent studies confirm this, and further indicate that the functional imprinting of *IGF2* is frequently lost in WTs, so that the even among tumours without LOH there are many cases with biallelic *IGF2* mRNA expression.[20,63] Thus, a majority of WTs have a functional double-dose of the active *IGF2* allele. Complicating this simple picture are the findings in two preliminary studies that, despite the high levels of *IGF2* mRNA, the amounts of immunoreactive Igf-2 protein in WTs appear to be quite low.[123,124]

The *H19* gene, closely linked to *IGF2*, is a candidate tumour–suppressor gene in WTs. This gene is paternally imprinted; expression is very low in undifferentiated cells, increases markedly in a wide array of fetal tissues at stages in which cells are differentiating and then declines in most differentiated tissues.[3] *H19* is transcribed to yield a spliced and polyadenylated RNA, which accumulates in the cytoplasm but which contains only very short translational reading frames[57] and while there is overall conservation of intron/exon structure and nucleotide sequence between *H19* genes of human, mouse and rat, the reading frames are not conserved.[125] Based on this it has been proposed that this gene might function directly at the level of its RNA product, perhaps as the RNA component of a ribonucleoprotein.[58] Transcription of *H19* is high in normal fetal kidney, adrenal and liver but is significantly repressed in a majority of cases of WT[112,126–128] and in at least some ADCCs[112] and HBs.[129] In tumours in which the gene is silenced there is CpG-hypermethylation of its promoter and transcribed region.[112,126–128] The fact that some patients with WT also show this hypermethylation in their non–neoplastic kidney cells[112] indicates that it is not caused by widespread alterations of DNA methylation in tumour cells, but rather is likely to be of specific importance in the tumorigenic pathway. Consistent with enhancer competition between these two genes, *H19* transcriptional silencing and DNA hypermethylation in WTs is linked to biallelic activation of *IGF2*.[112,126–128]

In contrast to WTs, adult carcinomas, including those from lung[130] and bladder,[131] can frequently express high levels of *H19* RNA and also show high *IGF2* mRNA. At least for lung cancers, it has been shown that there is no preferential loss of maternal 11p15.5 alleles,[132] suggesting that genomic imprinting is not relevant in these tumours, and there is uncoupling between *H19* and *IGF2* allelic expression,[130] possibly reflecting severe alterations in DNA methylation and chromatin structure in these genetically unstable neoplasms.

Evidence for direct trans growth-inhibitory activity of *H19* RNA is contradictory. *H19* transgenic mice, which expressed the transgene at high levels and in ectopic sites died in utero at a late fetal stage, thus suggesting a direct effect of the *H19* RNA;[133] however, this effect has subsequently been attributed to the structure of the particular expression construct used, rather than to the *H19* RNA itself (S. Tilghman, personal communication). When an expression vector containing the human *H19* gene was introduced into G401 cells, a line derived from a WT or a malignant rhabdoid tumour of the kidney, the cells expressed high levels of *H19* RNA and became non-clonogenic in soft agar and non-tumorigenic in nude mice and transection of this same expression construct into an ER cell line yielded a high percentage of growth- retarded clones, while the construct had no effect on growth or clonogenicity of the cervical cancer line SiHa.[134] A recent report of *H19* 'knock-out' mice has shown that the lack of *H19* RNA expression is compatible with normal development and *H19* deletion appears to have growth-promoting effects only by cis-activation of *Igf2*.[51] A lack of tumours in these mice did not support a tumour-suppressor role for *H19*. But because mice have never been observed to develop embryonal kidney tumours resembling WTs, even in the setting of hemizygous *WT1* deletions,[135] it is possible that the lack of tumorigenesis might reflect this species peculiarity.

If chromosome 11p15.5 imprinting is in fact regional, then it may be that multiple imprinted genes are co-ordinately disregulated in BWS and in the associated embryonal tumours. A tumour-suppressor locus centromeric to *H19* and *IGF2* has been proposed based on growth suppression after subchromosomal transfers into rhabdomyosarcoma cells[136] and based on the apparent coincidence of this region with some of the BWS-associated chromosomal breakpoints.[118,119] *Kip2*, encoding a cyclin-cdk inhibitor, has recently been proposed as a candidate 11p15.5 tumour-suppressor gene based on its paternal imprinting in mice,[32] but whether the human homologue is imprinted in kidney and inactivated in WTs remains to be seen. Further analysis of the 11p15.5 chromosomal region should soon resolve the uncertainties concerning the genes whose altered expression is responsible for BWS and the associated embryonal tumours.

Acknowledgements

This work was supported by grants CA60765 from the N.I.H. and JFRA-482 from the A.C.S.

REFERENCES

1 Efstratiadis A. Parental imprinting of autosomal mammalian genes. Curr Opin Genet Dev 1994; 4: 265–280

2 Driscoll DJ. Genomic imprinting in humans. Mol Genet Med 1994; 4: 37–77

3 Tycko B. Genomic imprinting: mechanism and role in human pathology. Am J Pathol 1994; 144: 431–443

4 Surani MAH, Barton SC, Norris ML. Development of reconstituted mouse eggs suggests imprinting of the genome during gametogenesis. Nature 1984; 308: 548–550

5 Barton SC, Surani MAH, Norris ML. Role of paternal and maternal genomes in mouse development. Nature 1984; 311: 374–376

6 McGrath J, Solter D. Completion of mouse embryogenesis requires both the maternal and paternal genomes. Cell 1984; 37: 179–183

7 Searle AG, Beechey CV. Complementation studies with mouse translocations. Cytogenet Cell Genet 1978; 20: 282–303

8 Cattanach BM, Kirk M. Differential activity of maternally and paternally derived chromosome regions in mice. Nature 1985; 315: 496–498

9 Searle AG, Beechey CV. Genome imprinting phenomena on mouse chromosome 7. Genet Res Camb 1990; 56: 237–244

10 Searle AG, Peters J, Lyon MF, et al. Chromosome maps of man and mouse IV. Ann Hum Genet 1989; 53: 89–140

11 Cattanach BM, Barr JA, Evans EP, et al. A candidate mouse model for Prader-Willi syndrome which shows an absence of Snrpn expression. Nature Genet 1992; 2: 270–274

12 Hadchouel M, Farza H, Simon D, et al. Maternal inhibition of hepatitis B surface antigen gene expression in transgenic mice correlates with de novo methylation. Nature 1987; 329: 454–456

13 Reik W, Collick A, Norris ML, et al. Genomic imprinting determines methylation of parental alleles in transgenic mice. Nature 1987; 328: 248–251

14 Sapienza C, Peterson AC, Rossant J, et al. Degree of methylation of transgenes is dependent on gamete of origin. Nature 1987; 328: 251–254

15 Swain JL, Stewart TA, Leder P. Parental legacy determines methylation and expression of an autosomal transgene: A molecular mechanism for parental imprinting. Cell 1987; 50: 719–727

16 DeChiara TM, Robertson EJ, Efstratiadis A. Paternal imprinting of the mouse insulin-like growth factor II gene. Cell 1991; 64: 849–859

17 Barlow DP, Stoger R, Hermann BG, et al. The mouse insulin-like growth factor type-2 receptor is imprinted and closely linked to the Tme locus. Nature 1991; 349: 84–87

18 Bartolomei MS, Zemel S, Tilghman SM. Parental imprinting of the mouse *H19* gene. Nature 1991; 351: 153–155

19 Zhang Y, Tycko B. Monoallelic expression of the human *H19* gene. Nature Genet 1992; 1: 40–44

20 Rainier S, Johnson L, Dobry CJ, Ping AJ, Grundy PE, Feinberg AP. Relaxation of imprinted genes in human cancer. Nature 1993; 362: 747–749

21 Zhang Y, Shields T, Crenshaw T, Hao Y, Moulton T, Tycko B. Imprinting of human *H19*: allele-specific CpG methylation, loss of the active allele in Wilms' tumor and potential for somatic allele switching. Am J Hum Genet 1993; 53: 113–124

22 Ohlsson R, Nystrom A, Pfeifer-Ohlsson S, et al. *IGF2* is parentally imprinted during human embryogenesis and in the Beckwith-Wiedemann syndrome. Nature Genet 1993; 4: 94–97

23 Giannoukakis N, Deal C, Paquette J, Goodyer CG, Polychronakos C. Parental genomic imprinting of the human *IGF2* gene. Nature Genet 1993; 4: 98–101

24 Leff SE, Brannan CI, Reed ML, et al. Maternal imprinting of the mouse Snrpn gene and conserved linkage homology with the human Prader-Willi syndrome region. Nature Genet 1992; 2: 259–264

25 Glenn CC, Porter KA, Jong MTC, Nicholls RD, Driscoll DJ. Functional imprinting and epigenetic modification of the human *SNRPN* gene. Hum Mol Genet 1993; 2: 2001–2005

26 Jong MTC, Carey AH, Stewart CL, et al. The *ZNF127* gene encodes a novel C3HC4

zinc-finger protein and its expression is regulated by genomic imprinting. Am J Hum Genet 1993; 53: Abstract 697

27 Driscoll DJ, Waters MF, Williams CA, et al. A DNA methylation imprint, determined by the sex of the parent, distinguishes the Angelman and Prader-Willi syndromes. Genomics 1992; 13: 917–924

28 Kalscheuer VM, Mariman EC, Schepens MT, Rehder H, Ropers H-H. The insulin-like growth factor type-2 receptor gene is imprinted in the mouse but not in humans. Nature Genet 1993; 5: 74–78

29 Xu Y, Goodyer CG, Deal C, Polychronakos C. Functional polymorphism in the parental imprinting of the human *Igf2R* gene. Biochem Biophys Res common 1993; 197: 747–754

30 Moore T, Haig D. Genomic imprinting in mammalian development: a parental tug of war. Trends Genet 1991; 7: 45–49

31 Hatada I, Mukai T. Genomic imprinting of p57KIP2, a cyclin-dependent kinase inhibitor, in mouse. Nature Genet 1995; 11: 204–206

32 Hayashizaki Y, Shibata H, Hirotsune S, et al. Identification of an imprinted U2af binding protein related sequence on mouse chromosome 11 using the RLGS method. Nature Genet 1994; 6: 33–40

33 Kaneko-Ishino T, Kuroiwa Y, Miyoshi N, et al. Peg1/Mest imprinted gene on chromosome 6 identified by cDNA subtractive hybridization. Nature Genet 1995; 11: 52–59

34 Orlando V, Paro R. Chromatin multiprotein complexes involved in the maintenance of transcription patterns. Curr Opinion Genet Dev 1995; 5: 174–179

35 Carlson LL, Page AW, Bestor TH. Properties and localization of DNA methyltransferase in preimplantation mouse embryos: implications for genomic imprinting. Genes Dev 1992; 6: 2536–2541

36 Monk M, Boubelik M, Lehnert S. Temporal and regional changes in DNA methylation in the embryonic, extraembryonic, and germ cell lineages during mouse development. Development 1987; 99: 371–382

37 Frank D, Keshet I, Shani M, Levine A, Razin A, Cedar H. Demethylation of CpG islands in embryonic cells. Nature 1991; 351: 239–241

38 Howlett SK, Reik W. Methylation levels of maternal and paternal genomes during preimplanatation development. Development 1991; 113: 119–127

39 Kafri T, Ariel M, Brandeis M, et al. Developmental pattern of gene-specific DNA methylation in the mouse embryo and germ line. Genes Dev 1992; 6: 705–714

40 Sanford JP, Clark HJ, Chapman VM, Rossant J. Differences in DNA methylation during oogenesis and spermatogenesis and their persistence during early embryogenesis in the mouse. Genes Dev 1987; 1: 1039–1046

41 Driscoll DJ, Migeon BR. Sex difference in methylation of single-copy genes in human meiotic germ cells: implications for X chromosome inactivation, parental imprinting, and origin of CpG mutations. Somatic Cell Mol Genet 1990; 16: 267–282

42 Tremblay KD, Saam JR, Ingram RS, Tilghman SM, Bartolomei MS. A paternal-specific methylation imprint marks the alleles of the mouse *H19* gene. Nature Genet 1995; 9: 407–413

43 Stoger R, Kubicka P, Liu C-G, et al. Maternal-specific methylation of the imprinted *Igf2r* locus identifies the expressed locus as carrying the imprinting signal. Cell 1993; 73: 61–72

44 Ferguson-Smith AC, Sasaki H, Cattanach BM, Surani MA. Parental-origin-specific epigenetic modification of the mouse *H19* gene. Nature 1993; 362: 751–755

45 Brandeis M, Kafri T, Ariel M, et al. The ontogeny of allele-specific methylation associated with imprinted genes in the mouse. EMBO J 1993; 12: 3669–3677

46 Bartolomei MS, Webber AL, Brunkow ME, Tilghman SM. Epigenetic mechanisms underlying the imprinting of the mouse *H19* gene. Genes Dev 1993; 7: 1663–1673

47 Eversole-Cire P, Ferguson-Smith AC, Sasaki H, et al. Activation of an imprinted *Igf2* gene in mouse somatic cell cultures. Mol Cell Biol 1993; 13: 4928–4938

48 Li E, Beard C, Jaenisch R. Role for DNA methylation in genomic imprinting. Nature 1993; 366: 362–365

49 Guillemot F, Caspary T, Tilghman SM, et al. Genomic imprinting of Mash2 a mouse gene required for trophoblast development. Nature Genet 1995; 9: 235–241

50 Zemel S, Bartolomei SM, Tilghman SM. Physical linkage of two mammalian imprinted genes, *H19* and insulin-like growth factor 2. Nature Genet 1992; 2: 61–65

51 Leighton PA, Ingram RS, Eggenschwiler J, Efstratiatis A, Tilghman SM. Disruption of imprinting caused by deletion of the *H19* gene region in mice. Nature 1995; 375: 34–39

52 Villar AG, Pedersen RA. Parental imprinting of the Mas protooncogene in mouse. Nature Genet 1994; 8: 373–379

53 Wevrick R, Kerns JA, Francke U. Identification of a novel paternally expressed gene in the Prader-Willi syndrome region. Hum Mol Genet 1994; 3: 1877–1882

54 Sutcliffe JS, Nakao M, Christian S, et al. Deletions of a differentially methylated CpG island at the SNRPN gene define a putative imprinting control region. Nature Genet 1994; 8: 52–58

55 Riggs AD, Pfeifer GP. X-chromosome inactivation and cell memory. Trends Genet 1992; 8: 169–174

56 Kitsberg D, Selig S, Brandeis M, et al. Allele-specific replication timing of imprinted gene regions. Nature 1993; 364: 459–463

57 Tsang P, Gilles F, Yuan L, et al. A novel L23-related gene 40 Kb downstream of the imprinted *H19* gene is biallelically expressed in mid-fetal and adult human tissues. Hum Mol Genet 1995; 4: 1499–1507

58 Byrne JA, Smith PJ. The 11p15.5 ribonucleotide reductase M1 subunit locus is not imprinted in Wilms' tumour and hepatoblastoma. Hum Genet 1993; 91: 275–277

59 Brannan CI, Dees EC, Ingram RS, Tilghman SM. The product of the *H19* gene may function as an RNA. Mol Cell Biol 1990; 10: 28–36

60 Brown CJ, Hendrich BD, Rupert JL, et al. The human Xist gene: analysis of a 17 kb inactive X-specific RNA that contains conserved repeats and is highly localized within the nucleus. Cell 1992; 71: 527–542

61 Davies SM. Developmental regulation of genomic imprinting of the *IGF2* gene in human liver. Cancer Res 1994; 54: 2560–2562

62 Vu TH, Hoffman AR. Promoter-specific imprinting of the human insulin-like growth factor-II gene. nature 1994; 371: 714–717

63 Ogawa O, Eccles MR, Szeto J, et al. Relaxation of insulin-like growth factor II gene imprinting implicated in Wilms' tumour. Nature 1993; 362: 749–751

64 Giddings SJ, King CD, Harman KW, Flood JF, Carnaghi LR. Allele-specific inactivation of insulin 1 and 2 in the mouse yolk sac, indicates imprinting. Nature Genet 1994; 6: 310–313

65 Jinno Y, Yun K, Nishiwaki K, et al. Mosaic and polymorphic imprinting of the WT1 gene in humans. Nature Genet 1994; 6: 305–309

66 Mutter GL, Stewart CL, Chaponot ML, Pomponio RJ. Oppositely imprinted genes *H19* and insulin-like growth factor 2 are coexpressed in human androgenetic trophoblast. Am J Hum Genet 1993; 53: 1096–1102

67 Jinno Y, Ikeda Y, Kankatsu Y, et al. Establishment of functional imprinting of the *H19* gene in human developing placentae. Nature Genet 1995; 10: 318–324

68 Sapienza C, Paquette J, Tran TH, Peterson A. Epigenetic and genetic factors affect transgene methylation imprinting. Development 1989; 107: 165–168

69 Allen ND, Norris ML, Surani MA. Epigenetic control of transgene expression and imprinting by genotype-specific modifiers. Cell 1990; 61: 853–861

70 Forejt J, Gregorova S. Genetic analysis of genomic imprinting: an Imprintor-1 gene controls inactivation of the paternal copy of the mouse Tme locus. Cell 1992; 70: 443–450

71 Hall JG. Genomic imprinting: Review and relevance to human diseases. Am J Hum Genet 1990; 46: 857–873

72 Knoll JHM, Nicholls RD, Magenis RE, Graham JM Jr, Lalande M, Latt SA. Angelman and Prader-Willi syndromes share a common chromosome 15 deletion but differ in parental origin of the deletion. Am J Med Genet 1989; 32: 285–290

73 Nicholls RD, Knoll JHM, Butler MG, Karam S, Lalande M. Genetic imprinting suggested by maternal heterodisomy in non-deletion Prader-Willi syndrome. Nature 1989; 342: 281–285

74 Malcolm S, Clayton-Smith J, Nichols M, et al. Uniparental paternal disomy in Angelman's syndrome. Lancet 1991; 337: 694–697

75 Wagstaff J, Knoll JHM, Glatt KA, Shugart YY, Sommer A, Lalande M. Maternal but not paternal transmission of 15q11–13-linked nondeletion Angleman syndrome leads to phenotypic expression. Nature Genet 1992; 1: 291–294

76 Buiting K, Dittrich B, Gross S, et al. Molecular definition of the Prader-Willi syndrome chromosome region and orientation of the *SNRPN* gene. Hum Mol Genet 1993; 2: 1991–1994

77 Buiting K, Saitoh S, Gross S, et al. Inherited microdeletions in the Angelman and Prader-Willi syndromes define an imprinting centre on human chromosome 15. Nature Genet 1995; 9: 395–400

78 Ozcelik T, Leff S, Robinson W, et al. Small nuclear ribonucleoprotein polypeptide N (SNRPN), and expressed gene in the Prader-Willi syndrome critical region. Nature Genet 1992; 2: 265–269

79 Glenn CC, Nicholls RD, Robinson WP, et al. Modification of 15q11–q13 DNA methylation imprints in unique Angleman and Prader-Willi patients. Hum Mol Genet 1993; 2: 1377–1382

80 Warram JH, Krowlewski AS, Gottlieb MS, Kahn CR. Differences in risk of insulin-dependent diabetes in offspring of diabetic mothers and diabetic fathers N Engl J Med 1984; 311: 149–152

81 Lucassen AM, Julier C, Beressi J-P, et al. Susceptibility to insulin dependent diabetes mellitus maps to a 4.1 kb segment of DNA spanning the insulin gene and associated VNTR. Nature Genet 1993; 4: 305–310

82 Pugliese A, Awdeh ZL, Alper CA, Jackson RA, Eisenbarth GS. The paternally inherited insulin gene B allele (1,428 FokI site) confers protection from insulin-dependent diabetes in families. J Autoimmun 1994; 7: 687–694

83 Lucassen AM, Screaton GR, Julier C, Elliott TJ, Lathrop M, Bell JI. Regulation of insulin gene expression by the IDDM associated, insulin locus haplotype. Hum Mol Genet 1995; 4: 501–506

84 Jansen G, Bartolomei M, Kalscheuer V, et al. No imprinting involved in the expression of DM-kinase mRNAs in mouse and human tissues. Hum Mol Genet 1993; 2: 1221–1227

85 Lawler SD, Povey S, Fisher RA, Pickthal VJ. Genetic studies on hydatidiform moles. II. The origin of complete moles. Ann Hum Genet 1982; 46: 209–222

86 Ko TM, Hsieh CY, Ho HN, Hsieh FJ, Lee TY. Restriction fragment length polymorphism analysis to study the genetic origin of complete hydatidiform mole. Am J Obstet Gynecol 1991; 164: 901–906

87 Linder D, McCaw BK, Hecht F. Parthenogenic origin of benign ovarian teratomas. N Engl J Med 1975; 292: 63–66

88 Stevens LC, Varnum DS. The development of teratomas from parthenogenetically activated ovarian mouse eggs. Dev Biol 1974; 37: 369–380

89 van der Mey AGL, Maaswinkel-Mooy PD, Cornellisse CJ, Schmidt PH, van de Kamp JJP. Genomic imprinting in hereditary glomus tumors: evidence for a new genetic theory. Lancet 1989; 2: 1291–1294

90 Heutink P, van der Mey AGL, Sandkuijl A, et al. A gene subject to genomic imprinting and responsible for hereditary paragangliomas maps to chromosome 11q23–qter. Hum Mol Genet 1992; 1: 7–10

91 Toguchida J, Ishizaki K, Sasaki MS, et al. Preferential mutation of paternally derived RB gene as the initial event in sporadic osteosarcoma. Nature 1989; 338: 156–158

92 Blanquet V, Turleau C, de Grouchy J, Creau-Goldberg N. Physical map around the retinoblastoma gene: possible genomic imprinting suggested by Nrul digestion. Genomics 1991; 10: 350–355

93 Greger V, Passarge E, Hopping W, Messmer E, Horsthemke B. Epigenetic changes may contribute to the formation and spontaneous regression of retinoblastoma. Hum Genet 1988; 83: 155–158

94 Sakai T, Toguchida J, Ohtani N, Yandell DW, Rapaport JM, Dryja TP. Allele-specific hypermethylation of the retinoblastoma tumor-suppressor gene. Am J Hum Genet 1991; 48: 880–888

95 Greger V, Debus N, Lohman D, Hopping W, Passarge E, Horsthemke B. Frequency and parental origin of hypermethylated RB1 alleles in retinoblastoma. Hum Genet 1994; 94: 491–496

96 Cheng JM, Hiemstra JL, Schneider SS, et al. Preferential amplification of the paternal allele of the N-myc gene in human neuroblastomas. Nature Genet 1993; 4: 191–193

97 Caron H, van Sluis P, van Hoeve M, et al. Allelic loss of chromosome 1q36 in neuroblastoma is of preferential maternal origin and correlates with N-myc amplification. Nature Genet 1993; 4: 187–190

98 Caron H, Peter M, van Sluis P, et al. Evidence for two tumour suppressor loci on chromosomal bands 1p35–36 involved in neuroblastoma: one probably imprinted, another associated with N-myc amplification. Hum Mol Genet 1995; 4: 535–539

99 Junien C. Beckwith-Wiedemann syndrome, tumourigenesis and imprinting. Curr Opin Genet Dev 1992; 2: 431–438

100 Mannens M, Hoovers JM, Redeker E, et al. Parental imprinting of human chromosome region 11p15.3-pter involved in the Beckwith-Wiedemann syndrome and various human neoplasia. Eur J Hum Genet 1994; 2: 3–23

101 Koufos A, Grundy P, Morgan K, et al. Familial Wiedemann-Beckwith syndrome and a second Wilms tumor locus both map to 11p15.5. Am J Hum Genet 1989; 44: 711–719

102 Ping AJ, Reeve AE, Law DJ, Young MR, Boehnke M, Feinberg AP. Genetic linkage of Beckwith-Wiedemann syndrome to 11p15. Am J Hum Genet 1989; 44: 720–723

103 Brown KW, Williams JC, Maitland NJ, Mott MG. Genomic imprinting and the Beckwith-Weidemann syndrome. Am J Hum Genet 1990; 46: 1000–1001

104 Turleau C, de Grouchy J, Chavin-Colin CF, Martelli H, Voyer M, Charlas R. Trisomy 11p15 and Beckwith-Wiedemann syndrome: A report of two cases. Hum Genet 1984; 67: 219–221

105 Henry I, Bonaiti-Pellié C, Chehensse V, et al. Uniparental disomy in a genetic cancer-predisposing syndrome. Nature 1991; 351: 665–667

106 Grundy P, Telzerow P, Paterson MC, et al. Chromosome 11 uniparental isodisomy predisposing to embryonal neoplasms. Lancet 1991; 338: 1079–1080

107 Ferguson-Smith AC, Cattanach BM, Barton SC, Beechey CV, Surani MA. Embryological and molecular investigations of parental imprinting on mouse chromosome 7. Nature 1991; 351: 667–670

108 Schroeder WT, Chao L-Y, Dao DT, et al. Nonrandom loss of maternal chormosome 11 alleles in Wilms' tumors. Am J Hum Genet 1987; 40: 413–420

109 Williams JC, Brown KW, Mott MG, Maitland NJ. Maternal allele loss in Wilms' tumor. Lancet 1989; 1: 283–284

110 Pal N, Wadey RB, Buckle B, Yeomans E, Pritchard J, Cowell JK. Preferential loss of maternal alleles in sporadic Wilms' tumor. Oncogene 1990; 5: 1665–1668

111 Scrable H, Cavenne W, Ghavimi F, Lovell M, Morgan K, Sapienza C. A model for embryonal rhabdomyosarcoma tumorigenesis that involves genome imprinting. Proc Natl Acad Sci USA 1989; 86: 7480–7484

112 Moulton T, Crenshaw T, Hao Y, et al. Epigenetic lesions at the *H19* locus in Wilms' tumor patients. Nature Genet 1994; 7: 440–447

113 Albrecht S, von Schweinitz D, Waha A, Kraus JA, von Deimling A, Pietsch T. Loss of

maternal alleles on chromosome arm 11p in hepatoblastoma. Cancer Res 1994; 54: 5041–5044

114 Montagna M, Menin C, Chieco-Bianchi L, D'Andrea E. Occasional loss of constitutive heterozygosity at 11p15.5 and imprinting relaxation of the IGFII maternal allele in hepatoblastoma. J Cancer Res Clin Oncol 1994; 120: 732–736

115 Ashton IK, Aynsley-Green A. Plasma somatomedin activity in an infant with Beckwith Wiedemann syndrome. Early Hum Dev 1978; 1: 4: 357–362

116 Spencer GS, Schabel F, Frisch H. Raised somatomedin associated with normal growth hormone. A cause of Beckwith-Wiedemann syndrome? Arch Dis Child 1980; 55: 151–153

117 Weksberg R, Shen DR, Fei YL, Song QL, Squire J. Disruption of insulin-like growth factor 2 imprinting in Beckwith-Wiedemann syndrome. Nature Genet 1993; 5: 143–150

118 Sait SNJ, Nowak NJ, Singh-Kahlon P, et al. Localization of Beckwith-Wiedemann and rhabdoid tumor chromosome rearrangements to a defined interval in chromosome band 11p15.5. Genes Chrom Cancer 1994; 11: 97–105

119 Redeker E, Hoovers JMN, Alders M, et al. An integrated physical map of 210 markers assigned to the short arm of human chromosome 11. Genomics 1994; 21: 538–550

120 Wilkins RJ. Genomic imprinting and carcinogenesis. Lancet 1988; i: 329–331

121 Reeve AE, Eccles MR, Wilkins RJ, Bell GI, Millow LJ. Expression of insulin-like growth factor-II transcripts in Wilms' tumour. Nature 1985; 317: 258–260

122 Scott J, Cowell J, Robertson ME, et al. Insulin-like growth factor-II gene expression in Wilms' tumour and embryonic tissues. Nature 1985; 317: 260–262

123 Haselbacher GK, Irminger J-C, Zapf J, Ziegler WH, Humbel RE. Insulin-like growth factor II in human adrenal pheochromocytomas and Wilms tumors: Expression at the mRNA and protein level. Proc Natl Acad Sci USA 1987; 84: 1104–1106

124 Baccarini P, Fiorentino M, D'Errico A, Mancini AM, Grigioni WF. Detection of anti-sense transcripts of the insulin-like growth factor-2 gene in Wilms' tumor. Am J Pathol 1993; 143: 1535–1542

125 Pachnis V, Brannan CI, Tilghman SM. The structure and expression of a novel gene activated in early mouse embryogenesis. EMBO J 1988; 7: 673–681

126 Steenman MJC, Rainier S, Dobry CJ, Grundy P, Horon IL, Feinberg AP. Loss of imprinting of *IGF2* is linked to reduced expression and abnormal methylation of *H19* in Wilms' tumor. Nature Genet 1994; 7: 433–439

127 Taniguchi T, Sullivan MJ, Osamu O, Reeve A. Epigenetic changes encompassing the *IGF2/H19* locus associated with relaxation of *IGF2* imprinting and silencing of *H19* in Wilms tumor. Proc Natl Acad Sci USA 1995; 92: 2159–2163

128 Moulton T, Chung W-Y, Yuan L, Hensle T, Waber P, Nisen P. Genomic imprinting and Wilms' tumor. Med Pediatr Oncol 1995; in press

129 Li K, Adam G, Cui H, Sandstedt B, Ohlsson R, Ekstrom TJ. Expression, promoter usage and parental imprinting status of insulin-like growth factor II (*IGF2*) in human hepatoblastoma: uncoupling of *IGF2* and *H19* imprinting. Oncogene 1995; 11: 221–229

130 Kondo M, Suzuki H, Ueda R, Osada H, Takagi K, Takahashi T. Frequent loss of imprinting of the *H19* gene is often associated with its overexpression in human lung cancers. Oncogene; in press

131 Kondo M, Suzuki H, Ueda R, Takagi K, Takahashi T. Parental origin of 11p15 deletions in human lung cancer. Oncogene 1994; 9: 3063–3065

132 Ariel I, Lustig O, Schneider T, Pizov G, Sappir M, de-Groot N, Hochberg A. The imprinted *H19* gene as a tumor marker in bladder carcinoma. Urology 1995; 45: 335–338

133 Brunkow ME, Tilghman SM. Ectopic expression of the *H19* gene in mice causes prenatal lethality. Genes Dev 1991; 5: 1092–1101

134 Hao Y, Crenshaw T, Moulton T, Newcomb E, Tycko B. Tumour-suppressor activity of *H19* RNA. Nature 1993; 365: 764–767

135 Krieder JA, Sariola H, Loring JM, et al. WT-1 is required for early kidney development. Cell 1993; 74: 670–691

136 Koi M, Johnson LA, Kalikin LM, Little PF, Nakamura Y, Feinberg AP. Tumor cell growth arrest caused by subchromosomal transferable DNA fragments from chromosome 11. Science 1993; 260: 361–364

14

Simplifying the spleen: a new look at splenic pathology

B. S. Wilkins

For many pathologists, the spleen is alternately tedious and frustrating. Tedious, because splenectomy is frequently incidental and no obvious pathology is present. Frustrating, because overt pathology may correlate poorly with clinical symptoms or seem impossible to attribute with confidence to a specific cause. Pathological changes which would cause no diagnostic problem in another tissue may seem less straightforward when encountered in the spleen. So, why is splenic pathology perceived to be difficult?

First, however big or small, whether suspected to be pathological or not, spleens usually arrive in histopathology departments having spent several hours immersed in fixative but otherwise untouched. The result is immediately apparent when the first cut is made through the organ: a rind of tissue 0.5 cm thick beneath the capsule is fixed, while all deeper tissue is red and partly autolysed owing to inadequate penetration of formalin. Left to fix further after slicing, the red areas oblige by turning an appealing shade of muddy grey over the next 24 h, but the damage has been done and the resulting histological sections will show good tissue preservation only in the immediate subcapsular areas.

Second, spleens sent for histopathological analysis are usually accompanied by minimal clinical details, or none at all, particularly in cases where removal has been considered by the surgeon to be incidental to the major surgical purpose of nephrectomy, gastrectomy, abdominal aneurysm repair, or whatever. When the spleen has been traumatized, there may be no indication of whether minor intraoperative trauma or a major road traffic accident was the cause. In cases of splenic trauma due to major abdominal injury, the pathologist is rarely told how long after the injury splenectomy was performed. These pieces of information are of fundamental importance. Most of our impressions of 'normal' splenic appearances are derived from such specimens and, just as a skin wound may be insignificant or extensive and will undergo reparative changes during the days following injury, so does an injury to the spleen.

Third, in part due to the foregoing problems, many pathologists lack a clear understanding of normal splenic anatomy and physiology. We rarely see genuinely normal spleens as surgical specimens and rapid post mortem autolysis results in generally poor morphological preservation of the spleen at autopsy. Normal spleens from experimental animals and spleens obtained at defined time-points following immunological challenge or injury in such animals offer insight into splenic pathophysiology. However, the anatomy and functions of the spleen differ considerably between species and data from experimental animals cannot be assumed to reflect accurately processes occurring in humans. For instance, the spleen in rodents is a major haemopoietic organ throughout life, while there is little evidence to support such a function in fetal or normal adult human spleen. Rodent spleens also differ significantly in structure from those of humans, particularly in the organization of white pulp marginal zones and the perifollicular vasculature. The spleens of cats and dogs have an important physiological role as a reservoir for blood cells. They have considerable amounts of capsular and trabecular smooth muscle to assist this function, and normal spleen volume may vary widely in these species. Such reservoir activity in human spleen is usually evidence of underlying pathology causing undesirable sequestration of blood elements, for example, hereditary spherocytosis.

To overcome these problems, we must encourage our surgical colleagues to send all spleens to the histopathology laboratory unfixed and accompanied by informative clinical details. We must be prepared to measure, weigh and describe the spleen promptly upon its arrival in the department and slice it at 0.5–1.0 cm intervals before submerging it in 10% neutral-buffered formalin (or other fixative, according to local practice) for 24–48 h. If the spleen is large, the formalin should be changed after 24 h. It is advisable (for diagnostic and self-educational purposes), even in the case of an incidental splenectomy, to take more than one tissue block for histological examination and to perform Giemsa, reticulin, Perls' and periodic acid–Schiff's stains on one block in addition to routine H&E staining.

Provided with high quality histological material it is then possible to make a rational assessment of spleen structure and any pathological changes present. What follows is information which, it is hoped, will useful for this purpose. It is not an exhaustive account of splenic pathology, but highlights some common and topical aspects of disease in this organ.

Normal microanatomy of the spleen

Red and white pulp components of the spleen are enclosed within a thin fibrous capsule from which trabeculae extend into the splenic parenchyma towards the hilum. Branches of the splenic artery and vein can frequently be identified within these trabeculae.

White pulp consists of periarterial and periarteriolar lymphoid sheaths (PALS), expanded at intervals by nodular lymphoid follicles.[1] The PALS is an organized T-cell compartment, which is clearly demarcated from the adjacent red pulp. Cells within the PALS are predominantly CD4-positive T cells: relatively few CD8-positive cells are normally found here. White pulp B-cell follicles are normally enclosed within the PALS, although the latter is highly attenuated over the follicular surface (Fig. 14.1). An unstimulated B-cell follicle consists of a nodule of small B lymphocytes surrounded by rim of marginal zone B cells, which are larger and have more abundant cytoplasm than the central cells. Marginal zones are not unique to the spleen, but in other lymphoid tissues they are generally inconspicuous. Marginal zone B cells are functionally heterogeneous, but a major subpopulation is responsible for generating T-independent immune responses to carbohydrate antigens such as bacterial capsular polysaccharides.[2,3] Small numbers of T cells are also present within marginal zones.

Red pulp consists of filtering areas, composed of sinusoids and cords, and non-filtering areas occupied by capillaries, venules and small amounts of supporting connective tissue.[1] Sinusoids are lined by endothelial cells, so-called littoral cells (from the Latin *littoralis* = by the shore), which are unique among endothelia in expressing the T-cell associated antigen CD8 (Fig. 14.4).[4] These endothelial cells are supported by 'barrel hoop' fibres of reticulin and separated by cords of Billroth. The resident cells of splenic cords are dendritic macrophages and small numbers of fibroblasts. Cords contain, in addition, varying numbers of transitory cells, including red blood cells, polymorphonuclear leukocytes, monocytes, lymphocytes and plasma cells. T cells expressing CD8 are present as a normal constituent of red pulp cords, scattered singly amongst cordal macrophages. Red pulp should therefore be considered as a distinctive T zone within the spleen, even though the CD8-positive T cells are not organized into a compact structure like the zone represented by the PALS.

At the interface between red pulp and marginal zones, sinusoids are replaced by an indistinct network of perifollicular capillaries (Fig. 14.3), which surrounds each white pulp nodule.[1,5] This site is probably important for antigen presentation to lymphocytes of the white pulp. It appears to be unique to human spleen, but it is not known whether it represents a direct equivalent of the well-defined capillary network found internal to the marginal zone in rodents. We have also demonstrated a reticular meshwork of dendritic cells expressing α-smooth muscle actin at this site[6,7] (Fig. 14.1b), possibly corresponding with a previously reported population of cytokeratin-positive perifollicular cells.[8]

Studies by van Krieken and colleagues, employing morphometric analysis of splenic tissue embedded in methyl methacrylate resin, have raised interesting questions about what constitutes normality in splenectomy specimens.[9–12] Spleens ruptured as a result of major trauma are often

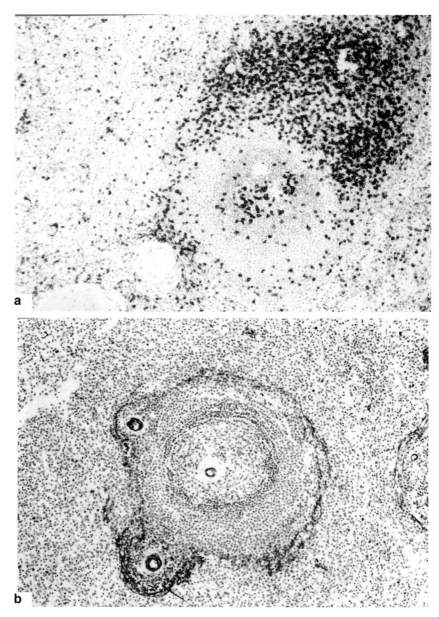

Fig. 14.1a Normal white pulp nodule immunostained using OPD4 (anti-CD45RO, available commercially from Dako, High Wycombe, UK) to highlight the periarterial and periarteriolar lymphoid sheaths (PALS). The T zone is sharply defined around a small arteriole (the tiny central defect in the immunostained area, top right) and extends to enclose, albeit incompletely, the B-cell nodule. CD45RO-positive T cells are also scattered in the centre of the B-cell nodule, reflecting the presence of a small, indistinct germinal centre. A prominent feature of this nodule is the pale marginal zone at its periphery.
b. PALS with an enclosed B-cell nodule, immunostained for α-smooth muscle actin, showing a dense reticular meshwork underlying periarteriolar T zones (two are represented in this picture, on the left side of the central B-cell nodule), which becomes attenuated as it extends around the outer aspect of the B-cell nodule.

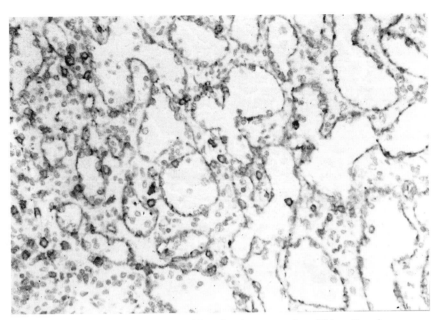

Fig. 14.2 Red pulp immunostained for CD8, showing expression of this antigen by sinusoidal endothelial cells as well as by scattered T lymphocytes within cords.

regarded as normal apart from any parenchymal disruption present, but they were found to differ significantly from spleens removed incidentally during abdominal surgery. Larger amounts of white pulp and expansion of the perifollicular capillary network were seen in trauma cases relative to incidental splenectomy cases. Whether such differences reflect pre-existing changes, which may have predisposed the spleen to rupture as a consequence of abdominal injury, or whether they reflect a reaction to parenchymal damage, is unknown at present. Availability of details of the nature of the injury and the relative timing of injury and splenectomy is essential if these questions are to be answered. Meanwhile, faced with a spleen removed for trauma (other than incidental, intraoperative injury), pathologists should be aware that the histology is likely to show quite marked reactive features.

Reactive changes in individual compartments of the spleen

Upon antigenic stimulation, splenic lymphoid follicles undergo enlargement and develop germinal centres, similar to follicles in lymph nodes. The central small lymphocytes of the follicle are displaced peripherally to form a mantle zone. In addition, the marginal zone frequently expands, becomes more cellular and often is seen to contain occasional blast cells resembling centroblasts. The PALS also expands and may gain small numbers of blast cells, but changes in this compartment are often difficult to appreciate in

Fig. 14.3a H&E stained section of spleen with highly reactive white pulp nodules, showing pale germinal centres surrounded by narrow mantle zones (inner dark rings), wide marginal zones and peripheral darkly stained rings representing the perifollicular capillary network. In colour these peripheral rings would appear as red `flares' owing to congestion with red blood cells.
b. Similar field to that shown in Fig. 14.3a, immunostained for α-sialoglycoprotein (glycophorin A), a glycoprotein expressed abundantly on red cell surface membranes, to illustrate congestion of the perifollicular capillary network with red blood cells. (Immunostained using monoclonal antibody BRIC101, the generous gift of Dr D. Anstee, South West Blood Transfusion Service, Bristol.)

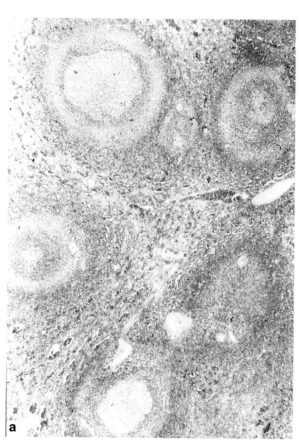

a

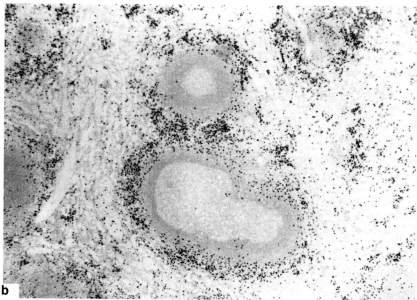

b

H&E stained sections. The relative predominance of germinal centre formation, marginal zone expansion or T-zone enlargement varies greatly between specimens, but is usually consistent throughout the parenchyma of an individual spleen. The variable nature of the changes presumably reflects differences in the precise nature and timing of the stimulus between cases. In the spleen, white pulp changes presumed to represent late stages and involution of immune responses are frequently seen,[13] which are unfamiliar to most pathologists because lymph nodes are rarely biopsied in the waning stages of reactive lymphadenopathy.

Red pulp changes are also heterogeneous and some of the features that correlate with specific pathological processes are described below. Non-specific reactive changes include plasmacytosis and CD8-positive T-cell lymphocytosis within cords, accompanying immune stimulation of the white pulp, congestion of perifollicular red pulp capillaries by neutrophils and red blood cells and cuboidal enlargement of endothelial cells lining sinusoids. Cords will become thickened and fibrotic in conditions of prolonged portal hypertension.

Alterations accompanying mechanical and autoimmune blood cell destruction by the spleen

Although primary pathology of the spleen is uncommon, splenectomy is sometimes performed for control of symptoms in disorders where the spleen is responsible for excessive destruction of blood cells. These include hereditary dyserythropoietic states such as spherocytosis and elliptocytosis, in which abnormal red blood cells are removed prematurely from the circulation by splenic sequestration. In autoimmune haemolytic anaemia (AIHA) and idiopathic thrombocytopenia (ITP), antibody-coated red cells and platelets are phagocytosed by splenic macrophages. Variable cytopenias may also occur in association with splenic enlargement from any cause, although the mechanism underlying hypersplenism in splenomegaly is often unclear.

In hereditary spherocytosis (HS) and other abnormalities of red cell shape/metabolism leading to reduced red cell lifespan, the predominant splenic change is widening of cords by sequestered red cells (Fig. 14.4, a and b). Most of these red cells are retained in the loose meshwork of the cords and relatively few of them are found as phagocytosed particles within macrophage cytoplasm. Sinusoidal lumens are often relatively empty, by contrast with AIHA, in which phagocytosis of antibody-coated red cells occurs predominantly within sinusoids (Fig. 14.4c) and to a lesser extent within the adjacent cords.[14] The phagocytosis of antibody-coated platelets in ITP has a different pattern again, occurring within cordal macrophages (Fig. 14.4d). Cordal macrophages in ITP are converted from their normal dendritic morphology into rounded cells, with superficial resemblance to the abnormal macrophages found in a variety of metabolic storage disorders.

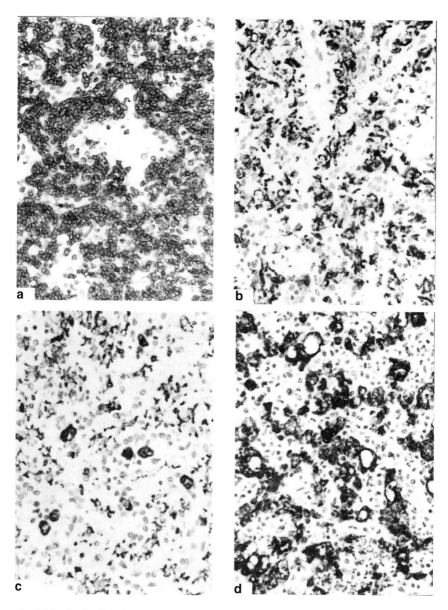

Fig. 14.4a Red pulp in hereditary spherocytosis (HS). Immunostained for α-sialoglycoprotein to show empty sinusoidal lumens and sequestered red blood cells expanding splenic cords.
b. Red pulp in HS. Immunostained for CD68 (antibody PG-M1, available from Dako, High Wycombe, UK) to demonstrate cordal macrophages, which are prominent in the widened cords and retain dendritic morphology.
c. Red pulp in autoimmune haemolytic anaemia (AIHA). Immunostained for CD68, showing prominent rounded, phagocytic macrophages within sinusoids in addition to dendritic cordal macrophages.
d. Red pulp in idiopathic thrombocytopenia (ITP). Immunostained for CD68, showing conversion of cordal macrophages from dendritic to rounded, vacuolated cells, reflecting intense platelet phagocytosis.

White pulp changes in HS, AIHA and ITP can be very confusing. One might predict absence of white pulp reactive changes in HS, this being a mechanical rather than an immune disorder, while spleens in AIHA and ITP might be expected to show evidence of immune stimulation. In fact, cases of HS may show florid white pulp reactive changes, particularly marginal zone expansion. The reason for this is unknown, but it may be that sequestered red cells, held in prolonged contact with splenic antigen-presenting cells, provoke an immune reaction to their highly carbohydrate-rich surface antigens.

Spleens from patients with ITP or AIHA may have floridly reactive white pulp but, in many cases, may appear unstimulated or even show white pulp atrophy. This variation reflects differences in disease activity between individuals, often further modified by steroid therapy. Patients in whom splenectomy is performed are usually those for whom medical therapy has been unsuccessful. Therefore, steroids may have been used in high doses for prolonged periods in attempts to control disease symptoms before splenectomy.

It must also be remembered that AIHA and, less commonly, ITP, are associated with underlying lymphoma in a significant proportion of cases.[15] The lymphoma is usually a low-grade non-Hodgkin's lymphoma and there may or may not be direct involvement of the spleen itself by neoplastic cells. The autoantibodies responsible for cytopenias are generally polyclonal and represent immunological dysregulation occurring as a result of the neoplasm, rather than a product of the neoplastic cell clone itself. The antigens against which such reactions are directed have proved difficult to characterize: Rhesus antigens are involved in at least some cases of AIHA.

Vaccination before splenectomy

Recently, another pre-splenectomy intervention has been introduced in the shape of vaccination for *Streptococcus pneumoniae*, type B *Haemophilus influenzae* and *Neisseria meningitidis* groups A and C.[16] In future, it is likely that inoculation against *N. meningitidis* group B will also be undertaken, as soon as an appropriate vaccine becomes available. These developments are significant for histopathologists because the vaccines specifically stimulate immune reactions for which the spleen is important (directed against bacterial capsular polysaccharides, as discussed above). They are therefore likely to produce morphological alterations in the spleen unrelated to those caused by the pathology for which splenectomy is being undertaken. Pathologists must learn to recognize vaccine-related changes in order to avoid attributing them to underlying splenic pathology. As yet, insufficient data exist to permit accurate distinction between vaccine and pathological effects in most cases. For many patients, a record has not been kept of whether and how long prior to splenectomy vaccination was performed, nor of precisely which vaccine(s) have been used (vaccines against *S. pneumoniae* became available before those against *H. influenzae*). The clinical parameters for vaccination are now becoming better standardized and, for any elective splenectomy, combined vaccine is usually administered 2 weeks preoperatively.[16] We are currently performing a comparison of known prevaccine splenectomies with vaccinated cases for which the vaccine history has been documented clearly, in order to assess vaccine-associated alterations in a variety of splenic pathologies.

The anticipated histological alteration in the spleen from such vaccination is marginal zone expansion with increased blast cell numbers. Preliminary data from our study show that these features in HS are no more marked in vaccinated than in non-vaccinated patients, supporting our hypothesis that the marginal zone response in HS is caused by red cell surface antigens rather than iatrogenic or incidental phenomena.

Splenic extramedullary haemopoiesis

Many standard texts of anatomy, embryology and pathology make reference to physiological extramedullary haemopoiesis in the spleen occurring during fetal life. This can conveniently be linked to the propensity in adult life for pathological extramedullary haemopoiesis preferentially to involve the spleen. Two alternative explanations for the latter occurrence have been hypothesized. First, it is suggested that haemopoietic stem cells remain dormant in the spleen from fetal life onwards and can be reactivated under a variety of conditions. Second, haemopoietic stem cells may be displaced into the circulation under conditions of marrow 'stress', including fibrosis from a variety of causes, and home to the spleen where they find a supportive microenvironment for subsequent proliferation and differentiation.

The data from which a role for the human spleen in fetal haemopoiesis has been inferred come mainly from animal studies, predominantly studies of rodents. Haemopoiesis in rodents is organized very differently from that in humans, with the spleen acting as a haemopoietic organ throughout life. It is inappropriate, therefore, to assume that data correct for rats and mice are equally correct for humans.

In fact, there is little evidence to support a significant role for the spleen in human fetal haemopoieis, and there is some evidence directly to the contrary.[17,18] We performed a quantitative analysis of early and late granulocyte and erythroid precursor cells in fetal spleens of appropriate gestational age (17–25 weeks). Only late erythroid cells (mid- and late normoblasts) were present in significant numbers, suggesting that the spleen filters some nucleated red cells from the circulation, actively or passively, and permits their terminal differentiation only. We found no evidence to suggest that earlier stages of erythropoiesis, or any stages of differentiation of other haemopoietic lineages, occurs in human fetal spleen. By contrast, abundant multilineage haemopoiesis could be detected in liver from the same fetuses (unpublished data). Moreover, splenic red pulp structure at this period of human gestation is primitive.[18,19] Barely vascularized, it lacks organization into cords and sinusoids and has few resident dendritic cordal macrophages.

Finally, the overall size of the fetal spleen is tiny in comparison with the liver and would offer only a very small volume of tissue from which to supply the haemopoietic needs of the fetus.

In adult life, however, splenic extramedullary haemopoiesis undoubtedly does occur. It takes two forms, one essentially insignificant and one highly pathological. In the first case, a spleen enlarged and/or reactive for any reason may be found to contain small foci of erythropoiesis within the red pulp, with occasional megakaryocytes and, less commonly, foci of granulopoiesis also present. In such spleens, the appearances of the differentiating haemopoietic cells are essentially normal.[20] Maturation to terminally differentiated erythrocytes and granulocytes is seen. Megakaryocytes have normal numbers of nuclei (approximately 5–10) and are dispersed singly. Similar, incidental, foci of extramedullary haemopoiesis may be found in liver, lung and probably other tissues as well. This should not be surprising because small numbers of haemopoietic stem cells are normally present in the circulation and presumably these become lodged in capillaries at a variety of sites. What factors determine whether they survive at these sites or undergo apoptosis are unknown, but include the activity of intrinsic cell processes as well as signals provided by the external microenvironment.

The second type of adult extramedullary haemopoiesis is essentially a form of metastasis. It is found in patients with chronic myeloproliferative disorders, including myelofibrosis, and also in some cases of myelodysplastic syndrome. In these disorders, splenic involvement may be extensive and appearances of the haemopoietic cells variable.[18,21] With the exception of advanced myelofibrosis, in which little intramedullary haemopoiesis remains for comparison, haemopoietic cells in the spleen appear similar to those found in the bone marrow, and the different lineages are present in approximately the same proportions. Therefore, predominance of immature granulocytic and erythroid cells, megaloblast-like erythroid dysplasia and megakaryocyte abnormalities are found in the spleen just as in the bone marrow. Megakaryocytes in chronic myeloproliferative disorders (particularly primary thrombocythaemia) are larger than normal with very high ploidy (often 20 or more nuclei, sometimes widely differing in size) and tend to form clusters. In the spleen, interaction between megakaryocyte clusters and sinusoidal endothelium may give rise to foci of peliosis (Fig. 14.5). Megakaryocyte clusters may be large enough to be detectable macroscopically as dark red nodules within the splenic parenchyma. Such megakaryocyte tumour formation is rare at other sites of extramedullary haemopoiesis and the splenic microenvironment may somehow favour neoplastic megakaryocyte proliferation.

Occasionally, splenic extramedullary haemopoiesis in chronic myeloproliferative disorders or myelodysplastic syndromes does not appear similar to the patient's bone marrow, but shows less maturation, more cytological atypia and possibly acute leukaemic transformation. In these cases, progression of disease has occurred preferentially within the spleen. Splenectomy in such cases, usually performed to relieve pain or discomfort caused by a

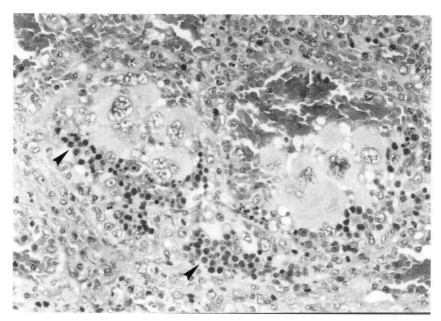

Fig. 14.5 Red pulp in extramedullary haemopoiesis associated with a chronic myeloproliferative disorder (H&E staining). The underlying diagnosis in this case was polycythaemia rubra vera, but megakaryocyte proliferation and atypia were prominent in the patient's bone marrow. Two clusters of atypical megakaryocytes are shown, one lying in a blood-filled space representing a focus of peliosis. Adjacent erythropoietic cell clusters are also shown (arrowheads), and other cells present include granulocyte precursors.

massively enlarged spleen, does not prevent progression of the disease in the bone marrow or other sites. Myeloproliferative or myelodysplastic disorders that transform to frank leukaemia in the spleen are almost certainly going to transform elsewhere, if they have not already done so.

Non-Hodgkin's lymphomas involving the spleen

There is probably no aspect of splenic pathology more topical at present than the characterization of non-Hodgkin's lymphomas (NHL), which appear to originate in the spleen or show preferential splenic involvement.[22-27] An excellent overview of the subject is given in Isaacson and Norton's recently published book on extranodal lymphomas.[28] It is a difficult area of pathology, in which classification is likely to be imperfect for some time, while knowledge of the nature and distribution of splenic lymphoid cells increases and understanding is gained of lymphocyte circulatory pathways through the spleen. Meanwhile, we need to apply a rational and pragmatic approach to diagnosis of NHL involving the spleen, in order to ensure that patients are given appropriate treatment.

Such an approach requires knowledge of the patient's history and clinical details. Of particular importance are details of any previous or concurrent evidence of NHL at another site (including bone marrow) and the presence or absence of a peripheral blood lymphocytosis. The precise cytology of any circulating abnormal lymphocytes is important: small lymphocytes, prolymphocytes, lymphoplasmacytoid cells, centrocyte-like cells or blast cells.

Any previous or concurrent lymph node or bone marrow trephine biopsy should be examined with care, because patterns of NHL may be more straightforward to interpret at these sites. Many NHL, including follicle centre lymphoma (FCL), chronic lymphocytic leukaemia/lymphoma (CLL), lymphoplasmacytoid lymphoma (LPL) and mantle cell lymphoma (MCL) will have nodal, marrow and/or peripheral blood characteristics which aid diagnosis. Care should always be taken, when selecting tissue blocks from a splenectomy specimen, to sample any hilar lymph nodes present because these are likely to contain the NHL and may permit clarification of a difficult splenic diagnosis.

Spleen size is of little value in diagnosis of NHL, as the spleen may be minimally or massively enlarged. Macroscopic appearances of the parenchyma may be more informative. Fine, miliary, white nodularity throughout the parenchyma usually indicates expansion of individual white pulp nodules and may be caused by FCL, MCL or marginal zone lymphoma (MZL). However, large, reactive, white pulp nodules can be visible macroscopically and diffuse granuloma formation should also be considered. The presence of small, irregular white tumour deposits adjacent to trabecular blood vessels, with or without a miliary background, occurs commonly in CLL. Large white nodules, several cm in diameter, with or without necrosis, usually represent high-grade B-cell lymphomas (diffuse large cell NHL with centroblastic or immunoblastic cytology).[29] Metastases from non-lymphoid malignancies, although rare in the spleen, should obviously be considered in the differential diagnosis of such lesions. Large nodules representing areas of high-grade transformation may also occur against a background of finely nodular low-grade lymphoma.

Uniformly red-brown splenic parenchyma with complete effacement of white pulp structures is rare in NHL with the exception of hairy cell leukaemia (HCL). Such appearances are more commonly associated with massive red pulp expansion by extramedullary myeloid proliferation. Partial architectural effacement may also occur in other NHL if red pulp involvement is extensive. Cases of HCL may have less uniform splenic parenchyma if there is extensive peliosis, but the latter causes cysts and haemorrhagic foci rather than white nodules. Some cases of high-grade lymphoma, particularly those of T-cell origin, also appear macroscopically to infiltrate diffusely throughout the splenic parenchyma, usually imparting a generalized pallor to the tissue.

Microscopic appearances of NHL in the spleen similarly reflect the extent of white and red pulp involvement (Fig. 14.6). Most low-grade NHL will tend to appear follicular because of predominant involvement of white pulp B-cell nodules. Therefore, follicularity alone is not a good indicator of follicle centre cell origin. Appreciation of cytological detail is fundamental

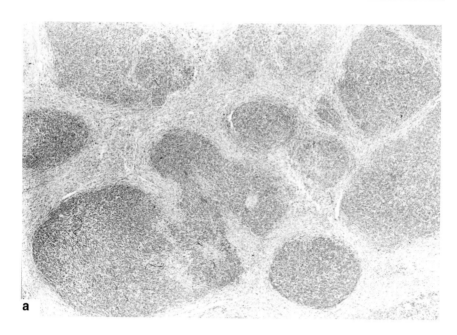

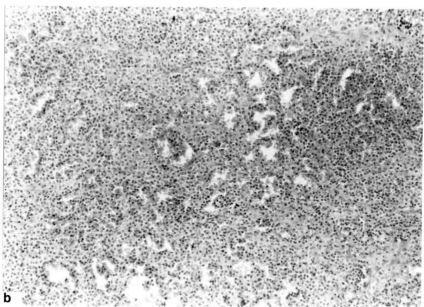

Fig. 14.6a Expansion of white pulp nodules with absence of red pulp spread in a case of follicle centre lymphoma (FCL) involving spleen. Nodules are sharply defined from the intervening red pulp.
b. By contrast with Fig. 14.6a, this case of hairy cell leukaemia (HCL) shows complete effacement of splenic architecture, so that red and white pulp cannot be distinguished from one another. The monotonous sheet of tumour cells is interrupted only by irregular spaces representing dilated, peliotic sinusoids.

to the correct diagnosis of such low-grade NHL in the spleen, reinforcing the need to achieve optimal fixation and high-quality tissue sections.

Nodules of FCL are composed of centrocytes and centroblasts, usually with centrocytes predominating, just as at nodal sites. Mantle and marginal zones may be present around the periphery of FCL nodules, but the pathology is essentially that of neoplastic germinal centre expansion. Red pulp involvement is minimal (Fig. 14.6a).

Nodules of MCL consist of a monotonous infiltrate of centrocyte-like cells or somewhat irregular lymphocytes. Small, residual germinal centres may be present in the centres of some nodules. Marginal zones are usually inconspicuous, but there is often extensive red pulp involvement, forming small satellite nodules around small venules and capillaries. Tumour cells will be abundant within sinusoids if the patient has leukaemic involvement of the peripheral blood, which is common in MCL. Unlike CLL, paraimmunoblasts and proliferation centres are absent from the infiltrates of MCL.

CLL, in addition to white pulp nodules, red pulp spread (which may be minimal or extensive), small lymphocyte cytology, paraimmunoblasts and proliferation centres, has a tendency to invade the walls of trabecular vessels, forming intramural nodules. Marginal zones are usually inconspicuous. LPL resembles CLL in many ways, but the infiltrate can be shown to have a mature plasma cell or intermediate plasmacytoid cell component, generally accompanied by scattered, reactive mast cells. Many cases of splenic LPL present in the clinical context of Waldenström's macroglobulinaemia, as does LPL at other sites. Some overlap may exist between LPL and so-called 'splenic lymphoma with villous lymphocytes' (SLVL).

White pulp nodules of MZL are usually dominated by their expanded marginal zone, but they are not necessarily very large because any residual germinal centres, mantles or primary (small lymphocytic) follicles may be extremely atrophic.[30-32] Immunoblast-like cells are present among the neoplastic marginal zone cells in varying numbers, as in reactive marginal zones. Red pulp involvement is generally extensive, with satellite nodules around small venules and capillaries and abundant intrasinusoidal spread. The satellite nodules are often accompanied by small epithelioid granulomas.[31] Many patients diagnosed on the basis of clinical and haematological parameters as having SLVL have splenic appearances of MZL.[33]

T-cell lymphomas may also arise in or preferentially involve the spleen. Classification of T-cell NHL is an area of much current debate and few clear conclusions, and splenic T-cell lymphomas are not exempt from this difficulty. Examples of T-CLL and T-PLL involving the spleen generally resemble their B-cell counterparts, but show greater cytological irregularity. T-cell NHL composed of pleomorphic, mixed medium-sized and large blast cells may present with splenomegaly and stage IE disease, possibly representing a clinico-pathological entity.[29] A lymphoma of γδ-T cells has also been described with predominant hepatosplenic involvement.[34] Diagnosis of these lymphomas generally requires immunophenotypic and/or molecular genetic evidence of T-cell origin, but morphological clues may be present that point towards T-cell NHL in the spleen. The PALS, being a defined T zone, may be preferentially infiltrated by the neoplastic cells. Normal white pulp B-cell nodules may be preserved: this can be recognized best when the neoplastic infiltrate is cytologically pleiomorphic and blastic, offering considerable contrast with normal mantle and marginal zone cells. Infiltration may be diffuse throughout the red pulp, with sparing or atrophy of white pulp structures, suggesting leukaemia or myeloproliferative disorder. This is particularly the case in hepatosplenic γδ-T cell NHL, and reflects the fact that red pulp is a normal compartment for preferential localization of γδ-T cells.[35]

Immunohistochemical analysis of the spleen

Reference is made throughout this chapter to the immunophenotypes of cell populations within red and white pulp of the spleen. A number of studies have been conducted using frozen sections and, more recently, paraffin sections to characterize cell populations within the various compartments of the human spleen.[4,6,36] These have demonstrated aspects of normal splenic architecture and cell distribution, increasing our understanding of normal and pathological splenic function. Immunohistochemistry for the differential diagnosis of splenic lymphomas remains somewhat confusing. The T-cell or B-cell lineage of a lymphoma can be determined readily in spleen and, in fresh tissue or well-fixed specimens, immunoglobulin light and heavy chains can be demonstrated. All of the many antibodies which can be used for lymphoma diagnosis in other tissues can be employed with spleen, but ability to achieve specific demonstration of marginal zone cells is currently imperfect. One antibody, UCL4D12, reacts specifically with marginal zone cells in frozen sections[37] but is unreactive with fixed tissue, even after microwave heating. A monoclonal antibody reactive with CD35, E11, usually employed with frozen sections to demonstrate follicular dendritic cells and some types of macrophage, also reacts with marginal zone B cells in formalin-fixed spleen tissue following microwave heating in citrate buffer, pH 6.0.[38] Another antibody, DND. 53,[39] immunostains marginal zone cells in formalin-fixed tissue, requiring no enzyme or microwave pretreatment.[6] Unfortunately, none of these antibodies appears entirely reliable in the discrimination of MZL from other low-grade splenic B-cell lymphomas.

In the absence of specific reagents for the demonstration of neoplastic marginal-zone B cells, differential diagnosis of splenic NHL is aided by use of antibodies reactive with B cells of other compartments. Particularly valuable is the demonstration of immunoglobulin D (IgD), which is normally expressed in the mantle zone and in rare cells within the marginal zone. It is absent from germinal centres. In FCL, partial preservation of IgD-positive mantle zones permits appreciation of the fact that neoplastic expansion of white pulp nodules is largely contained within the mantle zone. In some cases of MZL, the neoplastic expansion can be seen to be predominantly outside preserved IgD-positive mantles enclosing small, atrophic germinal centres. Unfortunately, a proportion of MZL express IgD, and in these cases no mantle zone can be distinguished from the neoplastic cells. Other antibodies preferentially reactive with normal mantle zone cells, including DBA. 44 (which reacts with the cells of hairy cell leukaemia[39]) and AT13/3,[6,38] have not yet been evaluated fully in the context of splenic MZL.

The availability of antibodies reactive with cyclin D1 should improve our ability to distinguish MCL from CLL, FCL and MZL in the spleen. Cyclin D1 is a cell cycle-associated protein whose expression is deregulated by rearrangements of the bcl-1 gene locus, typified by the translocation t(11;14), which occurs in most cases of MCL. Studies published to date indicate that immunohistochemical detection of nuclear cyclin D1 is highly specific for MCL.[40] Antibodies reactive with CD75 (e.g. LN1 and DNA. 7) demonstrate germinal centre cells, work in formalin-fixed tissue and can be used to show germinal centre expansion or atrophy as a further adjunct to differential diagnosis of splenic NHL. CD75 is also expressed by immunoblast-like cells in reactive and neoplastic marginal zones. The architecture of germinal centres can also be demonstrated using antibodies reactive with CD21 (1F8, Dako, High Wycombe, UK) or CD23 (BU38, The Binding Site, Birmingham, UK), antigens expressed by follicular dendritic cells (FDC). Therefore, expansion of the FDC network in the enlarged germinal centres of FCL can be contrasted with shrinkage and atrophy in most cases of MCL and MZL. In occasional cases of MZL, disruption and peripheral condensation of the FDC network is seen, suggesting a process of follicular colonization analogous to that seen in lymphomas of mucosa-associated lymphoid tissue (MALT).[41] This is of considerable interest in view of the current belief that MALT lymphomas are also of marginal zone cell derivation.[42]

The spleen in Hodgkin's disease

Staging laparotomy, including splenectomy, was regularly undertaken in Hodgkin's disease (HD) patients until the development of computerized tomography for imaging of the abdomen and retroperitoneum made this operation redundant. Splenic presentation of HD in the absence of disease elsewhere is extremely rare, and splenectomy specimens from HD patients are consequently seldom seen nowadays. If present in the spleen, HD forms one or several discrete nodules, with sizes varying from microscopic to massive. The macroscopic appearances are therefore more akin to those of high-grade B-cell NHL, which present as isolated masses, than to the majority of splenic NHL that show generalized involvement of the white pulp. Histologically and immunophenotypically, the features of HD at this site are essentially similar to those elsewhere in the body. Studies of non-involved spleens from HD staging laparotomies have shown no specific patterns of reactive change or other abnormalities.[4] Epithelioid granulomata may be found in red or white pulp, as in other tissues in HD patients, and their presence does not indicate actual involvement of the organ by HD deposits.

Acquired immunodeficiency syndrome (AIDS) and the spleen

Mild or moderate splenomegaly is not uncommon in individuals infected with human immunodeficiency virus (HIV). In many cases, the cause is unclear. It is increasingly recognized that secondary infections, including disseminated tuberculosis, *Mycobacterium avium-intracellulare* infection, histoplasmosis and cryptococcosis, may cause splenomegaly in acquired immune deficiency syndrome (AIDS) patients.[43,44] AIDS-associated lymphomas and Kaposi's sarcoma may also involve the spleen, although rarely presenting primarily at this site. A picture resembling ITP, usually with highly reactive white pulp, may be seen in early-stage HIV infection,[45] supporting the hypothesis that autoimmune platelet destruction contributes to the thrombocytopenia found in some HIV-positive individuals. Unlike ITP spleens, those from patients with HIV-associated thrombocytopenia frequently have increased numbers of CD8-positive T cells in the red pulp. Increased CD8-positive T cells have also been observed in red pulp and PALS of spleens from African individuals dying with advanced AIDS.[46] Comparison with spleens from African HIV-positive individuals without AIDS, who had died from incidental causes, showed that the increase in splenic CD8-positive cells correlated loosely with reduction in circulating CD4-positive T cells. In advanced AIDS, the spleen becomes severely atrophic as B-cell depletion follows loss of CD4-positive T cells. In some patients, expansion of CD8-positive T-cell numbers is sufficiently extreme to mimic neoplasia. Such severe reactions may be genetically determined, as association with several human leukocyte antigen (HLA) haplotypes has been shown (HLA-A1, HLA-B2, HLA-DR3 and HLA-DR5).[47,48]

It is interesting, but perplexing, to note that infections with capsulated bacteria, for which asplenic individuals are known to have an increased risk, are not increased in AIDS patients, and hyposplenism in AIDS remains poorly understood.[49]

Key points for clinical practice

- The spleen has few diseases of its own and most of the conditions discussed above represent splenic involvement as one component of processes affecting many tissues in the body.
- Primary disease diagnosis, as in hereditary spherocytosis, autoimmune haemolytic anaemia, idiopathic thrombocytopenic pupura or AIDS, is usually made on the basis of other investigations. In the pathology department, splenectomy appearances in such disorders are likely to be reported as either consistent with the diagnosis or normal and, possibly, dismissed as non-contributory.
- Recent interest in primary splenic non-Hodgkin's lymphoma has focussed attention on defining the normal histological appearances of

the spleen and understanding reactive changes that occur in its tissue compartments.

● The spleen, like many other tissues, has stereotyped patterns of response to disease. Careful analysis to confirm or exclude predicted changes associated with specific disorders makes rational interpretation of the spleen a rewarding exercise.

● Badly fixed splenic tissue is difficult or impossible to analyse. The key to appreciation of spleen pathology lies in obtaining adequate clinical information and ensuring optimal fixation of the tissue.

REFERENCES

1 Chamberlain JK. The microanatomy of the spleen in man. In: Bowdler AJ, ed. The spleen – structure, function and clinical significance. Chapter 2. London: Chapman and Hall, 1990

2 Kopp WC. The immune functions of the spleen. In: Bowdler AJ, ed. The spleen – structure, function and clinical significance Chapter 5. London: Chapman and Hall, 1990

3 Bruyn GAW, Zegers BJM, van Furth R. Mechanisms of host defence against infection with Streptococcus pneumoniae. Clin Infect Dis 1992; 14: 251–262

4 Timens W, Poppema S. Lymphocyte compartments in human spleen: an immunohistologic study in normal spleens and noninvolved spleens in Hodgkin's disease. Am J Pathol 1985; 120: 443–454

5 Kashimura M, Fujita T. A scanning electron microscopy study of human spleen: relationship between the microcirculation and functions. Scan Microsc 1987; 1: 841–851

6 Wilkins BS, Jones DB, Treasure JM, Delsol G. Alpha smooth muscle actin expression and white pulp compartmentalisation in normal and reactive spleen. J Anat 1995; 187: 206

7 Wilkins BS, Westwick R, Green A, Jones DB. Alpha-smooth muscle actin is expressed by a perifollicular cell network in normal and reactive human spleen. J Pathol 1995; 176: 37A

8 Doglioni C, Dell'Orto P, Zanetti G, Iuzzulino P, Coggi G, Viale G. Cytokeratin-immunoreactive cells of human lymph nodes and spleen in normal and pathological conditions. Virchows Archiv A Pathol Anat 1990; 416: 479–490

9 van Krieken JHJM, te Velde J, Hermans J, Cornelisse CJ, Welvaart C, Ferrari M. The amount of white pulp in the spleen; a morphometrical study done in methacrylate-embedded splenectomy specimens. Histopathology 1983; 7: 767–782

10 van Krieken JHJM, te Velde J, Hermans J, Welvaart K. The splenic red pulp; a histomorphometrical study in splenectomy specimens embedded in methylmethacrylate. Histopathology 1985; 9: 401–416

11 van Krieken JHJM, te Velde J, Kleiverda K, Leenheers-Binnendijk L, van te Velde CJH. The human spleen: a histological study in splenectomy specimens embedded in methylmethacrylate. Histopathology 1985; 9: 571–585

12 van Krieken JHJM, te Velde J. Normal histology of the human spleen. Am J Surg Pathol 1988; 12: 777–785

13 Wolf BC, Neiman RS. Non-neoplastic proliferations of splenic lymphoid tissue. In: Disorders of the Spleen. Major Problems in Pathology. Volume 20, Philadelphia: chapter 5. WB Saunders & Co., 1989

14 Schiffman FJ, Weiss L, Cadman EC. Erythrophagocytosis by venous sinus endothelial cells of the spleen in autoimmune hemolytic anemia. Hematol Rev 1988; 2: 327–343

15 Sokol RJ, Booker DJ, Stamps R. The pathology of autoimmune haemolytic anaemia. J Clin Pathol 1992; 45: 1047–1052

16 Mayon-White R. Protection for the asplenic patient. Prescrib J 1994; 34: 165–170

17 Wolf BC, Luevano E, Neiman RS. Evidence to suggest that the human fetal spleen is not a hematopoietic organ. Am J Clin Pathol 1983; 80: 140–144

18 Wilkins BS, Green A, Wild AE, Jones DB. Extramedullary haemopoiesis in fetal and adult human spleen: a quantitative immunohistological study. Histopathology 1994; 24: 241–247

19 Timens W, Rozeboom T, Poppema S. Fetal and neonatal development of human spleen: an immunohistological study. Immunology 1987; 60: 603–609

20 O'Keane JC, Wolf BC, Neiman RS. The pathogenesis of splenic extramedullary hematopoiesis in metastatic carcinoma. Cancer 1989; 63: 1539–1543

21 Wolf BC, Banks P, Mann RB, Neiman RS. Splenic hematopoiesis in polycythemia vera. A morphologic and immunohistologic study. Am J Clin Pathol 1988; 89: 69–75

22 Narang S, Wolf BC, Neimann RS. Malignant lymphoma presenting with prominent splenomegaly: a clinicopathologic study with special reference to intermediate cell lymphoma. Cancer 1985; 55: 1948–1957

23 van Krieken JHJM, Feller AC, te Velde J. The distribution of non-Hodgkin's lymphoma in the lymphoid compartments of the human pleen. Am J Surg Pathol 1989; 13: 757–765

24 Falk S, Stutte HJ. Primary malignant lymphomas of the spleen; a morphologic and immunohistochemical analysis of 17 cases. Cancer 1990; 66: 2612–2619

25 van Krieken JHJM. Histopathology of the spleen in non-Hodgkin's lymphoma. Histol Histopathol 1990; 5: 113–122

26 Brox A, Bishinsky JI, Berry G. Primary non-Hodgkin lymphoma of the spleen. Am J Hematol 1991; 38: 95–100

27 Coad JE, Matutes E, Catovsky D. Splenectomy in lymphoproliferative disorders: a report on 70 cases and review of the literature. Leukemia Lymphoma 1993; 10: 245–264

28 Isaacson PG, Norton AJ. Malignant lymphomas of the spleen. Chapter 12. In: Extranodal lymphomas. Edinburgh: Churchill Livingstone, 1994

29 Stroup RM, Burke JS, Sheibani K, Ben-Ezra J, Brownell M, Winberg CD. Splenic involvement by aggressive malignant lymphomas of B-cell and T-cell types: a morphologic and immunophenotypic study. Cancer 1992; 69: 413–420

30 Schmid C, Kirkham N, Diss T, Isaacson PG. Splenic marginal zone lymphoma. Am J Surg Pathol 1992; 16: 455–466

31 Pawade J, Wilkins BS, Wright DH. Low-grade B-cell lymphomas of the splenic marginal zone: a clinicopathological and immunohistochemical study of 14 cases. Histopathology 1995; 27: 129–137

32 Rosso R, Neiman RS, Paulli M, et al. Splenic marginal zone lymphoma: report of an indolent variant without massive splenomegaly presumably representing an early phase of the disease. Hum Pathol 1995; 26: 39–46

33 Isaacson PG, Matutes E, Burke M, Catovsky D. The histopathology of splenic lymphoma with villous lymphocytes. Blood 1994; 84: 3828–3834

34 Farcet J-P, Gaulard P, Marolleau J-P, et al. Hepatosplenic T-cell lymphoma: sinusal/sinusoidal localization of malignant cells expressing the T-cell receptor $\gamma\delta$. Blood 1990; 75: 2213–2219

35 Falini B, Flenghi L, Pileri S, et al. Distribution of T cells bearing different forms of the T cell receptor γ/δ in normal and pathological human tissue. Blood 1989; 143: 2480–2488

36 van Krieken JHJM, te Velde J. Immunohistology of the human spleen: an inventory of the localization of lymphocyte subpopulations. Histopathology 1986; 10: 285–294

37 Smith-Ravin J, Spencer J, Beverley PCL, Isaacson PG. Characterisation of two monoclonal antibodies (UCL4D12 and UCL3D3) that discriminate between human mantle zone and marginal zone B cells. Clin Exp Immunol 1990; 82: 181–187

38 Cuevas EC, Bateman AC, Wilkins BS, et al. Microwave antigen retrieval in immunohistochemistry: a study of 80 antibodies. J Clin Pathol 1994; 47: 448–452

39 Al Saati T, Caspar S, Brousset P, et al. Production of anti-B monoclonal antibodies (DBB.42, DBA.44, DNA.7 and DND.53) reactive on paraffin-embedded tissues with a new B-lymphoma cell line grafted into athymic nude mice. Blood 1989; 74: 2476–2485

40 Zuckerberg LR, Yang W-I, Arnold A, Harris NL. Cyclin D1 expression in non-Hodgkin's lymphomas. Am J Clin Pathol 1995; 103: 756–760

41 Isaacson PG, Wotherspoon AC, Diss T, Pan L. Follicular colonisation in B cell lymphoma of mucosa associated lymphoid tissue. Am J Surg Pathol 1991; 15: 819–828

42 Harris NL, Jaffe ES, Stein H, et al. A revised European-American classification of lymphoid neoplasms: a proposal from the international study group. Blood 1994; 84: 1361–1392

43 Klatt EC, Meyer PR. Pathology of the spleen in the acquired immunodeficiency syndrome. Arch Pathol Lab Med 1987; 111: 1050–1053

44 Pedro-Botet J, Maristany MT, Miralles R, López-Colomés JL, Rubiés-Prat J. Splenic tuberculosis in patients with AIDS. Rev Infect Dis 1991; 13: 1069–1071

45 Marti M, Feliu E, Campo E, et al. Comparative study of spleen pathology in drug abusers with thrombocytopenia related to human immunodeficiency virus infection and in patients with idiopathic thrombocytopenic purpura. Am J Clin Pathol 1993; 100: 633–642

46 Chandler Z, Wilkins BS, Wild AE, Delsol G, Lucas S, Jones DB. Splenic appearances in early HIV infection and advanced AIDS; an immunohistochemical study of post-mortem tissue from the Ivory Coast. J Pathol 1994; 173: 204A

47 Itesku S, Brancato LJ, Buxbaum J, et al. A diffuse infiltrative CD8 lymphocytosis syndrome in human immunodeficiency virus (HIV) infection: a host immune response associated with HLA-DR5. Ann Int Med 1990; 112: 3–10

48 Oksenhendler E, Autran B, Gorochov G, D'Agay MF, Seligmann M, Clauvel J-P. CD8 lymphocytosis and pseudotumoral splenomegaly in HIV infection. Lancet 1992; 340: 207–208

49 Grotto HZW, Costa FF. Hyposplenism in AIDS. AIDS 1991; 5: 1538–1540

Index